Frontiers in Endocrinology
Volume 9

HIGHLIGHTS IN MOLECULAR AND CLINICAL ENDOCRINOLOGY

Serono Symposia Publications

1. Metabolism in the Female Life Cycle. Diamond and Naftolin. 1993.
2. Reproductive Health. Campana, Dreifuss, Sizonenko, Vassalli and Villar. 1993.
3. Inhibin and Inhibin-Related Proteins. Burger, DeKretser, Findlay, Robertson and Petraglia. 1994.
4. Perspectives on Assisted Reproduction. Mori, Aono, Tominaga and Hiroi. 1994.
5. Cell and Molecular Biology of the Testis. Dufau, Fabbri and Isidori. 1994.
6. Developmental Endocrinology. Sizonenko, Aubert and Vassalli. 1994.
7. Molecular Basis of Endocrine Diseases. Isidori, New and Pavía. 1994.
8. Male Factor in Human Infertility. Tesarik. 1994.
9. Highlights in Molecular and Clinical Endocrinology. Andreoli and Shields. 1994.

Dust cover insert

see: M. Andreoli et al. p. 29 (cartoon modified from W.W. Chin, 1992): Putative receptor-mediated action of T_3 on central nervous system (CNS).

Frontiers in Endocrinology
Volume 9

Highlights in Molecular and Clinical Endocrinology

Edited by

Mario Andreoli
Scientific Editor
Professor of Endocrinology,
University of Rome La Sapienza
00161 Rome, Italy
President of the Italian Endocrine Society

Marian Shields
Coordinating Editor
Via Cosenza 8,
00161 Rome, Italy

ARES SERONO SYMPOSIA

Ares-Serono Symposia Publications

Ares-Serono Symposia, Via Ravenna 8, 00161 Rome, Italy

HIGHLIGHTS IN MOLECULAR AND CLINICAL ENDOCRINOLOGY
Ares-Serono Symposia Series - Frontiers in Endocrinology, Vol. 9

International Standard Book Number 88-85974-24-4

Printed in Rome, Italy - November 1994
by Christengraf, Via Anagnina 432/A

Foreword

As Chairman of the Organizing Committee of the 25th Congress of the Italian Endocrine Society, held in Rome, under the Patronage of the President of the Republic, on May 22-25 1994, I consider it a special privilege to also be serving as President of the Society, for this the 25th Anniversary of the biannual Meetings of the Society which has been operating continuously since its foundation in 1949. This special event, in my opinion, deserved to be celebrated with some really new initiatives, and it was with this in mind, that, as the abstracts received were submitted to peer review and anonymous selection in order to draw up the scientific program, I realized that the quality of the accepted papers was highly competitive. I, therefore, considered it might be worthwhile to publish a volume containing the selected Oral Communications, the Invited and Presidential Lectures, as well as the Clinical Symposium on Hormonal Contraception and the Workshops on selected topics, including also the Lecture delivered by the Winner of the Italian Endocrine Society 1994 Award, granted to investigations on experimental and clinical andrology.

The inspiration behind this very ambitious undertaking to produce a celebrative publication was threefold. Firstly, it was founded on my desire to dedicate to the International Community the striking efforts made by Italian Endocrinologists in achieving a high level in their scientific commitments in recent years; and this Volume reflects how the goals recently reached have been illustrated at the special edition of the "Silver" meeting.

Secondly, this Roman celebrative event represents an appropriate occasion to compare to-day's Italian Scientific contribution to Endocrinology with the scientific standard of the Congress held in Rome in 1970, organized then in symposial sessions dealing with Pathophysiology of Growth Hormone, Anterior Pituitary Tumours and Hirsutism, with the active participation of invited Italian and foreign Speakers, who presented, at the time, their pioneering studies with elementary and, nowadays, obsolete methodology. From this objective comparative analysis it is immediately obvious that progress has been made at an exponential rate. And I am very proud of the galvinizing and impressive itinerary made since then. My generation had the privilege of participating in the astonishing metamorphosis from Endocrinology conceived as a clinical "art" to the modern endocrinologist who is constantly faced with problems referring to the clinical implications of the continuous expansion of new information derived from the impressive cellular and molecular achievements on the biological substrates and the alteration of the endocrine system and its function. In this regard, in my Presidential Lecture* on the

*Dedicated to the memory of Piergiorgio Chiodini who actively participated in the life of the Italian Endocrine Society and, in particular, in the Scientific Program of the 1994 Meeting.

Pathophysiology of Hypothyroidism, which introduces the Thyroid Section, I stressed how this alteration in thyroid function represents an example of the continuous interaction between biological and clinical science. I take this opportunity to thank Dr. Clark T. Sawin who kindly made me a most welcome gift of a facsimile edition, printed in 1991, of the Report of the Special Committee nominated by the Clinical Society of London to investigate myxoedema, and first published in 1885. The hypotheses made by that prestigious Committee are an outstanding example of the usefulness of cooperation between experimental and clinical medicine. Thanks to the reciprocal and integrated cooperation, future perspectives are very exciting and we can truly envisage the possibility, in the not too distant future, of gene therapy. These promising forecasts, based on the headspinning progress made in the understanding of the molecular mechanisms involved in the transduction of the hormone message, are not without some very dramatic bioethical implications, as stressed in the Introductory Section.

Thirdly, I thought that Italian Endocrinology should pay a debt of gratitude to our foreign colleagues, particularly to scientists from the United States and, namely, from the famous Clinical Endocrinology Branch, at the National Institutes of Health, in Bethesda, with whom we have established a profitable collaborative exchange program which dates back to 1961. During those 30 years or more, the Italians attending the Branch have produced some 69 papers, and the journals where these have been accepted for publication give a clear indication of the very high standard of these articles: 17 in "Endocrinology" and 9 in the "Journal of Biological Chemistry". But, independently of the scientific results that have emerged, the final product, in terms of triggering off new lines of research and founding of new groups of young scientists, is greater by far than the mere assembly of the initial individual components. And Italy is proud to have earned, since the early sixties, a privileged relationship with this very important Laboratory which has moulded some 47 scientists, some 50% of whom, are currently holders of professorships in various Italian Universities.

In 1964 Dr. Jacob Robbins succeeded to Dr. Joseph Edward Rall, as Director of the renowned Clinical Endocrinology Branch founded in 1955 in the prestigious National Institutes of Health in Bethesda, one of the world sanctuaries of biomedical science. In recognition of his merits, both human and scientific, the Italian Endocrine Society, at this historic celebration, therefore, unanimously nominated Dr. Robbins Honorary Member, as a sign of gratitude for the dedication with which, regardless of his commitments, he has constantly supervised his young trainees, always with distinguished tact, guiding them in complex research programs, both as a teacher and in the finer experimental phases.

Furthermore, if we consider all the scientific papers produced by Italian basic and clinical Endocrinologists in collaboration with other prestigious Institutions, the list of publications appearing in outstanding Journals increases steeply. Therefore, I am convinced that Italian Endocrinology today, with the significant contribution of the younger generation of research workers, plays a determinant role in the International Scientific Community. In fact, the standard of the Italian Scientific production today has been guaranteed by the continued dedication of those research workers from numerous academic or scientific Institutions who had the opportunity of becoming actively involved in specific training programs, reaching, during their sabatical, an authorative personality, and upon returning to Italy, leaders of qualified groups in keeping with their international background and maintaining Italian basic and clinical endocrinology highly productive and competitive.

I take this opportunity to express my heartfelt gratitude to Professor Alessandro Beretta Anguissola, Honorary President of the Congress, who in the Opening Session, addressed the audience, underlining the important evolution of Endocrinology as a unique biomedical speciality which has, at the same time, an aggregating and unifying role between the various sectors of internal medicine. I should like to extend my warmest thanks to the Members of the Scientific Committee, Chaired by Sebastiano Filetti, as well as to the Referees who were assigned the task of processing the abstracts by deep and critical review. Sincere thanks are due to the Members of the Organizing Committee and Secretariat for the tremendous efforts made in coordinating the scientific program and the technical aspects of the Congress, attended by more than 1,000 participants.

The Authors kindly prepared their manuscripts without delay according to the editorial instructions asking for a mini-review format outlining the state of the art in the specific topics covered by their contribution. To all of them my warmest appreciation for their cooperation in rapidly submitting for publication the final revised text. Marian Shields graciously accepted the burden of Co-Editor on the basis of our common long-standing fruitful editorial engagements, having produced, in 1965, the Volume "Current Topics in Thyroid Research" published by Academic Press, and in 1981, "Advances in Thyroid Neoplasia", respectively, the Proceedings of the Fifth International Thyroid Conference and an International Colloquium held in Rome, Satellite of the European Thyroid Association Meeting. Her revision of the English language is, without altering the individual style, meticulous throughout, providing excellent editing which has resulted in a final amended text, structured, whenever possible, in a fairly homogeneous rational sequence.

My compliments and gratitude to Leda Pallante for her untiring and patient handling of the secretarial work and to Pietro Bonadies and Antonio Mennella for adapting their computer expertise to our editorial needs.

The Volume could not have been produced without the generous support of the General Manager of the Ares Serono Symposia Foundation, Sergio Rossetti, to whom I am particularly indebted for kindly offering to include this publication in the new outstanding series of Frontiers in Endocrinology.

I hope that this compendium, providing an outline of the most advanced Italian endocrine research, will be helpful to the reader and that the enthusiastic approach profused in conceiving and producing it will be appreciated.

President of the Italian Endocrine Society
Mario Andreoli

Verbier, September 5th, 1994.

Editorial Comment

The rapidly expanding knowledge in molecular biology has made a tremendous impact on the approach to understanding the pathogenesis of endocrine disorders. And the clinical application of the exploding new information in basic science has led not only to the elucidation of the biochemical mechanisms underlying human endocrine diseases, but has also made available molecular diagnostic tools. The present advancements offer the possibility, in the foreseeable future, to reach the ultimate goal of gene therapy. The profusion of endocrinological Journals and books reflects the need for research worker and physician alike to keep up with the latest progress.

This Volume is not intended to provide a comprehensive coverage of the endocrine system, nor is it intended as a mere compilation of the papers presented at the 25th Congress of the Italian Endocrine Society held in Rome, May 22-25 1994. Its objective is rather to focus the reader's attention on the important role played by basic endocrine research on clinical science. An attempt has been made to summarize the recent progress made in new exciting areas of endocrinology giving a preview of the most advanced research fields.

The original contributions in this Volume provide a "state of the art" and reflect on the current status, and on the main endocrine fields in which Italian Scientists are currently engaged. The articles appearing in this monograph represent an expanded format of the abstracts submitted for presentation at the biannual National Endocrine Meeting. These papers were accepted for oral Communication after anonymous selection by the Scientific Committee of the Society, taking into account the suggestions made by at least three referees, each an expert in his our particular field. These selected original papers, intended as a "mini-review" on specific topics, appear together with the Lectures delivered by Invited Speakers offering an authorative and informative overall view on basic and clinical subjects.

To avoid, as far as possible, irritative organizational and stylistic differences between one paper and another, all have all been processed by a time-consuming editorial revision and the amended manuscripts resubmitted for the authors' approval. Even if the final published text would have benefited from more overall editing, our target to reach a rapid publication whilst the material was still original prevented us from proceeding with a more careful scrutiny, mainly centered on the formal and linguistic presentation. We preferred to produce a readily understandable book on captivating investigations, comprehensive of the technological innovations involving cell and molecular research, emphasizing the synergism between basic and clinical research.

The topics discussed at the Congress have been broken down into logical groupings and assembled in integrated sections with the aim of bridging the gap between the rapidly advancing understanding of subcellular biological processes and the clinical approach which will provide an even more adequate diagnostic work up and lead to better treatment of endocrine disorders.

The introductory section, dedicated to the current debate on ethical, moral, religious and legal problems arising from the new sophisticated genetic technology opening the frontiers of therapeutic molecular medicine, stresses that bioethics aims to seek a reflection on (and not between) biomedicine and philosophy.

Other sections focus on the latest studies on cell and molecular investigations and the clinical application of the more recent technology in the pathophysiology of the specific organs and endocrine functions: thyroid-parathyroid, hypothalamus-hypophysial axis, andrology, reproductive apparatus and infertility, endocrine pancreas and metabolism, adrenals. The Volume also incorporates the Clinical Symposium on "Hormonal Contraception" focusing on the benefits, risks, side effects and contraindications of estrogen-progestogen contraceptives, as well as the present trends and future perspectives of hormonal methods for male contraception.

Also included in the Volume are reports presented at the four Workshops on Pathophysiology, Diagnostic and Therapeutic Aspects related to: Neuroendocrine Tumors, Growth Hormone Deficiency, Alterations of Gametogenesis, and Thyroid Autoimmunity, as well as on Diagnostic Procedures thus providing a critical overview and update on the recent progress and fascinating perspectives in these specific areas.

We hope that our efforts centered on our intention to rapidly produce this Volume containing front-line research and a critical synthetic review, will fulfil the scope to provide a source of up-to-date information on the most advanced areas of molecular and clinical research.

Our target is to capture the attention of a broad audience interested in research at cellular and molecular levels with emphasis on clinical application, hoping that this Volume may represent a useful reference tool.

Verbier, August 21st, 1994

Mario Andreoli
Marian Shields

Contents

NEUROENDOCRINOLOGY - HYPOPHYSIS

Neuroendocrine Tumors: Diagnostic and Therapeutic Aspects Workshop

Diagnosis

Therapy

Use of GH in Hypopituitarism in the Adult Workshop

INFERTILITY

Alterations of Gametogenesis Workshop

ANDROLOGY

FEMALE REPRODUCTIVE SYSTEM

HORMONAL CONTRACEPTION
Clinical Symposium

ADRENALS

DIAGNOSTIC PROCEDURES

Management of Out-Patients in the Endocrine Laboratory: Use of the Fully Automated Random Access Assay System (AxSYM) Workshop

INTRODUCTION

Italian Endocrine Society
1992-1994

President: M. Andreoli

Vice Presidents: F. Camanni, G. Faglia

Secretary: G.F. Fenzi. *Treasurer:* M. D'Armiento.

Council: A. Bellastella, B. Busnardo, P.G. Chiodini†, M. Cignarelli, S. Filetti, V. Macchia, G. Menzinger, F. Minuto, C.M. Rotella, G.A. Zampa.

XXV National Congress of the Italian Endocrine Society
Rome - May 22-25, 1994
Patron
President of the Republic

Honorary President: A. Beretta Anguissola

Presidents: M. Andreoli, A. Isidori

Scientific Committee: S. Filetti - *Chairman*, M. Andreoli, P. Chiodini†, R. Cordera, M. Mannelli, F. Petraglia, D. Tramontano.

Referees: D. Agnusdei, B. Ambrosi, L. Benzi, C. Betterle, M. Boscaro, F. Celotti, D. Cocchi, A. Fabbri, D. Giugliano, E. Jannini, G. Lombardi, M. Maggi, C. Marcocci, S. Migliaccio, A. Pontecorvi, P. Pozzilli, E. Roti, A. Spada, V. Toscano, V. Trischitta, P. Vitti.

Organizing Committee: M. D'Armiento, G. Frajese, E.A. Jannini, R. Lauro, A. Pontecorvi, F. Sciarra, G. Spera, V. Toscano, C. Tosti-Croce.

Secretariat: M. Centanni, D. Danese.

BIOETHICS AND MOLECULAR PERSPECTIVES

p. 1 - 16

SOCIETA'
ITALIANA
DI ENDOCRINOLOGIA

Frontiers in Endocrinology
Volume 9 - 1994

Bioethics. A Bridge from the Past to the Future

M. Garavaglia

Institute for the Analysis of the Social State,
Via G. Giusti 3, 00185 Rome, Italy

An ethical debate is as ancient as medicine itself: respect for patients and life was derived from the high self-respect of the physician in Hippocratic medicine, including the Oath (1); instead of a State-good oriented moral of Plato, according to whom the demographic equilibrium should be preserved at all costs and abortion may be an extreme way to reach it, a consideration of an absolute value of "sensitive life" is present in Aristotle, according to whom "abortion is allowed… [in a very early stage] or prohibited if sensitivity and life are present" (2).

If *kalós* and *agathós* are coupled together as key-words of a nobility standard (3), the physician of Greek and Roman times should be *kalakagathos* or *medicus gratiosus* (perfect gentleman or agréeable): perfect (or moral) behaviour is assumed to maintain the prestige of both medicine and the physician. Christianity, even at the beginning, introduces the centrality of man (*philantropía*) and attention is focused on the suffering patient: *cum-patere* is the participation not only to the disease, but above all to the suffering man.

An early influx of Christianity, however, is evident in a passage by Scribonius Largus, a Roman pagan physician, living at the time of Claudius Emperor, who says about the physician's *misericordia*, which is pity and compassion "*…precipue medicis, in quibus nisi plenus misericordiae et humanitatis animus est secundum ipsius professionis voluntatem, omnibus diis et hominibus invisi esse debent*" (4).

For centuries medicine has been balanced between ethics (moral and religious principles) and law-deontology (rules stated by Governments and/or Associations and Colleges of Physicians). The principles of Aristotle and St. Thomas concerning the *final finality* of humans in the direction of the *absolute* or *God* (5) has exerted a marked influence. Since medicine has dramatically increased the possibility of intervention on the patient (diagnosis, rehabilitation, mechanical support to respiration, etc.) and on life (*in vitro* fertilization, embryo transfer, fetal tissue transplantation, genetic diagnosis, genetic therapy, etc.) classical ethics and deontology seem not to be enough and semantic is asked for new terms to support the ideology (e.g. pre-embryo to justify a different ethical evaluation of manipulations between early and advanced stages of embryonic life). In this field, general and legal issues may differ, as in the rules suggested by the Warnock Committee or applied in the Davis vs Davis trial (6), and physicians ask for rules and guidelines, to prevent the spreading of legal conflicts.

The frontiers of technology in medicine are broadening and these concern fertilization procedures and genetic modifications as well as death. Informed consent may not be enough (7) and the debate on "medicalization" continues to increase.

Thus, the term "bioethics", which was formulated first by Van Rensselaer Potter, is the search for a reflection *in* (and not *between*!) biomedicine and philosophy (8).

The need to reflect on the great values of humanity is increased since the physician seems to be able to manipulate death and life; so, we believe in agreement with Hippocrates, that *ietròs gàr philósophos isótheos* (De dec. orn. 5) which is: the physician who loves wisdom is like a god (9).

According to the global approach of Van Potter, as suggested by the title of his first volume on the subject ("Bioethics. Bridge to the Future", 1971), the critical and moral discussion of the frontiers of applied medicine sinks its roots in our past and bioethics represents the bridge from the past to the future.

SELECTED REFERENCES AND NOTES

1. Angeletti L.R. (1992): Le concept de vie dans la Grèce ancienne et le Serment d'Hippocrate. Rev. Philosoph (Louvain) 90: 156-179.
2. Aristotle, Politics 1335b15
3. Kudlien F. (1970): Medical ethics and popular ethics in Greece and Rome. Clio Med. 5: 91-121.
4. Scribonius Largus, *Compositiones medicamentorum* (Deichgräber ed., p. 24, lines 29-32).
5. Angeletti L.R. (1990): Final finality in livings from ancient philosophy and medicine to contemporary biomedicine. Medicina nei Secoli n.s. 2: 139-213.
6. Human life "begins" at the 14th day says the Warnock Committee (GB, 1984; before there is a stage called pre-embryo) or at conception says the Judge Dale Young of the Blount County at Maryville, Tenn. (trial Davis vs Davis, September 21 1989: The Times 1989; 173:10; see also Angeletti L.R., ref. 5). A debate in this field has recently been published by Forum - Trends in Experimental and Clinical Medicine (Human Sciences Issues) 1993-94, with articles by L.R. Angeletti, M. Mori and E. Agazzi.
7. Cassileth B.R. et al. (1980): Informed consent. Why are its goals imperfectly realized? N.E.J.M. 302: 896-902.
8. Spinsanti S. (1994): Medical Humanities. Meet Van R. Potter, Arco di Giano 2: 233-244.
9. Hippocrates: Decorum 5. Loeb classical Library. Harvard Univ. Press. Cambridge (1923).

Frontiers in Endocrinology
Volume 9 - 1994

Frontiers of Applied Bioethics

L.R. Angeletti and L. Frati[1]

Department of History and Philosophy, Section of History of Medicine, University of Cassino (FR), Italy;
[1]Department of Experimental Medicine, University of Rome La Sapienza, Rome, Italy

The dilemma of the next century as far as concerns medicine is if the "selective pressure" of the evolution ideas, science and technology is the absolute protagonist of the evolution of medicine or if the prevalence is preserved of the role of sick persons together with the physicians as protagonists of medicine.

The problems concerning *technological medicine* have had different or conflicting solutions, regarding when human life begins (1) or if/how human somatic/germ-line indentity may be modified or how to regulate the conditions of human death, including the *post mortem* availability of the body (e.g. for transplantations).

A dramatic change in medicine has occurred with the advent of molecular medicine which has introduced the possibility of identifying a disease at molecular level: the pioneering work of Pauling (1) was followed by the discovery of the genetic code and its point mutations; thus, at the beginning of the 1970's hopes and fears have foreseen the possibility of a repair of a gene disorder. A general change is on the horizon of mankind and Van Potter postulated a general "ecological view" of the human species, called bioethics, as a bridge to a technological future (2).

A clear example is given with the problems involved in new medical technologies, related to the debate regarding the dignity of human life; they concern:

i. the possibility of transplantation of fetal cells (to cure Parkinson's disease or diabetes, etc.). When, in November 1988, Donald Nelson became the first US fetal-cell recipient against Parkinson's disease (he regained the use of his left hand) the way to the use of fetal tissues as "spare parts" of the human body was opened and more than 150 transplantations of fetal cells have since been carried out. The project of a trial supported by the US National Institute of Neurological Disorders and Stroke, proposed in January 1994, has led to a new debate in this field and the frontiers of molecular medicine, including the possibility of gene therapy in hemopoietic stem cells (to cure genetic anemias) (3). Tissues or cells from abortive fetuses or the so-called pre-embryos (4) are used for this purpose.

ii. special procedures of fertilization. Fertilization techniques include FIVET and GIFT, but also surrogacy of maternity, maternity in older women, etc., with ethical and legal problems for the babies.

iii. the genome project, involving problems concerning the "property" of human genome and its partial sequences. The high value of human life seems to be confirmed by the decision not to patent human DNA products by the US NIH (5) and the dignity of human life is claimed by the pioneer of studies on molecular genetics Erwin Chargaff (6), who believes, that "if medicine persists in the path, it seems to have chosen at present, we shall soon hear that its great mission actually is the abolition of death".

iv. exasperated therapeutic procedures and euthanasia. Patients today ask to live and to be free of diseases, but also to be aided in a "soft death" (a procedure that has involved about 85% of physicians in Rotterdam, who have been asked for various forms of "medical decisions concerning the end of life" or MDEL, i.e. euthanasia (7) and doctors recognize it as a duty to inform patients (informed consent).

A new scene has been opened by gene therapy, somatic or germ-line. General problems on the use of Somatic Gene Therapy (SGT) are related to the severity of the disease and absence of comparable valid therapies, whereas specific problems are typical of any advanced method (reliability, effectiveness, safety, i.e. insertion and expression of the mini-gene, absence of induced mutations, approval by an Ethics Committee, informed consent).

Germ-line gene therapy (GLGT) not used in the management of diseases on account of the unpredictable consequences regarding the effects of the method (not safe today); evaluations of general ethics focus attention on the fact that GLGT performed on an individual affects not only the individual, but also future generations (problem of informed consent, individual, by society, etc.), with violation of the "rights of future generations to inherit a genetic patrimony that has not been intentionally modified" (European Parliament, Recomm. 934/1993). The general aim of medicine (improvement of therapies), the respect of autonomy of a procreating couple (to be free from predicted genetic diseases) and the liberty of science represent arguments in favour of GLGT (8).

Thus, the "aegroti suprema voluntas" of classical medicine is under siege, because *self-determination* and *beneficence* principles may sometimes be in conflict: the "medical good" may differ from the "self-determined good". Thus, the exhortation of Harvey Cushing to reaffirm the adherence to traditional medical ethics (*anthropocentric*) may be a guide-line regarding the problems of technological medicine (9).

ACKNOWLEDGEMENTS

Supported by a grant to L.R.A. from the Italian Research Council CNR (93.01169.CT13).

SELECTED REFERENCES AND NOTES

1. Pauling L. et al. (1949): Sickle cell anaemia, a molecular disease. Science 110: 543.
2. van Potter R. (1970): Bioethics. The science of survival. Persp. Biol. Med. 14: 127.
3. Jonsen A.R. (1988): Transplantation of fetal tissues: an ethicist's viewpoint. Clin. Res. (1988): 36: 215-219.
4. Science (1994): 263: 909; New Scientist (1994); 1913: 4.
5. Hansen S. jr., (1989): Fetal research. Science; 246: 775; Pre-embryo: before the 14th day says the Lady Mary "Warnock Committee Report", GB, 1984.
6. Chargaff Erwin, Former Professor of Biochemistry at the Columbia University, N.Y., was Austrian by birth, but he was forced to leave Europe by the rise of the Nazis; in the late 1940s he demonstrated that the ratios of bases in DNA are constant, a concept which was crucial for the Watson and Crick's DNA model. For the ethics of molecular biology, see: Chargaff E., Engineering a molecular nightmare. Nature 1987; 327: 199-200.
7. Gunning K.F. (1991): Euthanasia. Lancet 338: 1010.
8. Berger E.M. and Gert B.M. (1991): Genetic disorders and the ethical status of germline gene therapy. J. Med. Philos. 16: 667-683.
9. Pellegrino E.D. (1983): The common devotion. Cushing's legacy and medical ethics today. J. Neurosurg. 59: 567-573.

Frontiers in Endocrinology
Volume 9 - 1994

Gene Manipulation by Homologous Recombination: Impact on Endocrine Research

D. Accili

The Diabetes Branch, National Institute of Diabetes and Digestive and Kidney Diseases National Institutes of Health, Bethesda, MD 20892, USA

INTRODUCTION

In recent years, recombinant DNA techniques have made a substantial impact on medical research. Endocrine sciences have also been greatly affected by this conceptual and technical revolution. First and foremost, this approach has been used to clone DNA sequences, identify genes, and direct expression of their protein products. Moreover, techniques of site-directed mutagenesis have greatly facilitated the task of understanding how genes work. Here, we review the area of gene manipulation in the living organism: homologous recombination in mouse embryonic stem cells.

HOMOLOGOUS RECOMBINATION

Introducing genes into cells via homologous recombination provides a powerful tool to understand gene function. Homologous recombination is a process whereby DNA introduced into a cell finds its way into the nucleus and replaces the corresponding sequence in the cell's genome (28). Specific mutations can be introduced in a cloned DNA fragment and then, via homologous recombination, into the genome of a living cell. As we will see, this technology can be used in mouse embryo-derived stem cells to generate mice of virtually any genotype. This approach is distinct from, and in many ways superior to, conventional mutagenesis and transgenic animal technology. In fact, mutations introduced in this fashion will be expressed with exactly the same tissue-specificity and developmental regulation as the endogenous gene.

Furthermore, by understanding the mechanisms of homologous recombination, it will be possible to apply this approach to site-specific mutagenesis of genes in human somatic stem cells, and, by doing so, to the therapy of many human genetic disorders.

Homologous recombination occurs through a reaction in which the ends of a DNA molecule are paired with the homologous regions in the target gene by virtue of a double-stranded break in the sequence (3, 5, 14, 21, 31). It should be emphasized, however, that mammalian homologous recombination is a complex reaction, probably involving multiple steps and multiple enzymes. To this date, it has not been possible to isolate the individual components of this system *in vitro*, so that all the evidence referred to herein is inferential. Most investigators will agree that multiple pathways can be active in determining a successful recombination reaction, and that they need not be mutually exclusive.

A DNA molecule engineered to achieve homologous integration at the target locus is generally referred to as a "targeting vector". It generally consists of genomic DNA sequences derived from the gene of interest in which a specific mutation has been introduced by site-directed mutagenesis. Considerable efforts have been devoted, so far, at generating animal models of total gene inactivation. Therefore, most investigators have chosen to introduce a mutation by interrupting the coding sequence of the gene with an exogenous DNA sequence. In most instances, this has been achieved by cloning the bacterial transposon Tn5, encoding the Neomycin phosphotransferase gene (Neo^r), in the coding sequence of the gene to be inactivated (18, 34).

Homologous DNA is required to perform efficient homologous recombination reactions. Early work of Capecchi and Thomas showed that the frequency of homologous recombination is, to some extent, related to the length of the homologous region (33). However, a linear relation is observed only in the range between 3 and 15 kilobase-pairs (kbp)(33, 9); longer constructs do not appear to further increase the frequency of the reaction. Other workers have suggested that the minimal extent of homology required to accomplish homologous recombination is indeed much smaller (13-29). However, extrapolation of these data should be done with some caution. The current consensus is that targeting vectors should include between 5 and 15 kbp of homologous DNA. The source of homologous DNA is obviously genomic DNA of the same species in which targeting experiments are to be performed.

It has been shown that different loci can be targeted with different efficiencies: it is not clear to date whether the observed differences depend upon the locus itself and the type of DNA constructs used, or whether the presence of certain sequences represents a predictor of how efficiently homologous recombination will be performed (31, 33).

Because of its intrinsically low frequency, gene replacement by homologous recombination involves only one of the two alleles of a euploid cell. This property has both advantages and disadvantages. The main advantage is represented by the ability to introduce mutations in mice in a heterozygous fashion through the use of embryo-derived stem cells. Experiments of complete gene inactivation may potentially be lethal at various points of development or interfere with the reproductive abilities of the animals (20, 35). In these cases, the presence of heterozygote mutants greatly simplifies the maintenance of a livestock of animals. Furthermore, heterozygote animals provide a model to understand gene dosage effects (8).

The main disadvantage of allele inactivation experiments are evident in aneuploid cells. For example, most somatic cell lines established from mouse become aneuploid as a result of prolonged *in vitro* culture. In these cell lines, gene inactivation experiments by homologous recombination are very problematic. In fact, some of these cell lines may have eight or ten copies of the same chromosome (1). Interestingly, this feature does not appear to interfere with the ability to obtain a measurable effect from gene replacement by homologous recombination. We and others have shown that inactivation of a single copy of a gene can be associated with a decrease in the levels of expression of that gene (1, 16). This intriguing observation can be explained by the fact that most cultured cells are functionally hemizygous, i.e. they actively express only one copy of any given gene. Furthermore, some evidence suggests that actively expressed genes are better targets for the recombination reaction than their inactive counterparts, probably by virtue of the fact that their chromatin structure is potentially more accessible to the recombination machinery (1, 2, 15, 24, 25, 29, 30, 36).

As homologous recombination techniques have become more sophisticated, several investigators have reported double-inactivation strategies, whereby both alleles of a gene can be disrupted in embryo-derived stem cells prior to reintroduction into a blastocyst (7, 12, 22, 23, 32). In one variant of this technique, cells in which one allele has been inactivated are subjected to a second round of homologous recombination, using a different selectable marker for isolation of transfected clones (7, 22, 32). Alternatively, it has been suggested that double-allele inactivations may be derived from clones harboring a single-allele inactivation by means of selection in the presence of high concentrations of G418 (23).

The large number of non-homologous integrations has long represented a formidable obstacle *en route* to applying homologous recombination to the mutagenesis of non-selectable genes. However, several screening procedures are now available to detect cells in which recombination has occurred in a "targeted" fashion (hence the popular term of "gene targeting").

The breakthough came in 1988, when Capecchi's laboratory at the University of Utah proposed the so-called "positive-negative selection" procedure, a means by which any gene could be targeted using a biochemical procedure to enrich for clones of cells in which homologous recombination had occurred (18). The idea behind it is based on the early observation that the ends of a DNA construct introduced into the nucleus are essential in order to catalyze homologous recombination. Surprisingly, however, the presence of a large region of non-homology at the end of the vector will not affect the efficiency with which homologous recombination is carried out by the cellular machinery.

Positive-negative selection exploits these features in the following way: a positive selection marker (e.g., Neo^r) is cloned within the targeting construct, thus conferring onto recipient cells the ability to grow in medium containing the neomycin analogue G418. At one end (or, in a more recent modification of the technique, at either end) of the targeting vector, sequences of the herpes simplex virus (HSV) thymidine kinase (TK) gene are added.

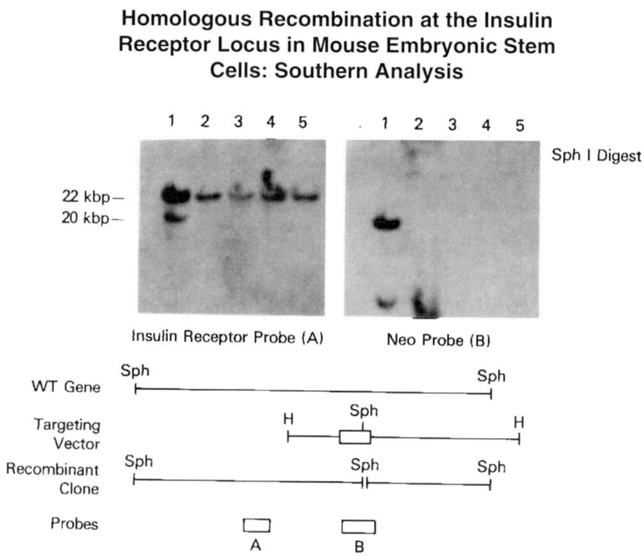

FIG. 1. Southern blotting analysis of homologous recombination events. After introduction of DNA into the cells and clonal selection, proof of successful targeting is acquired through Southern blotting analysis. Integration of vector sequences at the target locus will result in a recognizable and predictable alteration of the restriction pattern of the target gene. This picture shows integration of a targeting vector in exon 1 of the insulin receptor gene in ES cells (Accili and Taylor, unpublished). The normal pattern after digestion with Sph I is represented by a 22 kbp band. Upon homologous recombination, however, an additional Sph I site derived from the Neo^r gene is introduced in this region of the insulin receptor gene. Thus, two bands are now visible, a wild-type band at 22 kbp and a recombinant band at 20 kbp. Ideally, the intensities of the two bands should be equal; however, since ES cells are grown on layers of feeder cells, the wild-type band is more intense, due to contribution from DNA co-purified from the feeder cells. To further confirm the origin of the additional band, the same blot is stripped and reprobed with a Neo probe (panel B). The lower band derives from a 3' fragment of the Neo gene downstream of the Sph I site. Lane 1: targeted clone; lanes 2 through 5: wild-type clones.

Cells are then selected in the presence of the thymidine analogue ganciclovir (18), which is poorly metabolized by the mammalian TK gene, but is efficiently phosphorylated by the HSV-TK. Therefore, cells actively expressing HSV-TK will incorporate ganciclovir in their DNA. This drug prevents elongation of the DNA strand and causes cell death. When random integration occurs, expression of the TK gene derived from the targeting construct will render cells sensitive to ganciclovir, so that random integration events can be selected against by the use of this drug. However, when homologous integration occurs, the TK gene is removed by cellular recombinases because it represents a region of non-homology. These cells will be resistant to ganciclovir ($ganc^r$). Therefore, a double selection strategy will detect cells in which homologous recombination has occurred. These cells will be $ganc^r/G418^r$. Because during the transfection procedure random inactivation of the TK gene occurs, only a fraction of doubly resistant cells will be produced as a result of homologous recombination. However, the ratio of homologous to non-homologous recombinants will be considerably higher in doubly resistant clones than in clones that have been selected with G418 only. This difference is also referred to as "enrichment".

To determine that homologous integration has occurred as expected, Southern blotting analysis is performed. In fact, integration of sequences derived from the Neo^r gene is likely to alter the pattern on Southern blotting in a predictable fashion (Fig. 1). However, because many clones have to be analyzed in order to detect homologous recombinants, faster screening procedures have also been devised. Analysis of recombinant clones can be facilitated by the use of PCR-based techniques. PCR amplification is carried out on cells transfected with the targeting construct using two oligonucletoide primers: one is complementary to sequences located in the Neo^r gene, while the other primer is complementary to sequences of the target gene outside of the recombination boundaries (1).

MOUSE EMBRYO-DERIVED STEM CELLS

In the early eighties, Evans and Kaufmann (11) and Martin (19) independently developed methods to establish primary cultures of mouse embryo-derived cells. This develpoment marks the beginning of a new era in mouse genetics. In fact, as shown later by other workers, mouse embryonic stem cells possess two most important features: they can be grown *in vitro* for many passages without losing their totipotentiality, that is to say their ability to differentiate into virtually any cell type present in an adult mouse; furthermore, they retain this capability when reintroduced into a mouse blastocyst (4, 10). This feature can be exploited to generate chimeric mice which are partly derived from the strain of the host blastocyst, and partly from the strain of embryonic stem cells introduced into it. Embryonic stem cells introduced this way will colonize several tissues of the developing embryo, including the germ line. If the germ line of the offspring derives from exogenously introduced stem cells, the ensuing generations of mice will be phenotypically similar to the strain from which embryonic stem cells are derived. In order to facilitate the analysis of the degree of chimerism in mice, the recipient strain (i.e., the strain from which the host blastocyst is derived) has a different coat color from that of the embryonic stem cells. For all practical matters, embryonic stem cells are derived from the 129/ter SV strain. The fur of this strain is agouti, a greyish brown color. Recipient or "foster" strains are generally black or albino mice. Therefore, animals can be scored for their degree of chimerism by simple visual inspection after birth (Fig. 2) (other markers, like eye pigmentation or presence of specific isozymes of glucose-6-phosphate dehydrogenase can be used as well) (6). Furthermore, to analyze germ line transmission, chimeric mice are back-crossed with mice of the recipient strain. If germ line transmission of exogenous ES cells has occurred, the mice will have the same agouti color fur as the wild-type 129 strain, whereas, if chimerism is not associated with colonization of the germ line, the animals will revert to the original fur color of the host strain (6).

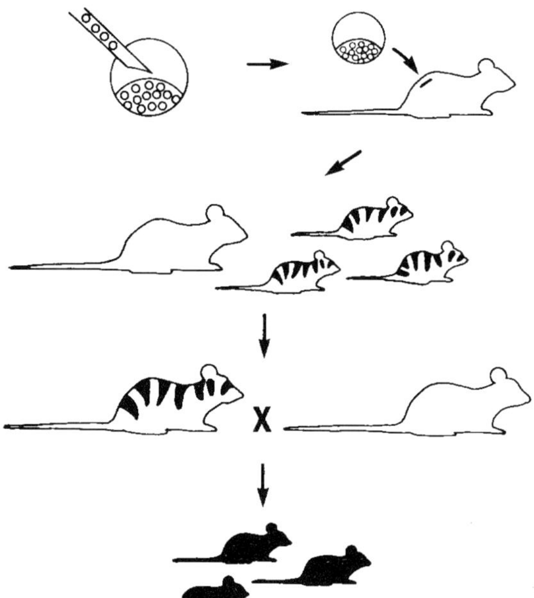

Fig. 2. Generation of transgenic mice by blastocyst injection of ES cells. ES cells are microinjected into a 3.5 - day-old blastocyst of a suitable recipient strain. Following injection, the blastocyst is reintroduced into the uterus of a pseudo-pregnant (foster) mouse. ES cells will colonize the developing embryo, including the germ line. Pups are screened by coat color. If an albino mouse is used as a recipient strain, an agouti color will signal contribution from ES cells. The degree of chimerism is variable, and is generally a good predictor of the efficiency with which the blastocyst has been colonized. Germ line transmission is assessed by back-crossing chimeras with wild-type animals of the recipient strain. If ES cells have colonized the germ line, some of the F_1 animals will be completely agouti; if the germ line has not been colonized, F_1 animals will revert to the original coat color. If a mutation has been introduced in ES cells by homologous recombination, the animals will be heterozygous carriers of the mutation. By appropriately breeding heterozygotes, homozygotes for the desired mutation can be derived (Reproduced with permission from Capecchi MR. "The new mouse genetics: altering the mouse genome by homologous recombination." Trends in Genetics 5: 72,1989. Copyright® Elsevier Press, Oxford).

From this preamble, it follows that a mutation can be introduced in embryonic stem cells via homologous recombination, and then be expressed in a living mouse without altering the remainder of the mouse genome. This property has revolutionized transgenic mouse technology: in fact, mutations can be introduced by homologous recombination in mouse embryonic stem cells, and their effects can be studied in the living animal.

APPLICATION OF GENE TARGETING BY HOMOLOGOUS RECOMBINATION

Gene targeting by homologous recombination has been applied extensively in conjunction with embryonic stem cell technology to generate null alleles in mice. Fewer efforts have been directed at utilizing gene targeting in cells other than ES. Certainly, in cells of proven karyotype stability, this approach is most valuable to generate null variants or to introduce specific mutations (1, 12, 15, 16).

Examples of gene knock-outs in mice are numerous at this point in time, as more and more investigators successfully apply these techniques (17, 26, 27). Efforts have mainly been directed at utilizing gene targeting as a way of improving our understanding of the exact role of certain genes in mammals. It is conceivable that a second phase will follow, in which gene targeting will be applied to introduce more subtle mutations, in order to dissect more specifically structure/function relationships in genes. The latter approach could be referred to as "*in vivo* site-specific mutagenesis". Its main implication is the idea of using homologous recombination as a way of delivering gene therapy. Two main obstacles have hindered progress in this direction: the lack of somatic stem cells to be used for gene restoration experiments, and the poor efficiency with which mammalian cells carry out homologous recombination. Progress is now being made in the development of cloned somatic stem cells from organs like bone marrow, liver and muscle. With respect to the frequency of gene targeting in mammalian cells, efforts are underway to find better methods for DNA delivery and to improve the overall efficiency of this process. As our understanding of the mechanisms of mammalian homologous recombination improves, it is possible to envision more efficient procedures to target specific mutations in the mammalian genome through the use of more suitable targeting vectors or more efficient ways of delivering DNA molecules to the nucleus.

Homologous recombination is a fascinating field. As progress continues to be made in its applications, we are probably going to witness a major change in our understanding of biology and in our approach to the genetic manipulation of the living cell.

REFERENCES

1. Accili D. and Taylor S.I. (1991): Proc. Natl. Acad. Sci. USA 88: 4708-4712.
2. Blackwell T.K., Moore M.W. Yancopoulos G.D., Suh H., Lutzker S., Selsing E. and Alt F.W. (1986): Nature 324: 585-589.
3. Bollag R.J., Waldmann A.S. and Liskay R.M. (1989): Ann. Rev. Genet. 23: 199-225.
4. Bradley A. Evans M., Kaufman M.H. and Robertson E.J. (1984): Nature 309: 255-256.
5. Bradley A. (1991): Basic Life Sci. 57: 83-97.
6. Bradley A. (1987): In: EJ Robertson (Ed) Teratocarcinoams and embryonic stem cells, pp.113-151. IRL Press, Oxford, Washington DC.
7. Cruz A., Coburn C.M. and Beverley S.M. (1991): Proc. Natl. Acad. Sci. USA 88: 7170- 7174.
8. De Chiara T.M., Efstradiatis A. and Robertson E.J. (1990): Nature 345: 78-80.
9. Deng C. and Capecchi M.R. (1992): Mol. Cell. Biol. 12: 3365-3371.
10. Doetschman T., Gregg R.G., Maeda N., Hooper M.L., Melton D.W., Thompson S. and Smithies O. (1987): Nature 330: 576- 578.
11. Evans M.J. and Kaufman M.H. (1981): Nature 292: 154-6.
12. Farese R.V., Flynn L.M. and Young S.G. (1992): J. Clin. Invest. 90: 256-261.
13. Hasty P., Rivera-Perez J. and Bradley A. (1991): Mol. Cell. Biol. 11: 5586-91.
14. Holliday R.A. (1964): Genet. Res. 5: 282-304.
15. Jasin M., Elledge S.J., Davis R.W. and Berg P. (1990): Genes and Dev. 4: 157-166.
16. Jasin M. and Berg P. (1988): Genes and Dev. 2: 1353-1363.
17. Koller B.H. and Smithies O. (1992): Annu. Rev. Immunol. 10: 705-730.
18. Mansour S.L., Thomas K.R. and Capecchi M.R. (1988): Nature 336: 348-352.
19. Martin, G.R. (1981): Proc. Natl. Acad. Sci. USA 78: 7634-8.
20. McMahon, A.P. and Bradley, A. (1990): Cell 62: 1073-1085.
21. Meselson M.S. and Radding C.M. (1975): Proc. Natl. Acad. Sci. 73: 358-361.
22. Mortensen R.M., Zubiaur M., Neer E.J. and Seidman J.G. (1991): Proc. Natl. Acad. Sci. USA 88: 7036-7040.
23. Mortensen R.M., Conner D.A., Chao S., Geisterfer-Lowrance A.A.T. and Seidman J.G. (1992): Mol. Cell. Biol. 12: 2391-2395.
24. Nickloff J.A. and Reynolds R.J. (1990): Mol. Cell. Biol. 10: 4837- 4845.
25. Nickloff J.A. (1992): Mol. Cell. Biol. 12: 5311-5318.
26. Robertson E.J. (1991): Biol. Reprod. 44: 238-245.
27. Piedrahita J.A., Zhang S.H., Hagaman J.R., Oliver P.M. and Maeda N. (1992): Proc. Natl. Acad. Sci. USA 89: 4471-4475.
28. Sedivy J.M. and Joyner A.L. (1992): Gene targeting. WH Freeman & Co. New York.
29. Shulman M.J., Nissen L. and Collins C. (1990): Mol. Cell. Biol. 10: 4466-4472.
30. Stewart S.E. and Roeder G.S. (1989): Mol. Cell. Biol. 9: 3464-3472.
31. Szostak J.W., Orr-Weaver T.L., Rothstein R.J. and Stahl F.W. (1983): Cell 33: 25-35.
32. te Riele H., Maandag E.R., Clarke A., Hooper M. and Berns A. (1990): Nature 348: 649-651.
33. Thomas K.R., Folger K.R. and Capecchi M.R. (1986): Cell 44: 419-28.
34. Thomas K.R. and Capecchi M.R. (1987): Cell 51: 503-12.
35. Thomas K.R and Capecchi M.R. (1990): Nature 346: 847-850.
36. Thomas B.J. and Rothstein R. (1989): Cell 56: 619-630.

THYROID - PARATHYROID

p. 17 - 132

Thyroid Autoimmunity: Recent Progress and Perspectives (Workshop)

p. 97 - 132

Frontiers in Endocrinology
Volume 9 - 1994

PRESIDENTIAL LECTURE

MARIO ANDREOLI
PRESIDENT ITALIAN ENDOCRINE SOCIETY 1992-1994

Hypothyroidism Today: from a Multisystemic Clinical Entity to an Experimental Model of Altered Expression of the Iodothyronine Message

M. Andreoli, A. Farsetti[1], S. Sciacchitano and A. Pontecorvi[2]

2nd Chair of Endocrinology, Department of Experimental Medicine, University of Rome La Sapienza;
[1]Institute of Experimental Medicine, CNR;
[2]Department of Internal Medicine, Catholic University; Policlinico Umberto I, V.le Regina Elena 324, 00161 Rome, Italy

Lecture delivered at the XXV National Congress - Rome, 22-25 May, 1994 and dedicated to the memory of Piergiorgio Chiodini.

HISTORICAL BACKGROUND

At the end of the last Century it was observed that the clinical picture of the devastating syndrome produced by struma excision, and designated by the Swiss surgeons Kocher (15) and Reverdin (26) as "cachessia strumipriva", was similar to that of the rare spontaneous condition first observed by Gull (12) in 1874, and called "cretinoid state" and defined, by Ord (19) in 1878, as "myxoedema"; these conditions were also seen to resemble both endemic and sporadic cretinism, described by Curling in 1850.

On the basis of these pioneering observations, the Clinical Society of London appointed a Special Committee "to investigate the subject of myxoedema". After almost five years of careful clinical and morphological studies, integrated by experimental observations on the effect of thyroidectomy in several animal species, Ord, Chairman of the Committee, concluded, at the crowded Meeting of the Society held on May 25th 1888, that "these several conditions are dependent on, or associated with, destruction or loss of the function of the thyroid gland" (20).

These remarkable and clear-cut conclusions, crystallized in the Final Report published in the Transactions* of the Society, should be considered a milestone in the understanding of thyroid physiology, since they represented the starting point of the incessant investigations that led to the identification and synthesis of thyroid hormone.

On the grounds of the Committee's work, George Murray (18), three years later, made medical history with his extraordinary therapeutic success in the treatment of adult myxedema that represented, in those days, a fatal condition, by injecting an extract of sheep's thyroid into a female patient. This brilliant intuition, to correct a deficient and, at that time, unknown factor, causing a disease, inaugurated the era of thyroid pathophysiology, starting from the isolation of the active principle, thyroxine, realized in a crystallin form by Kendall on Christmas Day 1914 (14), to the recent understanding of the mechanism of action of thyroid hormones at molecular level.

DEFINITION

On the basis of our more recent knowledge in thyroid pathophysiology, hypothyroidism may be defined, today, as a plurisystemic clinical entity caused by an inadequate expression of the thyroid hormone signal at target cell level, due either to a reduced production of the hormone message by the

* The Authors are grateful to Dr. Clark T. Sawin for the generous and most welcome gift of a 1991 facsimile edition of the Clinical Society of London Report on Myxoedema first published in 1888.

thyroid gland, or to an impaired response of the cell structures mediating thyroid hormone action (2, 3, 25).

The present review deals not only with personal experience, since 1974, in over 23,000 thyroid patients, from Central and Southern Italy, observed in the Outpatient Section of the Department of Endocrinology of the University of Rome La Sapienza, but also the results of a congenital hypothyroidism screening program, initiated in Rome in 1977 as a pilot study and progressively extended to the entire national territory with examinations in over 6 million newborns.

Moreover, results will be reported of experimental studies, performed in our laboratory, to elucidate the pathophysiology of thyroid hormone action impairment and on the structural alteration of nuclear receptors in the Resistance to Thyroid Hormone (RTH) condition.

EPIDEMIOLOGY

It has been held that hypothyroidism is a rare condition, mostly referring to the overt hypometabolic state. However, an analysis of our cohort of thyroid patients, using an original software for storing and elaborating clinical records, showed a prevalence of hypothyroidism of 11.1%. Subclinical hypothyroidism represented the largest proportion, prevailing in 62.5% of hypothyroid patients, while overt hypothyroidism was observed in 37.5% of cases (Fig. 1). These data are in agreement with recent epidemiological studies (4, 27).

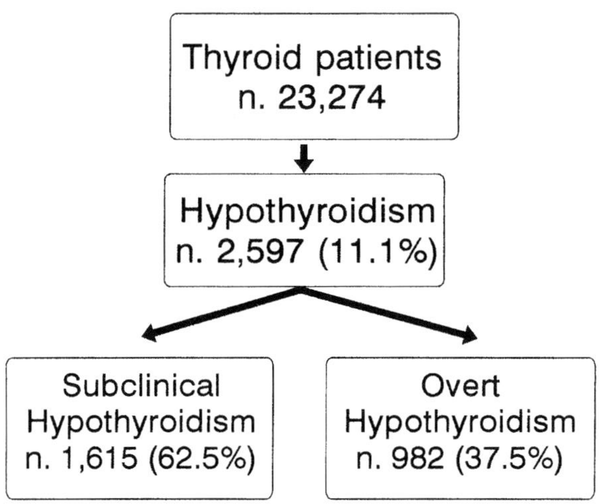

FIG. 1. Prevalence of hypothyroidism in our cohort of thyroid patients.

NOSOGRAPHY AND CLINICAL ASPECTS

Clinical classification

On the basis of its phenotypic appearance, the hypothyroid syndrome may be classified as overt, subclinical or homeostatic hypothyroidism.

Overt hypothyroidism refers to the taxonomic clinical picture of myxedema, characterized by a plurisystemic impairment that may show a variable degree of severity, related to the entity of the thyroid hormone deficiency and to the duration of the hypometabolic state. It should be stressed that the availability of increasingly sensitive diagnostic assays allows early detection of thyroid deficiency, thus preventing long-lasting impairment of target organ function and morphology. For this reason, the observation of the paradigmatic clinical stigmata of myxedema, described in the past, has become a rare entity. In this respect, the most typical feature of the myxedematous condition, the "non pitting edema", initially thought to be due to an excessive accumulation of mucine and responsible for most of the clinical signs and symptoms, including poor brain function, can be interpreted today on the basis of an excessive production of glycosaminoglycans. Similarly, myxedematous cardiopathy, initially interpreted as an interstitial myocarditis, is today referred to the molecular changes in myosin isoenzymes as well as to the modification in the type 2 Ca^{++}-ATPase of the sarcoplasmic reticulum resulting in a reduction of cardiac contractility and output efficiency (9).

Subclinical hypothyroidism is a clinical condition characterized by inadequate stimulation by thyroid hormones due either to a reduction of thyroid tissue or to inefficient hormonogenesis, as well as a defective target cell response to the thyroid hormone message. The inadequate thyroid hormone action results in an increased thyrotrophin reserve. Subclinical hypothyroidism prevails in about 3-10% of the general population, being more frequent in women (F/M= 5:1) and increasing with increasing age (27). In our patient population, the most frequent etiological factor of subclinical hypothyroidism is partial surgical removal of thyroid tissue, which represents about 45% of all cases, followed by autoimmune-induced thyroid damage (24%) (Fig. 2).

The laboratory profile is characterized by total and free iodothyronines within the normal limits, although T3 levels may even be at the higher limits of the normal range, in the attempt to compensate the initial thyroid hormone deficiency. TSH levels may be elevated or in the upper limits of the normal range, with an exaggerated response (maximum of 20μU/ml) to TRH challenge, which is diagnostic for this apparently asymptomatic condition.

The *clinical features* of subclinical hypothyroidism are characterized by *generalized systemic symptoms*, such as, for example, fatigue and anergia, cold intolerance, constipation, muscle cramps, dry skin and hair. The function of several organs may be affected by the reduced metabolic activity.

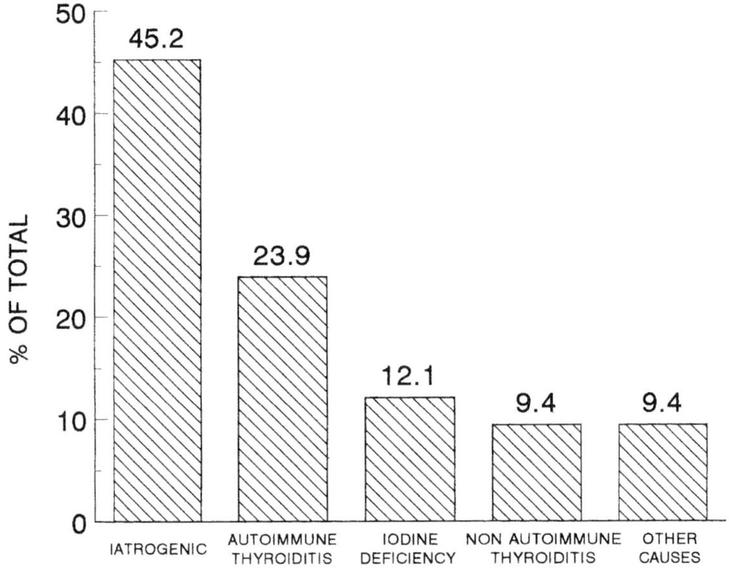

FIG. 2. Etiology of subclinical hypothyroidism in our cohort of thyroid patients (other causes refers to congenital, central and peripheral hypothyroidism).

Neuropsychiatric alterations (13), such as attention deficits, tendency to depression and melancholia, cognitive and behavorial disturbances, impaired concentration and memory, sleep disturbances, are frequently present but may be misdiagnosed or erroneously interpreted as "physiologic aging".

Cardiac parameters are also affected, as revealed by low ECG voltage and alterations in the repolarization phase together with changes in systolic time intervals, consistent with decreased myocardiac contractility (9). In addition, subclinical hypothyroidism may represent a risk factor for coronary heart disease. In this respect, alterations in the lipid metabolism frequently occur in patients with moderate hypothyroidism showing high cholesterol levels, and less commonly hypertriglyceridemia (33). Hypercholesterolemia is caused mainly by the decreased clearance of LDL-cholesterol, while HDL-cholesterol levels are reduced, thus increasing atherogenic risk. On the other hand, 6-10% of dyslipidemias are associated with an unsuspected and apparently asymptomatic hypothyroidism.

For this reason, the opportunity to screen all elderly patients with hypercholesterolemia to exclude subclinical hypothyroidism, prior to starting costly long-term treatment with lipid lowering drugs, should be considered. Conversely, in all patients diagnosed as having subclinical hypothyroidism, screening for the presence of alterations in the lipid profile appears mandatory as a valid preventive procedure for reducing the risk of coronary heart disease.

A variable hypocholesterolemic response to L-thyroxine therapy is common in hypothyroid patients (28). In about 25% of hypothyroid patients, in fact, L-T4 treatment fails to induce an increase in LDL receptors at the cell surface, therefore limiting the hypocholesterolemic response to hormone replacement. This finding has been correlated to a different polymorphic pattern of the LDL receptor gene, which allows us to identify a poor-responder subgroup of patients at greater risk for coronary heart disease (33).

Taken together, the results of our study confirm that subclinical hypothyroidism may not be as asymptomatic as initially thought, thus stimulating deeper inquiry and investigation by the physician (4). Therefore, on the basis of its high prevalence in the general population, particularly in the elderly, and the derangement caused on the function of several target organs, widespread biochemical screening for hypothyroidism is to be considered a valid method in preventive medicine.

Homeostatic hypothyroidism This biochemical profile refers to reduced thyroid hormone activity at cellular targets which could be present in non thyroidal illness (NTI) characterized by a derangement of the hormone plasma concentration depicting the so-called low-T3 syndrome. In this chronic and debilitating disease, the reduction of the thyroid hormone stimulating effect on cell metabolism and fuel consumption may be interpreted as a compensatory mechanism, involving a decreased intracellular deiodinating enzymatic activity as well as a reduced intracellular transfer of the active hormonal molecules. In this respect, our experimental data show that free fatty acids, which are released into the circulation in NTI (6), are able to inhibit intracellular and intranuclear T3 transport (Fig. 3). The situation of low-T3 (and in severe cases, also of a low-T4) syndrome, may, therefore, be referred to as a compensatory form of thyroid hormone insufficiency, which could be defined as "homeostatic hypothyroidism" (7).

In summary, the metabolic homeostasis of the thyroid hormone cell targets is modulated not only by the amount of circulating iodothyronine, but mainly it reflects the level of the active hormonal molecule in the various intracellular compartments (23).

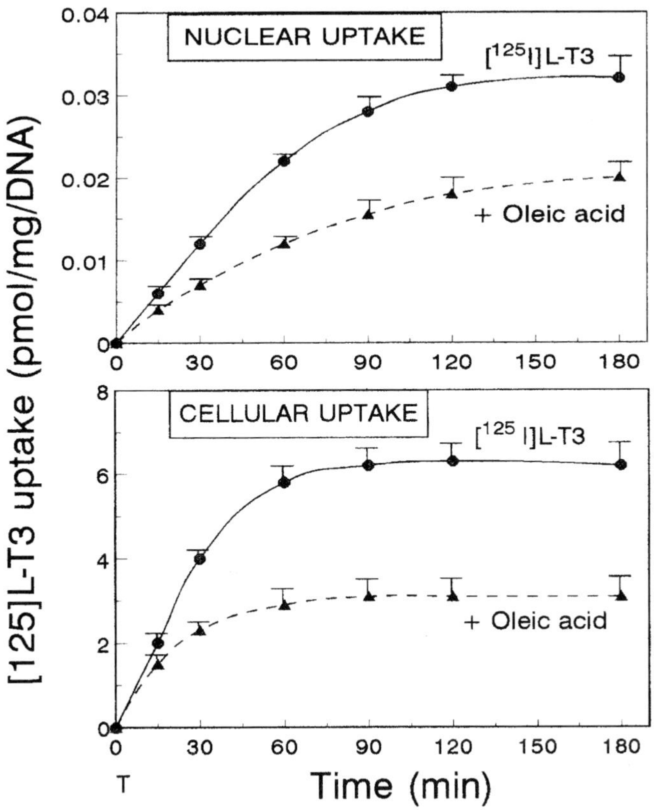

FIG. 3. Inhibition of L-T3 intracellular and intranuclear transport by oleic acid in rat skeletal muscle cells.

Pathophysiologic classification

On the basis of the structures involved in the genesis of thyroid hormone deficiency, it is possible to define a pathophysiologic classification of the various etiological factors responsible for hypothyroidism (Table 1). Hypothyroidism may, therefore, be classified as *primary*, due either to a quantitative reduction of thyroid tissue or to hormonogenetic defects (17); *central*, caused by the impairment of the hypothalamus-hypophysial tropic action on the thyroid gland, and *peripheral* (resistance to thyroid hormone), characterized by a reduced expression of the thyroid hormone message at the level of peripheral target tissues that may be due either to a defective intracellular transfer of the active hormonal molecule or to a defect of nuclear receptor structural and functional properties or to post-receptorial defects (Table 1).

Table 1. *Etiopathogenic classification of hypothyroidism*

PRIMARY		
	REDUCTION OF THYROID PARENCHYMA	
		Thyroid dysgenesia: agenesia, ectopia
		Iatrogenic: surgical or radioiodine treatment
		Chronic autoimmune thyroiditis
		Subacute thyroiditis: (transient hypothyroidism)
		Neoplasia
	HORMONOGENETIC ERRORS	
		Genetic defects of hormonogenesis
		Severe iodine deficiency
		Iatrogenic (antithyroid drugs, iodine, lithium, amiodarone)
CENTRAL		
	HYPOPHYSIAL	
		Hypophysial infarction
		Congenital defects (aplasia, or hypoplasia, Pit-1 defects)
		Ischemic necrosis (post-partum, vasculitis, severe shock)
		Traumatic events and iatrogenic causes
		Bioinactive TSH
	HYPOTHALAMIC	
		TRH deficiency (isolated or associated to other Releasing Hormones)
		Suprasellar neoplasia; cerebral tumors (primary or metastatic)
		Congenital defective formations; iatrogenic; sarcoidosis and histiochromatosis
PERIPHERAL OR RESISTANCE TO THYROID HORMONE (RTH)		
	PRE-RECEPTORIAL: Intracellular transport defects; intranuclear transport defects	
	RECEPTORIAL: Receptor abnormalities (affinity, capacity, hormone-receptor complex-DNA interactions)	
	POST-RECEPTORIAL: RNA maturation defects; translational and post-translational alterations	

The rare condition of *central hypothyroidism* is associated with a pronounced alteration of the lipid profile characterized by greater atherogenic risk. Recently, in familial cases of inadequate TSH production or of a more general pituitary hormone deficiency, mutations of the subunit of the TSH receptor or of the Pit-1 gene, whose products represent a primary stimulation of pituitary hormone synthesis, have been reported (31). In addition, in different physiologic and pathologic conditions, various TSH bioactive forms, characterized by a different carbohydrate moiety, may be secreted (21, 22).

Primary hypothyroidism, the most frequent form of thyroid deficiency, may be classified according to the age at onset of the disease. *Neonatal hypothyroidism* produces, if not detected early and treated promptly, severe and irreversible neuropsychiatric and somatic damage due to inadequate supply of the thyroid hormone message during the critical period of the initial postnatal life. In fact, iodothyronine plays a pivotal role in synchronizing and modulating the central nervous system maturation and differentiation (1).

A perinatal screening for early detection of congenital metabolic diseases, including congenital hypothyroidism, was initiated in 1977, by our group, undertaking a pilot study which was progressively extended to include large areas of Central and Southern Italy. Our screening program is now included in a national network that, at the present time, covers about 99% of the Italian newborn population (29).

Out of more than 6 million newborns screened in Italy, our group has contributed by 10% examining, at 31.12.93, a total of 624,086 newborns. Our results showed a prevalence of congenital hypothyroidism of 1/2,611, compared to an incidence of 1/2,977 over the whole National Territory (Table 2). The efficacy of the mass screening program is now evaluated from data elaborated by the National Registry of Congenital Hypothyroidism supported by the Ministry of Health (29).

Table 2. *Prevalence of congenital hypothyroidism in Italy (1977-1993)*

	25 National Centers	C.N.R. - Rome Center
Newborns screened	6,096,995	624.086 (≈10%)
Hypothyroid cases detected	2,048	239
Prevalence	1 / 2,977	1 / 2,611

Congenital impairment of thyroid hormone function is mainly due to embryogenetic derangements in thyroid gland development (agenesia, ectopia) but also to hormonogenetic defects, such as those affecting thyroglobulin and thyroid peroxidase genes (17).

Effects of thyroid hormone on Central Nervous System (CNS) In order to clarify the mechanism of the neurobiological damage produced by an inadequate supply of thyroid hormone, we have undertaken experimental studies aimed to investigate the molecular basis of thyroid hormone action on the CNS, during the "critical period" of postnatal cerebral differentiation and myelinogenesis (10).

An experimental neurobiological model, rendering rats hypothyroid pharmacologically, starting on the 16th gestational day with MMI (methimazole), was set up. The effect of T3 deficiency on the expression of the brain-specific myelin basic protein (MBP) gene, whose protein product represents about 30% of the total protein content of the myelin sheet, was studied during fetal and neonatal life (11). A dramatic decrease of MBP mRNA was observed in hypothyroid vs euthyroid animals, the maximal effect being at the 18th day of neonatal life. The reduction of cytoplasmic mRNA was caused by a decreased transcription of the MBP gene, but the prevalent effect observed on the 21.5 k and 18.5 k isoforms, originating from an alternative splicing of a common precursor RNA, suggested that thyroid hormone could also act at post-transcriptional level (11, 16).

Subsequent *in vitro* studies have led to the identification and characterization of a thyroid response element (TRE) in the MBP gene promoter. This finding represents the first identification of a TRE in a brain specific gene. Moreover, we demonstrated that, during cerebral differentiation, the induction of MBP transcription is mainly mediated by thyroid hormone receptor (TR) β, rather than α. This receptor selectivity was probably conferred by the TRE surrounding sequences, since the insertion of the MBP-TRE into a heterologous promoter was able to abolish thyroid receptor to preferential transactivation. Interestingly, MBP gene expression *in vivo* correlated with the peak of myelination and with a striking increase of TRβ expression in the developing neonatal brain, all these parameters reaching maximum levels at 18-19 days after birth.

The physiological significance of the multiplicity of thyroid hormone receptor subtypes, interacting with a uniform hormonal message, highlights new perspectives on the molecular basis of thyroid hormone action (Fig. 4). In this view, the different response to the hypothyroid condition of the adult brain, in comparison to neonatal brain, may be due to the differential cerebral distribution of the various thyroid hormone receptor subtypes, with a gradual increase of the variant isoform α2 with approaching adult life. The α2 isoform, in fact, is not able to bind T3, but may compete with the active forms of thyroid receptors in eliciting their transactivating action on target genes (Fig. 5).

Peripheral hypothyroidism The syndrome of RTH, characterized by clinical and biochemical manifestations due to reduced thyroid hormone action on peripheral target cells, reflects the condition known as "*peripheral hypothyroidism*" (24, 25). This syndrome is characterized by a persistent elevation of circulating T3 and T4 and inappropriately "non suppressed" TSH levels, in the absence of intercurrent acute illnesses, drugs or alteration of thyroid hormone binding to serum proteins. RTH is a rare genetic condition usually transmitted as an autosomal dominant character, first described by Refetoff in 1967, and so far identified in 296 cases belonging to 98 families (24, 25).

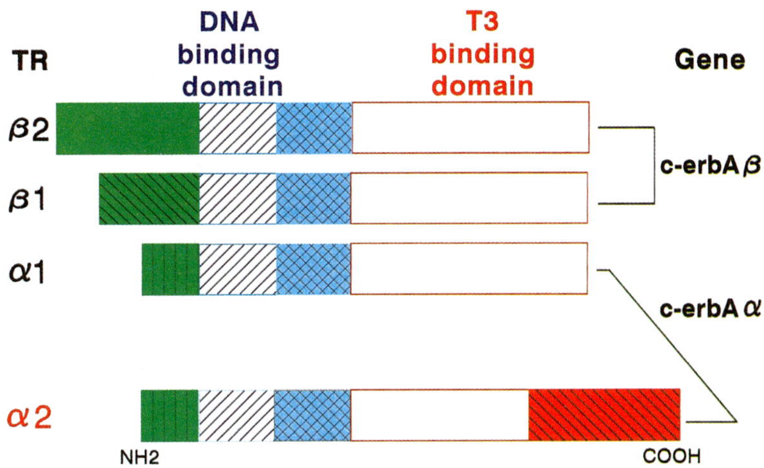

FIG. 4. Family of thyroid hormone receptors (TR).

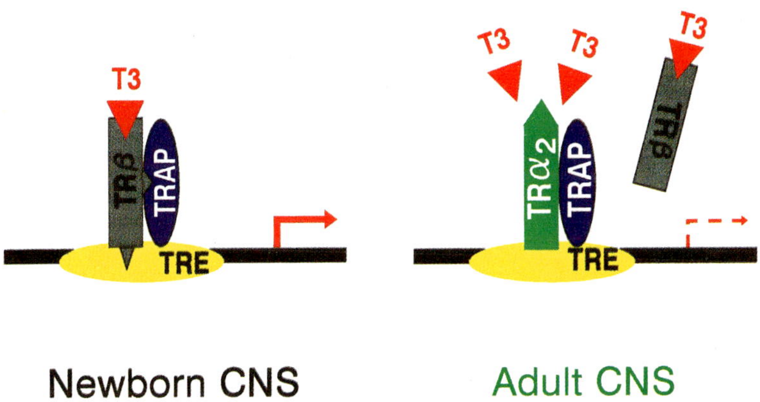

FIG. 5. Heterodimer formation involving Thyroid hormone Receptor, TR, or Thyroid hormone Receptor α2, TRα2 and Thyroid Receptor Auxiliary Protein, TRAP; heterodimers bind to Thyroid hormone Response Element (TRE). Arrows indicate the site of initiation and direction of transcription which are enhanced in the newborn and decreased in the adult CNS due to a rise in the TRα2 isoform levels. Modified from (8) Chin W.W. (1992): Thyroid Today Vol. 15: 3. 1-9.

The clinical picture of the syndrome is characterized by goiter, detected in 90% of cases and frequently requiring surgical removal, and a variable association of hypo- and hyperthyroid signs and symptoms which may vary between the various members of a same family and coexist in a same patient. This indicates the important role played by accessory factors in determining the clinical phenotype of the syndrome. For example, in the three affected subjects of the family D.G., studied by us, a decreased liver response to thyroid hormone action (ferritin and SHBG levels at the lower limit of the normal range) was observed (5). Liver parameters were not modified by T4 and/or TRIAC treatment. In contrast, osteocalcin levels appeared elevated, indicating an increased bone turnover that correlated with the high circulating T3 levels. This finding suggests a normal bone response to the thyroid hormone metabolic effect. In addition, systolic time intervals were reduced in one of the daughters, but normal in the mother, while showing a paradoxical increase after thyroid hormone administration in the other daughter (5).

After the first demonstration, by Usala et al. (32), of the *genetic linkage* of the syndrome with the thyroid receptor β gene, a large number of mutations of this gene have been identified as the molecular substrate of the syndrome. Interestingly, all mutations so far described, occurred at the level of the hormone binding domain of the receptor, altering thyroid hormone binding and transactivation properties. The mechanism responsible for the dominant mode of inheritance of the disease is the dominant negative action of the mutated receptor on the normal receptor synthesized by the unaffected allele. In a recent study, we have investigated three RTH families from Southern Italy and identified three new mutations of the thyroid hormone receptor β gene (5). In particular, one of the mutations occurred in the same codon, where another mutation, causing a different aminoacid substitution, was identified by a Japanese group (30). This codon defines, therefore, a new "hot spot" mutation region of the TR β gene.

CONCLUSIONS

Following the dramatic progress in the understanding of the molecular mechanisms of thyroid hormone action, as well as the improvement in diagnostic procedures, the multisystemic involvement due to thyroid deficiency can, today, be referred to a *reduced production of the hormonal signal, or to the inadequate expression of the thyroid hormone message at the level of the multiple intracellular target structures.*

Hypothyroidism should no longer be regarded as a rare clinical condition but, considering also the subclinical form which represents over 60% of the hypothyroid syndromes, it is a frequent situation, showing a prevalence in the general population ranging from 2.5 to 10%. This prevalence is similar to that of diabetes, representing 11% of all thyroid patients, increasing with age and showing a F/M ratio of 5:1. The apparently symptomless thyroid deficiency should no longer be considered a "laboratory disease", since it is not really asymptomatic, but may reveal clinical abnormalities consisting in generalized systemic symptoms as well as neuropsychiatric disorders, changes in cardiac parameters and in lipid metabolism.

Mass screening procedures are mandatory in newborns, to prevent irreversible damage to the CNS, but, in our opinion, screening should be taken into consideration in a selected adult population, to identify symptomless thyroid deficiency, in the attempt to avoid long-term intellectual complications and to prevent increased atherogenic risk and cardiovascular disease.

Our experimental contribution to the understanding of the mechanism of action of thyroid hormone, during CNS differentiation, demonstrates that the mediation of thyroid hormone action is exerted by a peculiar nucleotide sequence, the thyroid hormone response element (TRE), identified in the regulatory region of a brain specific gene. Moreover, we showed that thyroid hormone receptor β appears to play a predominant role during the development and maturation of the CNS, emphasizing the concept of thyroid receptor-dependent *differential regulation* of the neuronal gene expression. We have also confirmed that structural and functional alterations of the thyroid hormone receptor β causes insensitivity of target organs to thyroid hormone action.

In conclusion, the complexity of gene expression regulation by thyroid hormone, whether stimulatory or inhibitory, may be related to the existence of multiple isoforms of thyroid receptors, with specific space- and development-related distribution in target tissues.

Finally, it is tempting to suggest that the differential distribution, qualitative and quantitative, of thyroid hormone receptors, in the various target tissues, represents the molecular substrate of the heterogeneous clinical symptoms of overt and subclinical forms of thyroid deficiency, as well as of the different phenotypes of thyroid hormone resistance syndrome.

REFERENCES

1. Andreoli M. and Giacovazzo M. (1980): Neuropsichiatr. Inf. 224: 275-317.
2. Andreoli M., Pontecorvi A., Dominici R. and Antonozzi I. (1987): Med. Int. 3: 49-59.
3. Andreoli M. and Centanni M. (1991): Rec. Prog. Med. 82: 344-351.
4. Barnes D.J., O'Connor J.D. and Bending J.J. (1993): B.J.C.P. 47: 123-127.
5. Bartolone L., Regalbuto C., Benvenga S., Filetti S., Trimarchi F. and Pontecorvi A. (1994): J. Clin. Endocrinol. Metab. 79: 323-261.
6. Centanni M. and Robbins J. (1987): J. Clin. Invest. 80: 1068-72.
7. Centanni M., Sapone A., Taglienti A. and Andreoli M. (1991): Endocrinology 129: 2175-2179.
8. Chin W.W. (1992): Thyroid Today 15: 1-9.
9. Dillmann W.H. (1990): Am. J. Med. 88: 626-30.
10. Farsetti A., Mitsuhashi T., Desvergne B., Robbins J. and Nikodem V.M. (1991): J. Biol. Chem. 266: 23226-232.
11. Farsetti A., Desvergne B., Hallenbeck P., Robbins J. and Nikodem V.M. (1992): J. Biol. Chem. 267: 15784-788.
12. Gull W.W. (1874): Transactions of the Clinical Society of London 7: 180-85.
13. Haggerty J.J., Garbutt J.C., Evans D.L., Golden R.N., Pedersen C., Simon J.S. and Nemeroff C.B. (1990): Int'l. J. Psych. Med. 20: 193-208.
14. Kendall E.C. (1915): JAMA 64: 2042-43.
15. Kocher T. (1883): Archiv für Clinische Chirurgie 29: 254-337.
16. Lebel J.M. and Dussault J.H. (1994): Curr. Opin. Endocrinol. Diab. (1) 167-174.
17. Medeiros-Neto G., Targovnik M. and Vassart G. (1993): End. Rev. 14: 165-183.

18. Murray G. (1891): British Medical Journal 2: 796-797.
19. Ord W.M. (1878): Medico-chirurgical Transactions 61: 57-78.
20. Ord W.M. (1888): Transactions of the Clinical Society of London 21: 298-300.
21. Papandreou M.J., Persani L., Asteria C., Ronin C. and Beck-Peccoz P. (1993): J. Clin. Endocrinol. Metab. 77(2): 393-8.
22. Persani L., Asteria C., Tonacchera M., Vitti P., Krishna V., Chatterjee K. and Beck-Peccoz P. (1994): J. Clin. Endocrinol. Metab. 78(5): 1034-9.
23. Pontecorvi A. and Robbins J. (1989): Trends Endocr. Metab. 2: 90-94.
24. Refetoff S, DeWind L.T. and DeGroot L.J. (1967): J. Clin. Endocrinol. Metab. 27: 279-294.
25. Refetoff S., Weiss R.E. and Usala S.J. (1993): Endocr. Rev. 14: 348-399.
26. Reverdin J.L. (1882): Revue Medicale de la Suisse Romande 2: 539-540.
27. Robuschi G., Safran M., Braverman L.E., Gnudi A. and Roti E. (1987): Endoc. Rev. 8: 142-153.
28. Sawin C.T. (1990): Thyroid Today 13: 1-11.
29. Sorcini M., Balestrazzi P., Grandolfo M.E., Carta S. and Giovannelli G. (1993): J. Clin. Endocrinol. Invest. 16: 573-577.
30. Takeda K., Sakurai A., DeGroot L.J. and Refetoff S. (1992): J. Clin. Endocrinol. Met. 74: 49-55.
31. Tatsumi K., Miyai K., Notomi T., Kaibe K., Amino N., Mizuno Y. and Kohno H. (1992): Nat. Genet. 1(1): 56-8.
32. Usala S.J., Bale A.E., Gesundheit N., Weiberger C., Lash R.W., Wondisford F.E., McBride O.W. and Weintraub B.D. (1988): Mol. Endocrinol. 2: 1217-20.
33. Wiseman S.A., Powell T. J., Humphries S.E. and Press M. (1993): J. Clin. Endocrinol. Metab. 77: 108-112.

Frontiers in Endocrinology
Volume 9 - 1994

Mapping Thyroid Peroxidase Epitopes using Recombinant Protein Fragments

M. Tonacchera, F. Cetani, S. Costagliola, L. Alcalde, G. Vassart[1] and M. Ludgate

Institut de Recherche Interdisciplinaire (I.R.I.B.H.N.) and [1]Service de Genetique Medicale, Universitè Libre de Bruxelles, 808 Route de Lennik, 1070 Bruxelles, Belgium

INTRODUCTION

Thyroid peroxidase (TPO) is the major component of the thyroid "microsomal" antigen involved in thyroid autoimmune disease (3). TPO autoantibodies (TPOAb) are routinely used as markers for the diagnosis of thyroid autoimmune disease; a direct role of these antibodies in the destruction of the gland in atrophic thyroiditis has also been hypothesized.

The number and location of B cell epitopes within the TPO molecule is a matter of debate; some reports suggest that TPO antibodies bind only to conformational epitopes (6), while in our initial studies we showed the existence of two linear epitope domains (C2 amino acids 590-675; C21 651-750) (7-9); other authors showed the presence of multiple and linear epitopes using recombinant (2, 10) or other techniques (1, 4).

In order to clarify the number and type of TPO epitope domains we performed Western Blot analysis using four recombinant peptide fragments covering the whole molecule and sera from patients with different types of thyroid diseases and sera from normal healthy subjects with TPOAb.

MATERIAL AND METHODS

Patients Group 1: Fourteen patients with Graves' disease and nineteen patients with Hashimoto's thyroiditis or atrophic thyroiditis were diagnosed on the basis of the classical clinical data and laboratory findings.

Group 2: Seventeen patients with nodular goiter and focal thyroiditis were diagnosed by the presence of a nodular goiter, normal FT3, FT4, and TSH serum levels and evidence of thyroid peroxidase antibodies.

Group 3: Ten normal subjects were selected for the presence of thyroperoxidase antibodies in the absence of goiter and/or hyper/ hypothyroidism.

Controls: Sera from 30 normal healthy subjects and negative for TPOAb measured by RIA were used as controls.

Plasmid construction The cDNA of four overlapping fragments of human TPO (TPO 1 Gln 17-Ser 227), (TPO 2 Tyr 226-Thr 476), (TPO 3 Gln 471- Ser 720), (TPO 4 Phe 709-Leu 933) were amplified by PCR and subcloned into the expression vector p-MAL.

Each of these constructs encodes a fusion protein in which the aminoterminal portion is maltose binding protein followed by the sequence of the fragment of the human TPO. The plasmid constructs were transformed in Escherichia coli and, after growth, bacterial cells were harvested, lysed and the lysate was passed over an amylose affinity column and eluted with maltose. Purified proteins were loaded onto 10% sodium dodecyl sulfate polyacrylamide gels, stained with Coomassie blue or electrophoretically transferred to nitrocellulose membranes.

Western blots were performed by incubating 1:100 dilution of individual normal or patient's sera.

RESULTS

To optimize the production of each recombinant fusion protein in a soluble form from the bacterial lysate Escherichia coli were grown at a temperature of 30° and 0.05 mM of isopropylthiogalactoside (IPTG) was used for growth induction. These conditions yielded a fusion protein of the expected size for each construct.

To confirm the identity of the fusion protein an immunoblot was performed with the relevant rabbit antisera.

The results obtained, incubating human sera from individuals of the three groups, show that in the first group 91% of sera recognized TPO 3, 33% recognized TPO 4 while 21% and 18% reacted with TPO 1 and TPO 2, respectively.

Among the three sera negative for TPO 3, 2 sera did not recognize any other fragment, while one serum reacted with TPO 4 alone. In the second group of patients, 76% of sera recognized TPO 3, 35% recognized TPO 4, and 29% reacted with TPO 1 and 29% with TPO 2. Among the four sera negative for TPO 3, three sera did not react with any other fragment, while one recognized

TPO 1. In the group of normal healthy subjects, the single peptides were recognized at a similar frequency compared to the other groups.

CONCLUSIONS

In this work, we have optimized the production of large peptide fragments of TPO in bacteria which is useful to the investigation of B cell epitopes using a large number of patients' sera.

We have demonstrated that:

1) TPOAb are able to bind linear epitopes with a hot spot in TPO 3 (known to contain the linear epitopes (C2 and C21));

2) TPOAb recognize other epitopes in the aminoterminal and close to the carboxyterminal part of the protein;

3) no difference is observed, comparing the levels of antibodies and the number or type of peptide fragments recognized;

4) there are no disease specific epitopes, and sera from normal healthy subjects with TPOAb recognize the same epitopes in a similar percentage.

REFERENCES

1. Banga J.P., Doble N., Tomlison R.W.S., Odell E. and McGregor A.M. (1989): Immunology 67: 197-204.
2. Banga J.P., Barnett P.S., Ewins D.L., Page M.J. and McGregor A.M. (1990): Autoimmunity 6: 257-68.
3. Czarnoscka B., Ruf J., Fernand M., Carayon P. and Lissintzky S. (1985): FEBS Lett. 190: 147-52.
4. Doble N.D., Banga J.P., Pope R., Lalor E., Kilduff P. and McGregor A.M. (1988): Immunology 64: 23-29.
5. Elisei R., Mariotti S., Swillens S., Vassart G. and Ludgate M. (1990): Autoimmunity 8: 65-70.
6. Finke R., Seto P. and Rapaport B. (1989): J. Clin. Endocrinol. Metab. 71: 53-59.
7. Libert F., Ruel J., Ludgate M., Swillens S., Alexander N., Vassart G. and Dinsart C. (1987): EMBO J. 6: 4193-96.
8. Libert F., Ludgate M., Dinsart C. and Vassart G. (1991): J. Clin. Endocrinol. Metab. 713: 857-60.
9. Ludgate M., Mariotti S., Libert F., Dinsart C., Piccolo P. and Santini F. (1988): J. Clin. Endocrinol. Metab. 68: 1091-96.
10. Maastricht J., Koenig R.J., Kaplan M.M., Arscott P., Thompson N. and Baker J.R. (1992): J. Clin. Endocrinol. Metab. 75: 121-26.

Frontiers in Endocrinology
Volume 9 - 1994

Specific Autoantibody Binding to Thyroid Peroxidase: Dominant Role of the Light Chain in Determining Epitope Recognition

G. Costante, S. Portolano, S.M. McLachlan and B. Rapoport

Thyroid Molecular Biology Unit, Veterans' Administration Medical Center, University of California, San Francisco, CA 94121, USA

INTRODUCTION

Circulating autoantibodies directed against thyroid peroxidase (TPO) are typically present in patients with autoimmune thyroid disease. These autoantibodies are polyclonal, as indicated by the contribution of different immunoglobulin G subclasses (IgG1, IgG4) and light chain types (κ–λ) to TPO binding in the same patient serum (reviewed in 3). Recently, a panel of recombinant human IgG class antigen binding fragments (Fab) with high affinity (10^{-10} M Kd) for TPO has been isolated using the combinatorial heavy (H) and light (L) chain library approach (1, 4). The TPO-specific Fabs recognize a limited number of epitopes grouped in 2 major domains (domain A and B) on TPO molecule (1). The genes coding for the H and L chains of the TPO-specific Fabs have also been characterized. Analysis of the nucleotide sequences of these genes showed a restricted gene usage (4 H chains and 3 L chains), with only 5 different H-L chain combinations (1).

Aim of the present study was to investigate the roles of H and L chains in determining autoantibody binding to different TPO epitopes.

MATERIAL AND METHODS

Preparation of soluble Fab fragments Fabs were expressed as soluble proteins in XL1-blue cells as previously described (1, 4).

Direct binding of ^{125}I-TPO by Fab fragments Secreted recombinant human TPO (2) was labelled with ^{125}I to a specific activity of ~50μCi/μg by the Iodogen method (6). The Fabs, diluted in assay buffer (0.1 M NaCl - 10 mM Tris, pH 7.5 - 0.1 % Tween 20 - 0.5 % BSA) were incubated with ^{125}I-TPO (15.000 - 20000 cpm) and mouse monoclonal antibody to human-κ L chain (QE11, Recognition Sciences, Birmingham, UK) in a total volume of 200 μl. After 1 h at room temperature, Sac-cel (IDS, Boldon, Tyne and Wear, UK) was added and the incubation continued for an additional 30 min. The mixture was then diluted with 1 ml of assay buffer, centrifuged (5 min, 1000 x g) and the pellet counted to determine the percentage of ^{125}I-TPO bound. Nonspecific binding was 2-5 % of total counts.

Competition between Fabs for binding to TPO One Fab was immobilized with mouse monoclonal antibody to human-κ L chain (QE11). After 1 h at room temperature, Sac-cel was added and the incubation continued for an additional 30 min. The mixture was then washed, centrifuged (5 min, 1000 x g) and the pellet resuspended in normal human serum (1:30 in assay buffer). In a separate set of tubes, increasing concentrations of free Fabs were incubated with ^{125}I-TPO for 1 h, at room temperature. Aliquots (100μl) were then incubated for 30 min with the immobilized Fabs, washed in assay buffer, centrifuged and the radioactivity bound to Sac-cel counted. Nonspecific binding was ~2 %.

RESULTS

We selected two Fabs known to bind to non overlapping epitopes in the immunodominant region of TPO: clone TR1.9, which lies exclusively on domain B and clone WR1.7, the binding site of which resides only on domain A (Fig. 1). Both Fabs use H chain variable region genes (VH) most closely related to V1-3B germline gene, with minor amino acid changes throughout VH. However, the most striking amino acid differences between TR1.9 and WR1.7 are in the complementarity-determining region-3 (CDR3) (Fig. 1) and this could be relevant in determining epitope specificity. Nevertheless, the epitope specificity could result from the use of different L chain variable region (VL)

Clone	VH	CDR3	VL
TR1.9	V1-3B	DPYGGGKSE	A'
WR1.7	V1-3B	RGDSNIWYLG	KL012
TR1.10	V1-3B	VLGIIAADH	KL012
TR1.23	V1-3B	SGVGSNDFHFAL	KL012

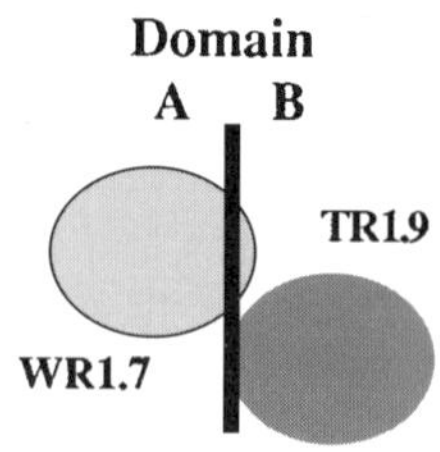

FIG. 1. VH and VL germline genes and aminoacid sequences of the H chain CDR3 regions of the four clones (left). Schematic representation of TPO domains A and B (right).

germline genes. In fact, WR1.7 uses a KL012-like VL while TR1.9 VL is mostly homologous to A' germline gene. Two other Fabs, TR1.23 and TR1.10, like WR1.7, use V1-3B VH and KL012 VL germline genes. However, the H chain CDR3 of these two Fabs differ from each other and from that of WR1.7.

We, therefore, compared the domains recognized by TR1.23 and TR1.10 with those recognized by TR1.9 (B domain) and WR1.7 (A domain). For this purpose, we determined the ability of increasing concentration of one Fab to inhibit the binding of ^{125}I-TPO by a second, immobilized Fab. As illustrated in Figure 2, TR1.9 did not inhibit TPO binding to immobilized WR1.7 and WR1.7 was completely ineffective in inhibiting TPO binding by immobilized TR1.9. Similarly, TR1.23 and TR1.10 even at very high concentrations did not inhibit TPO binding by immobilized TR1.9. On the contrary, both TR1.23 and TR1.10 were almost as effective as WR1.7 in inhibiting TPO binding to immobilized WR1.7. Therefore, the epitopes of TR1.10 and TR1.23 overlap with the TR1.7 epitope.

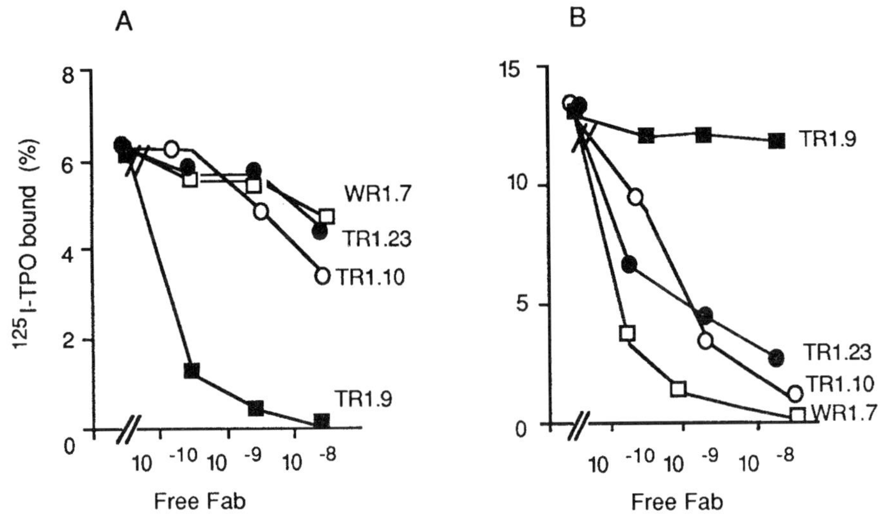

FIG. 2. Competition between Fabs for the binding of ^{125}I-TPO. Free Fabs were used to compete for TPO binding to immobilized TR1.9 (panel A) or to immobilized WR1.7 (Panel B).

DISCUSSION

Several studies indicate that the H chain, in particular its CDR3, plays a dominant role in determining antibody specificity (6, 7). However, another study has shown that the L chain may be involved in epitope specificity (5). In the present investigation, we examined the role of H and L chains in determining the binding of recombinant IgG autoantibody Fab fragments to different TPO epitopes. We took four Fabs which use V1-3B-like H chain with different CDR3 regions. Three of the four Fabs (WR1.7, TR1.10 and TR1.23) have a KL012-like L chain and one Fab (TR1.9) uses a completely different L chain (A'-like). Previously, we observed that WR1.7 (KL012-like L chain) binds to the A domain, while TR1.9 (A'-like L chain) recognizes the B domain in the immunodominant region of TPO (Fig. 2) (1). The present data show that the epitopes recognized by TR1.10 and TR1.23 (KL012-like L chain) overlap the WR1.7 epitope, suggesting that the KL012-like L chain and not the H chain CDR3 determines the domain specificity of the TPO-specific Fabs.

In conclusion, the L chain, rather than the H chain plays a dominant role in defining the epitope recognition of TPO binding Fabs.

REFERENCES

1. Chazenbalk G., et al. (1993): J. Clin. Invest. 92: 62-74.
2. Foti D., et al. (1990): Mol. Endocrinol. 4: 786-791.
3. McLachlan S. and Rapoport B. (1992): Endocr. Rev. 13: 192-206.
4. Portolano S., et al. (1992): J. Clin. Invest. 90: 720-726.
5. Ruff-Jamison S. and Glenny J.R. (1993): J. Immunol. 150: 3389-3396.
6. Salacinski P.R.P., et al. (1981): Anal. Biochem. 117: 136-146.
7. Smith-Gill S.J., et al. (1987): J. Immunol. 139: 4135-4144.

Frontiers in Endocrinology
Volume 9 - 1994

Transfection of a Poorly Differentiated Rat Thyroid Cell Line (FRT) with the cDNA of the Human Thyrotropin (TSH) Receptor

P. Vitti, R. Elisei, L. Chiovato, C. Mammoli, C. Romei, F. Santini, G. Bendinelli, P. Lapi, P. Agretti, A. Capaccioli and A. Pinchera

Institute of Endocrinology, University of Pisa, V.le del Tirreno, 64, 56018 Tirrenia, Pisa, Italy

INTRODUCTION

Thyroid cell cultures of different animal species have been developed in the last years and used for clinical and thyroid pathophysiology research. The differentiated rat thyroid cell line FRTL-5 (1, 5) allowed the studies of several thyroid specific cell functions such as TSH-dependent growth (10, 11) adenylate cyclase (12, 13), iodide uptake (7) and expression of thyroid specific proteins (3) using FRTL-5 cells. Clinical assays for thyroid stimulating antibodies (TSAb) (12, 13) and TSH-blocking antibodies (TSH-BAb) (4) present in sera of patients with thyroid autoimmune diseases were also developed.

More recently, cell clones expressing the human TSH receptor on the cell surface were developed by stable transfection of Chinese hamster ovary cells (CHO) with the cDNA of the human TSH receptor (hTSH-R) gene (6, 8, 9). With respect to FRTL-5 cells, CHO-R cells have the advantages of requiring less sophisticated culture conditions and of expressing the hTSH-R that offers species specificity (14). On the other hand, CHO-R cells have the disadvantage of not being suitable for studies that require the evaluation of steps occurring beyond the activation of the adenylate cyclase as they are not derived from thyroid cells.

In this study, we report the stable transfection with the hTSH-R cDNA of a cell line (FRT) that is derived from the rat thyroid (1), but has no functional TSH receptor, does not secrete thyroglobulin, nor express thyroperoxidase (2).

MATERIAL AND METHODS

FRT cells were grown in 10 cm Petri dishes to confluency in Coon's F12 medium and 5% calf serum. The hTSH-R pSVL expression vector (kindly provided by Dr. G. Vassart I.R.B.H.N., Bruxelles) and pSV2 NEO neomycin resistance gene vector were co-transfected into FRT cells using a modified calcium phosphate method (9). After 48 h, selection of transfected cells was initiated by addition of medium containing 0.4 g/L geneticin (Sigma Co, St Louis). Cells were fed fresh medium containing geneticin every 3 days. After 3 weeks, when all cells of a parallel nontransfected culture exposed to geneticin had died, the few nests of cells surviving the selection were gently scraped from the dish, subjected to limiting dilution and seeded into a 96 well dish (Costar, Cambridge MA). Cells growing in the 96 well dish were further amplified and tested for their ability to increase cAMP production in response to TSH.

RESULTS

FRT cells were tested for adenylate cyclase activity in basal conditions (hypochloric medium, in the presence of IBMX for 60 min at 37°C). TSH (0.1-1000 μU/mL) was unable to increase cAMP production (Fig. 1), while 1-100 nMol/mL forskolin elicited a cAMP stimulation of 12-100 fold with respect to the basal value (data not shown).

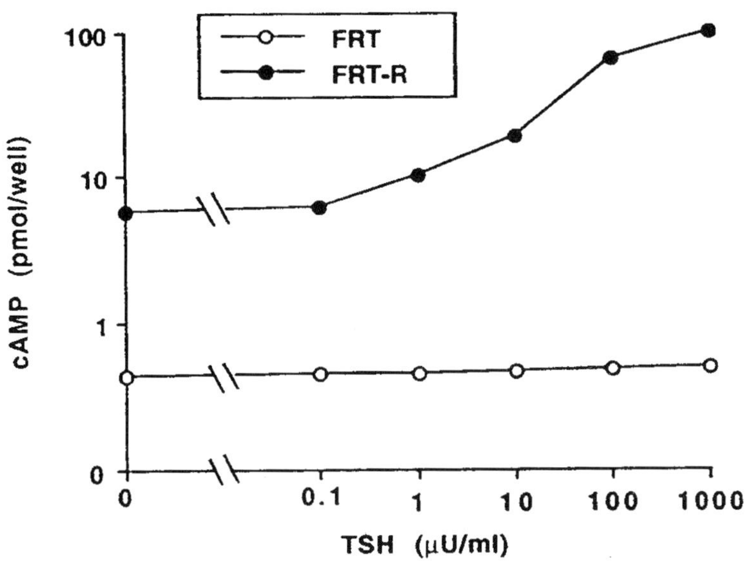

FIG. 1. cAMP production stimulated by TSH in FRT and FRT-R3 cells.

Co-transfection with the TSH-R gene vector and pSV2-NEO resulted in 7 clones of cells surviving to the geneticin selection. Two of these clones (FRT-R3 and FRT-R6) were able to increase cAMP production in response to TSH. In particular, the FRT-R3 clone showed the highest sensitivity to the hormone, the minimal amount of TSH able to elicit a significant response being 1 μU/mL, with a 12-fold cAMP increase with respect to the basal value at 100 μU/mL TSH (Fig. 1). This sensitivity is comparable to that displayed by the well differentiated rat thyroid cell line FRTL-5 and CHO-R (12-14). The ability to respond to TSH was unchanged after several splitting passages with Tripsin/EGTA mixture, showing that transfection was long-standing.

CONCLUSIONS

The data reported in this paper show that insertion of the hTSH-R cDNA in the genome of a nontumoral, but poorly differentiated rat thyroid cell line, results in the recovery of some properties of thyroid cells such as the TSH-dependent adenylate cyclase. More extensive studies on this, or potentially other cell lines constructed by the recombinant DNA technology, may be useful for a better understanding of the pathways activated via the TSH receptor.

REFERENCES

1. Ambesi-Impiombato F.S., Parks L.A.M. and Coons H.G. (1980): Proc. Natl. Acad. Sci. USA 77, 3455-3459.
2. Ambesi-Impiombato F.S., Picone R. and Tramontano D. (1982): In: Vol. 9 Sirbasku A., Sata G.H., Pardee A. (Eds), Cold Spring Harbor Conference on Cell Proliferation. Growth of cells in hormonally defined media. Cold Spring Harbor Laboratories, New York, p. 483-492.
3. Chiovato L., Vitti P., Lombardi A., Ceccarelli P., Cucchi P., Marcocci C., Carayon P. and Pinchera A. (1988): Endocrinology 123, 1140-1146.
4. Chiovato L., Vitti P., Santini F., Lopez G., Mammoli C., Bassi P., Giusti L., Tonacchera M., Fenzi G.F. and Pinchera A. (1990): J. Clin. Endocrinol. Metab. 71, 40-45.
5. Kohn L.D., Valente V.A., Grollman E.F., Aloj S.M. and Vitti P. (1986): US Patent 4, 609-622.
6. Libert F., Lefort A., Gerard C., Parmentier M., Perret J., Ludgate M., Dumont J.E. and Vassart G. (1989): Biochem. Biophys. Res. Commun. 165, 1250-1255.
7. Marcocci C., Valente W.A., Pinchera A., Aloj S.M., Kohn L.D. and Grollman E.F. (1983): J. Endocrinol. Invest. 6, 463-471.
8. Parmentier M., Libert F., Maenhaut C., Lefort A., Gerard C., Perret J., van Sande J., Dumont J.E. and Vassart G. (1989): Science 246, 1620-1622.
9. Perret J., Ludgate M., Libert F., Vassart G., Dumont J.E. and Parmentier M. (1990): Biochem. Biophys. Res. Commun. 171, 1044-1050.
10. Valente W.A., Vitti P., Kohn L.D., Brandi M.L., Rotella C.M., Toccafondi R., Tramontano D., Aloj S.M. and Ambesi-Impiombato F.S. (1983a:) Endocrinology 112, 71-79.
11. Valente W.A., Vitti P., Rotella C.M., Vaughan M.M., Aloj S.M., Grollman E.F., Ambesi-Impiombato F.S. and Kohn L.D. (1983b): New Engl. J. Med. 309, 1028-1034.
12. Vitti P., Valente W.A., Ambesi-Impiombato F.S., Fenzi G.F., Pinchera A. and Kohn L.D. (1982): J. Endocrinol. Invest. 5, 179-182.

13. Vitti P., Rotella C.M., Valente W.A., Cohen J., Aloj S.M., Laccetti P., Ambesi-Impiombato F.S., Grollman E.F., Pinchera A., Toccafondi R. and Kohn L.D. (1983): J. Clin. Endocrinol. Metab. 57, 782-791.
14. Vitti P., Elisei R., Tonacchera M., Chiovato L., Mancusi F., Rago T., Mammoli C., Ludgate M., Vassart G. and Pinchera A. (1993): J. Clin. Endocrinol. Metab. 76, 499-503.

Frontiers in Endocrinology
Volume 9 - 1994

Novel Mutations of Thyrotropin Receptor Gene in Thyroid Hyperfunctioning Adenomas. Rapid Identification by Fine Needle Aspiration Biopsy

A. Porcellini, I. Ciullo, L. Laviola, G. Amabile[1], L. Marzano, V.E. Avvedimento[2] and G. Fenzi[1]

Centre for Endocrinology and Experimental Oncology C.N.R., Department of Biology and Molecular and Cellular Pathology, II Faculty of Medicine, via S. Pansini 5, Napoli; [2]Department of Experimental Medicine, Faculty of Medicine in Catanzaro, via T. Campanella 3, Catanzaro; [1]Chair of Endocrinology, II Faculty of Medicine, via S. Pansini 5, 80131 Naples, Italy

INTRODUCTION

Hyperfunctioning adenomas of the thyroid are neoplasms characterized by autonomous growth and overproduction of thyroid hormones. The consecutive activation of growth, differentiation and oversecretion of thyroid hormones by these neoplasms inhibits pituitary secretion of TSH leading to suppression of the function in the contiguous non-adenomatous tissue.

Recently several somatic mutations have been reported in the TSH receptor (TSH-R) and Gs or Gi protein genes, all of them leading to clonal growth and activation of cAMP pathway, ultimately responsible for hyperthyroidism (4, 8 and refs. therein). These TSH-R mutations were rare (3 out of 11 patients), and were all located in the third cytoplasmic loop of the receptor (8).

MATERIAL AND METHODS

11 patients (3 males and 8 females, aged between 25 to 70 years) with hyperfunctioning thyroid nodules were selected. All had a single "hot" nodule revealed by ^{131}I scan and complete suppression of the remaining thyroid tissue observed at echotomography, undetectable TSH by ultrasensitive radioassay

(Incstar Corp, Stillwater, MN. - normal range 0.4-3.7 mU/L) normal or elevated total and free T_4 and T_3 levels.

Total RNA was extracted from fine needle aspiration biopsy samples using acid guanidinium thiocyanate-phenol-chloroform extraction (1). Single strand cDNA synthesis was performed on 1 µg of total RNA (denatured by heating at 75 °C for 5 min) in 20 µl of reaction buffer (50 mM Tris-HCl pH 8.3, 75 mM KCl, 15 mM $MgCl_2$, 10 mM DTT, 500 µM dNTP) containing 20 pmol of random primers and 200 U of M-MLV RNase H^- Reverse Transcriptase (Superscript-GIBCO BRL) at 42 °C for 2 h.

Five microlitres of the cDNA reaction (or 200 ng of genomic DNA obtained from PBL) was amplified in 100µl of PCR buffer (10 mM Tris-HCl pH 8.3, 50 mM KCl_2, 1.5 mM $MgCl_2$, 0.001% gelatine, 200 mM dNTP) containing 30 pmol of each oligonucleotide primer. One unit of Taq DNA polymerase was added after the first denaturation (5 min at 97 °C). Samples were then subjected to 31 cycles consisting of 1 min at 95 °C, 1 min at 60 °C and 1 min at 72 °C. The last extension was carried out for 12 min. The 3' region was amplified with primers: **D** 5'-ACCGAGACCCCTCTTGCTCT-3'; 5' end at 1720 and **F** 5'-CCCCTACCATTGTGAGTAGTG-3'; 5' end at 2326 (7, 2 and Fig. 1).

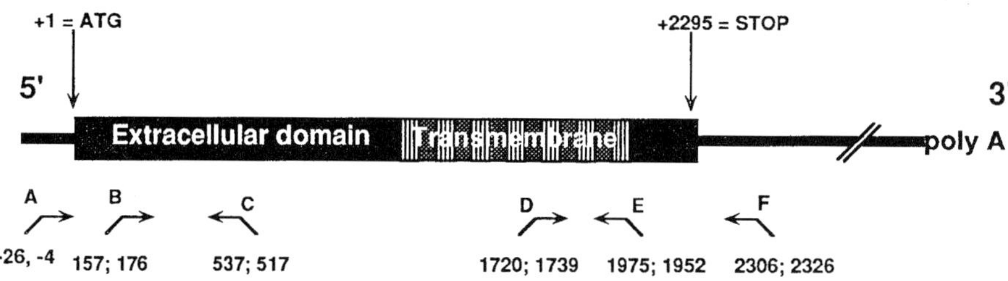

FIG. 1. Structure of human TSH-R mRNA and location of DNA primers used for amplification.

DNA sequencing was performed on double-stranded PCR products by modifyng a previously described procedure (T7 Sequencing Kit, Pharmacia). Briefly: one pmole of purified template DNA was mixed with 20 pmol of primer (oligo **E** 5'-AGTTGCTAACAGTGATGAGAGGCT-3'; 5' end at 1975) in 14 µl of 40mM Tris-HCl (pH 7.5), 25 mM $MgCl_2$, 50 mM NaCl, and 10% DMSO. After boiling for 3 min and cooling on ice, 3 µl of labeling mix, 10µCi (3.3 pmol) $\alpha[^{32}P]$dATP, and 2 µl of 1.5 U/µl T7 polymerase were added. The labeling reaction was incubated at 25 °C for 45 sec and then transferred (4.5 µl each) in four prewarmed tubes containing 2.5 µl each of termination mix and incubated at 37 °C for 5 min. Termination reactions were stopped by adding 5 µl of stop solution. Two microliters of each reaction was loaded onto a 5% denaturing polyacrylamide gel.

Plasmid constructions: TSH-R wild type has been cloned by PCR amplification of reverse transcribed RNA from normal thyroid with primers A and F (2). The amplified band was purified, ligated with Eco RI linkers and cloned in the Eco RI site of pUC19. To clone TSH-R mutants, the cDNAs from the FANB has been amplified with primers D and F, digested with Bgl II/Bst EII and cloned in the same sites of TSH-R wild type-pUC19. Clones containing the wild type and mutated inserts were selected by restriction and subcloned in the expression vector pBabe-puro (6). The clones were checked by DNA sequence analysis.

NIH 3T3 cells were transfected by calcium phosphate procedure (9) with 5 μg of pRSV-lacZ, CRE-CAT and TSH-R wild type or mutants, respectively. 24 hours later the calcium precipitate was removed, the dishes were washed and supplemented with DMEM medium containing 10% fetal calf serum. After 34 hours from the transfection the medium was changed and the serum was lowered to 0.5%. 10 hours later, in triplicate dishes, IBMX (0.5 mM), IBMX and TSH (1 mU/ml) or IBMX and forskolin 25 μM were added. The stimulation was maintained for 4 hours (50 hours from the transfection) and was then stopped by washing the cells with PBS. Total cell extracts were prepared as described (9). Lac-Z activity was measured and used to normalize for differences in transfection efficiency. CAT activity was measured as described (9).

RESULTS

We found 7 mutants all located in the sixth membrane-spanning domain of the TSH-R adjacent (4 to 5 residues) to the third intracytoplasmic loop, where other mutations have been found (8). The DNA sequence revealed the presence of 4 different aminoacid changes at residues 631-632-633 (Phe-Thr-Asp) of the receptor. All the mutations were present in one allele and were somatic, since the DNA from lymphocytes of the same patient did not present such changes. The most frequent mutation changes the residue 632 (Thr->Ile due to a G->A transition). This change has been found independently in three cases. The second most frequent mutation was located at the residue 633 and consisted in a Asp->Glu change (C->A) in two cases and in a Asp->Thy (G->A) in another patient. The mutation 631 (Phe->Cys) was found in one patient. To test the biological effects of these mutations we inserted the mutations in the wild type receptor, expressed them in mouse fibroblasts and analysed the cAMP dependent transcription. Figure 2 shows the activity of a reporter gene (E. coli cloramphenicol acetyl transferase) driven by cAMP responsive element (CRE) in cells expressing wild type or mutated receptors (residues 631 and 632). The activation of CRE driven transcription represents a very specific assay of cAMP dependent response, since it is downstream the cAMP cascade and it is extremely sensitive to the nuclear concentration of catalytic subunit of cAMP dependent kinase (3).

Transcription of CRE in 3T3 cells was induced only by forskolin, due to the absence of the TSH-R in these cells (control in Figure 2). The expression of wild type TSH-R conferred TSH induction to the CRE promoter (HTSH-R wt). The expression of the mutated receptor containing the Thr->Ile substitution (HTSH-R M632) significantly increased the basal value of the cAMP dependent transcription. Also the mutation 631 produced the same effects.

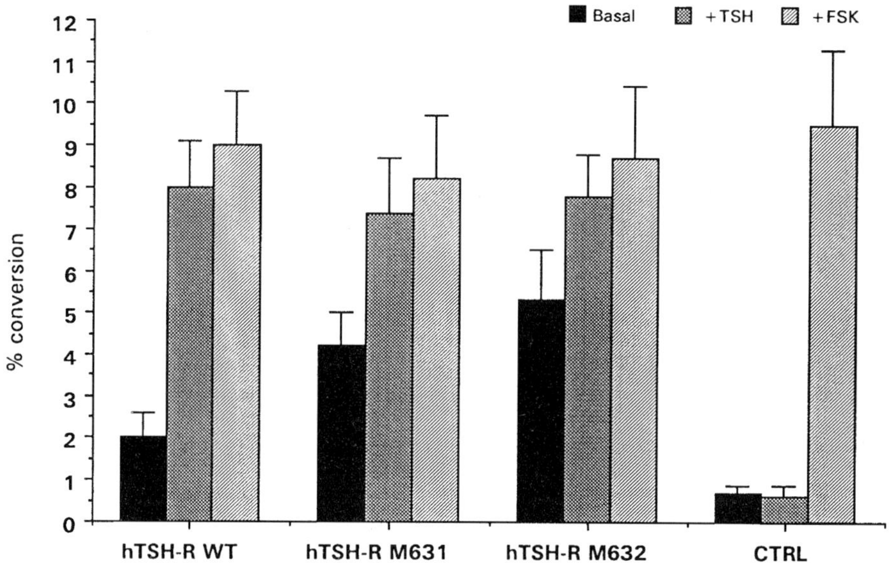

FIG. 2. Expression of mutated TSH-R at residues 631 (Phe->Cys) and 632 (Thr->Ile) constitutively activates cAMP dependent transcription in mouse fibroblasts. 3T3 cells were transiently transfected with plasmid constructs containing wild type TSH receptor (HTSH-R WT), mutated receptor at residue 631 (HTSH-R M631) and 632 (HTSH-R M632), and vector alone (control). In all transfections RSV-lac Z DNA was included. The cells were stimulated with TSH and forskolin (FSK) as indicated in Methods. Lac-Z activity was determined and comparable amounts of proteins, normalized for transfection efficiency were tested for CAT activity by thin layer chromatography, as described in Methods. The acetylated and non-acetylated chloramphenicol was quantitated by excising the spots from the rigid support and counted by liquid scintillation. The values are expressed as % of conversion from non-acetylated to acetylated chloramphenicol.

Most of the mutations lead to a gain or loss of a site of a restriction enzyme in this segment of TSH-R, as deduced by DNA sequence of the wild type and mutants. We tested this prediction by restriction analysis of the amplified fragments of TSH-R obtained from FNAB or from PBL of the patients. The results are summarized in Table 1. The restriction enzymes Taq I, Eco RI, Hph I and Asp718 can be used as tools for the rapid identification of these mutations. It is worth noting that this analysis is rapid and diagnostic of the molecular lesion causing hyperfunctioning adenoma.

Table 1. *Rapid identification of TSH-R gene mutations by restriction analysis*

Mutation	Enzyme	Fragments Wild-type	Fragments Mutant
632: T->I	Taq I ACCGAC->ATCGAC	606 bp	431 bp 175 bp
633: D->E	Eco RI GACTTC->GAATTC	606 bp	433 bp 173 bp
631: F->C	Hph I TCACC*->GCACC	285 bp 172 bp 150 bp	322 bp 285 bp
619: D->G(8)	Asp 718 GATACC->GGTACC	606 bp	472 bp 134 bp

* HphI site (5'-GGTGA-3' 8/7) reported here is on the (-) strand.

DISCUSSION

Our results show that in 11 independent thyroid hyperfunctioning adenomas, TSH receptor gene is mutated in a cluster of three aminoacids located in the IV membrane spanning domain of the receptor. These mutations are somatic, specifically present in the tumor tissue and absent in other cell types from the same individual.

Even though we did not formally prove that all the 4 mutations reported here have biological effects on cAMP dependent transcription, we believe that this is the case on the basis of the following considerations:

1. mutations at residues 631 and 632 significantly stimulate basal cAMP dependent transcription in the absence of TSH;
2. detailed mutagenesis of glycoprotein receptors indicates that the third cytoplasmic loop and the sixth membrane-spanning segment contain invariant residues and that any change in these areas results in constitutive activation of the receptor. The wild-type residues are uniquely suited to the task of keeping the receptor in its inactive state (4, 8, 5);
3. mutations of Aspartic residue (corresponding to position 633 in TSH-R) in glycine of LH receptor, has been shown to activate the receptor, leading to precocious puberty in the male (10);
4. the mutations reported here are somatic and unique in these two segments of the TSH-R required for G-protein interaction.

We did not find any of the three mutations recently reported in thyroid adenomas. We believe that this is due to the low frequency (3/11) of these changes, compared to those that we found (7/11). Conversely, the mutations reported here escaped detection due to the contiguity to the FTD residues of the oligonucleotides used as primers in the study (8).

CONCLUSIONS

In our opinion, the membrane spanning domain may be the hot spot of mutations causing hyperfunctioning adenomas of thyroid gland. If the frequency of these TSH-R mutations is confirmed, we speculate that most hyperfunctioning thyroid adenomas are caused either by mutations in TSH-R or in G-protein genes.

Clinical implications If the high frequency of the mutations reported here, are confirmed in higher number of hyperfunctioning adenomas, a new approach to hot nodules will have to be considered. Fine needle aspiration biopsy is a routine and initial procedure for screening many types of thyroid lesions. It will be of interest to test for the presence of the mutations reported here by restriction enzyme analysis of PCR products. This may provide early detection and possibly a new classification of lesions that will ultimately lead to hyperfunctioning adenomas.

REFERENCES

1. Chomczynski P. and Sacchi N. (1987): Anal. Biochem. 162: 156-159.
2. Feliciello A., Porcellini A., Ciullo I. et al. (1993): Lancet 342: 337-338.
3. Hagiwara M., Brindle P., Harootunian A., Armstrong R., Rivier J., Vale W., Tsien R. and Montminty M.R. (1993): Mol. Cell. Biol. 13 (8): 4852-9.
4. Lefkowitz, R.J. (1993): Nature; 365: 603-604.
5. Lefkowitz R.J., Cotecchia S., Samama P. and Costa T. (1993): Trends Pharmacol. Sci. 14 (8): 303-7.
6. Morgenstern J.P. and Land H. (1990): Nucleic Acid Res. 18 (12): 3587-96.
7. Nagayama Y., Kaufman K.D., Seto P. and Rapoport B. (1989): Biochem. Biophys. Res. Commun. 165: 1184-1190.
8. Parma J., Duprez L., Van Sande J. et al. (1993): Nature 365: 649-651.
9. Sambrook J., Fritsch E.F. and Maniatis T. (1989): Cold Spring Harbor Laboratory Press, Cold Spring Harbour, New York.
10. Shenker A., Laue L., Kosugi S. et al. (1993): Nature 365: 652-653.

Frontiers in Endocrinology
Volume 9 - 1994

Pathogenic Role for the cAMP Cascade in Thyroid Hyperfunctioning Adenomas

D. Russo[1], F. Arturi, U. Crocetti, M. Musella[2], E. Rocca[3], M. Schlumberger[4], H.G. Suarez[5] and S. Filetti

Chair of Endocrinology, Department of Experimental and Clinical Medicine; [1]Chair of Pharmacology, Faculty of Pharmacy, University of Reggio Calabria, 88100 Catanzaro; [2]Chair of Endocrine Surgery; [3]Ospedale Civile A. Pugliese, Catanzaro, Italy; [4]Institut de Recherches Scientifiques sur le Cancer, CNRS Villejuif; [5]Institut Gustave-Roussy, 94805 Villejuif, France

INTRODUCTION

Autonomously functioning thyroid adenomas are localized nodules, the function and growth of which are not dependent upon thyrotropin or any extrathyroidal stimulators.

These nodules may remain unchanged over years or progress slowly to become larger (diameter >3 cm) and they may cause thyrotoxicosis (2). Autonomous thyroid nodule was shown to have a higher prevalence in iodine deficient areas (4.4% in Europe vs 0.9% in USA (3), where they represent the most frequent cause of thyrotoxicosis.

The clinical picture is dominated by the presence of anxiety, insomnia, irritability, heat intolerance, tachycardia and palpitations, and, locally, a single hot nodule with an unlimited growth rate, unless spontaneous necrosis or surgical excision occur.

The diagnosis is based upon the presence of a "hot" nodule and suppression of the remaining tissue upon ^{131}I-thyroid scanning, associated with elevated serum levels of free thyroid hormones and low or undetectable TSH, even after the TRH stimulation test.

Biological characteristics (coexistence with quiescent TSH responsive cells) and experimental evidence (hyperactivity of the nodular cells transplanted in nude mice (2) support the hypothesis of the clonal expansion of genetically altered cells as the causative event of this disease. As far as concerns the dual role of cAMP in mediating the TSH effects in both proliferation and differentiation signals (1), the constitutive activation of the cAMP signal transduction system may be considered the pathogenic mechanism responsible for the disease. As shown in Figure 1, it may derive from the constitutive activation of either the Gαcs protein or the TSH receptor (TSHR) which may fully reproduce the condition of permanent TSH stimulation on growth and function of the thyrocytes.

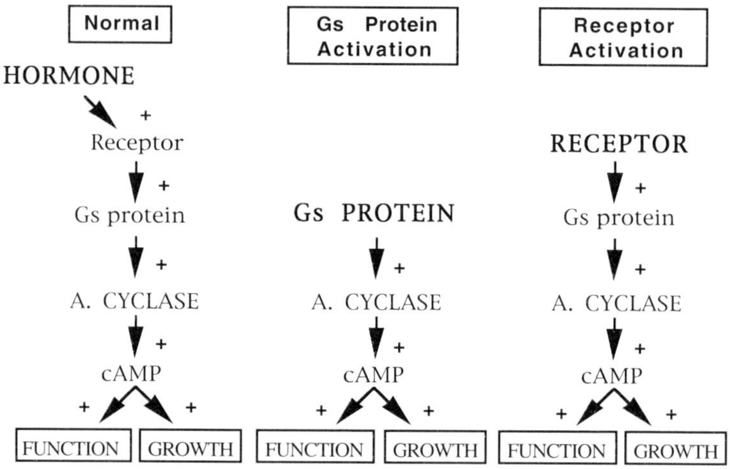

Fig. 1. cAMP cascade as possible oncogenic pathway.

Activation of the oncogene gsp due to point mutations in the Gαs protein gene, has been described in about 30% of thyroid autonomously hyperfunctioning adenomas in different studies (5, 7, 9). In the remaining 70% of gsp-negative tumors the same phenotype may be derived from alterations of other components of the cAMP pathways, first of all the TSH receptor (TSHR), a G-protein coupled receptor with seven transmembrane spanning regions (6). Indeed, activating alterations of G-protein coupled receptors, including the TSHR, have recently been described in human pathology (4, 8).

MATERIAL AND METHODS

Thyroid hyperfunctioning adenomas (n=37) removed at surgery were examined for the presence of mutations in the TSHR, Gαs and ras genes. PCR amplified fragments of the TSHR C-terminal part (exon 10), the Gs alpha protein (exons 8 and 9) genes and ras probes were obtained from the genomic DNA extracted by the tumors and the adjacent normal tissue. These samples were sequenced by the method of Sanger for detection of mutations in the TSHR gene or, alternatively, blotted in nitrocellular filters and hybridized with a series of wild-type and mutated oligonucleotides encompassing the areas containing the hot codons of gsp (201 and 227) or ras (12/13 and 61) genes (10, 11).

RESULTS AND DISCUSSION

Sequencing of parts of exon 10 of the TSHR gene revealed the presence of a single base substitution at residue 623 (TCC for GCC: Ser for Ala), together with the wild-type sequence, in 3 tumors (Table 1). The mutation, absent in the normal tissue from the same individuals, used as controls, is somatic and heterozygotic and consequently presumably dominant.

Table 1. *Mutations in thyroid hyperfunctioning adenomas*

Gene	% of mutated tumors	Codon	Amino acid changed
TSHR	9 (3 / 37)	GCC	Ala 623
Gαs	25 (9 / 37)	CGT CAG	Arg 201 Gln 227
Ha-ras	3 (1 / 37)	CAG	Gln 61

The substitution of an alanine, located in the C-terminal of the third intracellular loop of the receptor, by a serine represents a major change in the protein structure since a polar amino acid, putative target of phosphorylation, substitutes a neutral one. Besides, it is able to constitutively activate the receptor, as assessed by *in vitro* studies where increased basal cAMP levels were detected in CHO cells transfected with the cDNA of the TSHR gene carrying a serine at residue 623. This site, together with adjacent regions represents a "hot" spot for hosting activating mutations, as demonstrated by alterations reported in other studies (8). Only a complete analysis of all the TSHR gene in a larger number of samples will clarify the real frequency of these alterations in the hot nodules.

Screening of the same series of hyperfunctioning adenomas revealed the presence of a mutation in the two described 'hot' codons 201 and 227 of the Gαs protein gene in nine samples (Table 1). These data confirm those of previous reports (5, 7, 9) in assigning a prevalence of 25-35% of gsp activation in the autonomously hyperfunctioning thyroid adenomas. A mutation in codon 61 of the Ha-ras proto-oncogenes has also been detected in one tumor (Table l); a linkage between this genetic alteration and the hyperfunction of the hot nodule remains to be clarified. The simultaneous presence of more than one mutation was never detected in our tumors.

In conclusion, in thyroid hyperfunctioning adenomas, a tumorigenic role is played by the constitutive activation of the TSH Receptor and the Gs-protein, through an increase in the basal levels of cAMP.

Further studies are necessary to determine whether other induced and/or constitutive changes in other components of the cAMP cascade (Adenyl cyclase, Protein kinase A) participate in the pathogenesis of this type of thyroid tumors.

ACKNOWLEDGEMENTS

This work was supported by a grant from AIRC (Associazione Italiana per la Ricerca del Cancro).

REFERENCES

1. Dumont J.E., Vassart G. and Refetoff S. (1989): The Metabolic Basis of Inherited Diseases. McGraw-Hill. New York.
2 Ermans A.M. and Camus M. (1972): Acta Endocrinol. 70: 46.
3. Fumarola A., Sciacchitano S., Danese D. and Andreoli M. (1993): Min. Endocr. 18: 147.
4. Lefkowitz R.J. (1993): Nature 365: 603.
5. Lyons J., Landis C.A., Harsh G., Vallar L., Grunewald K., Feichtinger H., Duh Q.-J., Clark O.H., Kawasaki E., Bourne H.R. and McCormick F. (1990): Science 249: 655.
6. Nagayama Y. and Rapoport B. (1992): Mol. Endocrinol. 6: 145.
7. O'Sullivan C., Barton C.M., Staddon S.L., Brown C.L. and Lemoine N.R. (1991): Mol. Carcinogen. 4: 345.
8. Parma J., Duprez L., Van Sande J., Cochaux P., Gervy G., Mockel J., Dumont J.E. and Vassart G. (1993): Nature 365: 649.
9. Said S., Schlumberger M. and Suarez H.G. (1994): J. Endocrinol Invest. 17: 371.
10. Suarez H.G., Du Villard J.A., Caillou B., Schlumberger M., Parmentier C. and Monier R. (1991): Oncogene 6: 677-679.
11. Suarez H.G., Du Villard J.A., Severino M., Caillou B., Schlumberger M., Tubiana M., Parmentier C. and Monier R. (1990): Oncogene 5: 565-570.
12. Vignaud J.M., Duprez A., Bene M.C., Leclere J., Faure G., Dauchin N. and Burlet C. (1984): Am. J. Pathol. 117: 355.

Frontiers in Endocrinology
Volume 9 - 1994

Domain-Specific Polarization of Cell Adhesion Molecules is missing in Thyroid Carcinomas: an Applicative Hypothesis

G. Serini[1], F. Orlandi, E. Saggiorato, L. Trusolino[1] and P.C. Marchisio[1, 2]

Department of Clinical and Biological Sciences, University of Torino; San Luigi Gonzaga Hospital, Regione Gonzole 10, 10043 Orbassano (TO); [1]Department of Biomedical Sciences and Human Oncology, University of Torino, Corso Massimo D'Azeglio 52, 10126 Torino; [2]DIBIT, Department of Biological and Technological Research, San Raffaele Scientific Institute, Via Olgettina 58, 20132 Milan, Italy

Normal and differentiated thyrocytes, like many other epithelia, are endowed with a specific structural, functional and biochemical polarization because of their separating two distinct environments: the apical pole faces the follicle with microvilli, the basal pole interacts with extracellular matrix components surrounding the follicle, whereas the lateral domain is mainly involved in maintaining the identity and the compartmentalization between the apical and the basal poles as well as the three-dimensional scaffold of thyroid follicles, presumably under hormonal influences. Thyroid follicular cells take up hormone precursors basally, synthesize thyroglobulin intracellularly and secrete it apically into the follicle space. Inactive hormone is apically taken up and further processed to release basally active iodothyronines. The latter process involves unique reversal of secretory polarity. The induction and maintenance of this polarized and differentiated epithelial phenotype lies upon the expression, membrane sorting, and function of surface adhesion molecules that modulate cell-substratum and/or cell-cell interactions (14). Among these molecules, cadherins (11, 12) represent a family of integral monomeric membrane glycoproteins that mediate homotypic Ca^{2+} dependent intercellular adhesion, whilst integrins

(2, 7) are a superfamily of transmembrane glycoprotein α/β heterodimers that play a major role in cell-substratum as well as in cell-cell contacts. The integrin family comprises 14 α and 8 β subunits, which form at least 20

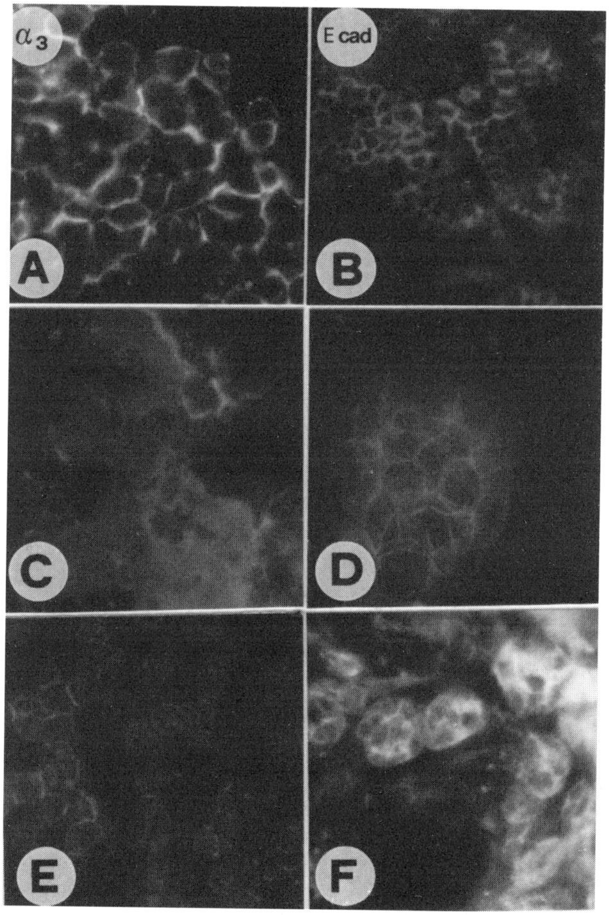

FIG. 1. Conventional indirect immunofluorescence (IIF) analysis of α3 and E-cadherin in FNA (fine-needle aspiration) biopsies. Briefly, after aspiration the specimen was smeared onto a polylysine-coated slide, air-dried for 2h, prefixed in absolute methanol and stored at -80°C. For IIF analysis smears were fixed in a chloroform-acetone mixture, air dried, and saturated with TBS-BSA 0.4%. Slides were incubated with mAb F2 (kind gift of L. Zardi, IST, Genova, Italy) to α3 and HECD-1 (from Takara Shuzo Co., Kyoto, Japan) to E-cadherin and then with the appropriate rhodamine-tagged secondary antibody (Dakopatts, Copenhagen, Denmark). In follicular adenomas the α3 chain displayed a diffuse peripheral and basal staining (A), whereas E-cadherin was exclusively enriched at cell-cell contacts (B). Follicular carcinomas appeared as three-dimensional structures (C, D), surrounded by monostratified thyrocytes at times resembling abortive follicles (E, F). In follicular cancer α3 was subverted laterally (E), while E-cadherin was localized mainly at the basal aspect of the cells (D, F).

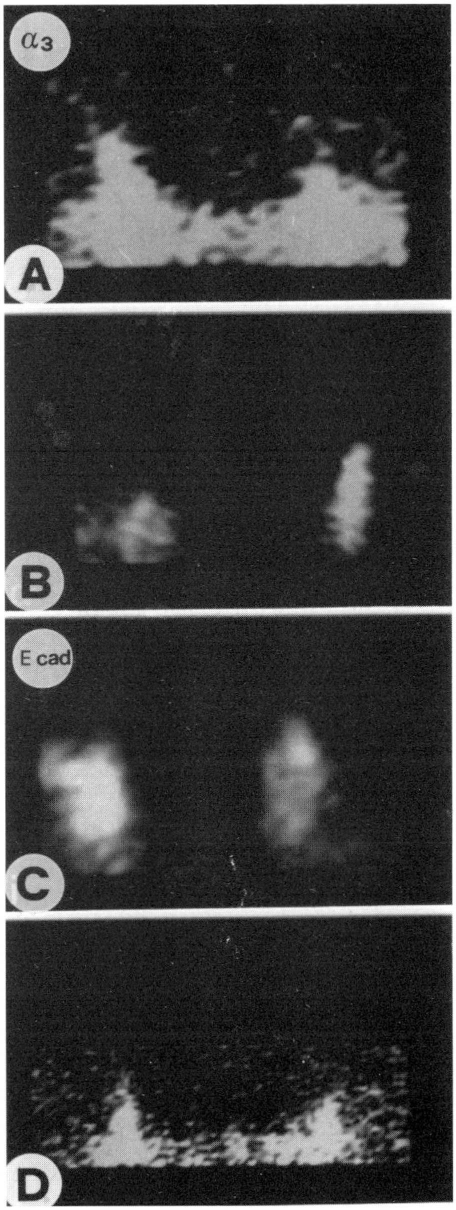

FIG. 2. Confocal microscope analysis of α3 and E-cadherin in FNA biopsies. Briefly, a stack of serial optical sections, every 0.7 μm along the z-axis, were obtained by scanning with the Sarastro 2000 (Molecular Dynamics, Sunnyvale, CA, USA) laser scanning system attached to a Zeiss Axioskop fluorescence microscope. Image processing and three-dimensional reconstruction analyses were performed using a Vanis™ program running in a Silicon Graphics Personal Iris computer. The basal location of α3 (A) and the lateral enrichment of E-cadherin (B) in follicular adenomas were confirmed. The confocal microscope analysis showed intercellular redistribution of α3 (C) and basal diffusion of E-cadherin (D).

integrin combinations. These molecules, which are exposed at discrete domains of the plasma membrane of epithelial cells (1, 3, 4), cooperate in establishing a so-called *adhesion asymmetry* (5) that takes place early in the sequence of aggregation events. In keratinocytes, for example, the basal domain is responsible for recognition and attachment to the basement membrane zone (BMZ) via the α6β4 heterodimer (4, 8), which has been shown to be located in hemidesmosomes (9, 10), whereas the lateral domain mediates cell reciprocal aggregation by means of several classes of membrane adhesion molecules including cadherins and integrins of the β1 subfamily, namely the α3β1 complex (3, 4). This asymmetric integrin distribution may be a prerequisite for the onset of most specialized epithelial functions (5), like possibly correct thyroid hormone synthesis and release.

Little is known about the progression of normal thyroid tissue to the dedifferentiated and malignant phenotype, and whether follicular adenomas must be considered precurring lesions or stable local masses (13).

In the present investigation morphololological and biochemical techniques were used to study the adhesive mechanisms controlling the acquisition of the polarized phenotype of thyrocytes both along the basal and the lateral axis and tried to observe the potential topographical rearrangements of the adhesion molecules during neoplastic progression.

It was shown that normal thyrocytes lack hemidesmosomes so that the co-operative role in basal adhesion of α6β4 and kalinin, a component of the anchoring filaments (6), is missing and attachment to the basal lamina is modulated by α3β1, which is not found at cell-cell contacts; this integrin topography is kept in adenomas but is severely altered in carcinomas regardless of their histotype or differentiation. E-cadherin, a member of the Ca^{2+}-dependent intercellular adhesion molecules mainly expressed in human epithelia, is consistently found at cell-cell contact domains in normal and adenomatous thyroid, but it undergoes pericellular diffusion in carcinomas. To our knowledge, this is the first report in which loss of lateral polarization of E-Cadherin, without reduced expression of the molecule, is described in the progression from benign to malignant lesions.

The positional rearrangement of adhesion molecules in thyroid malignancies, in contrast with their preserved pattern in follicular adenomas, was consistently observed in materials obtained from fine-needle aspiration biopsies (Fig. 1 a-f) and confirmed in the confocal microscope (Fig. 2 a-d). If this result is confirmed by a large-scale applicative study (experiments in progress), a new tool will be available for the pre-operative differential diagnosis of adenomas versus follicular carcinomas.

ACKNOWLEDGEMENTS

Supported by CNR target project “Applicazioni Cliniche della Ricerca Oncologica” and AIRC to P.C.M., and MURST to F.O.

REFERENCES

1. De Luca M., Tamura R.N., Kajiji S., Bondanza S., Rossino P., Cancedda R., Marchisio P.C. and Quaranta V. (1990): Proc. Natl. Acad. Sci. USA 87: 6888-6892.
2. Hynes R.O. (1992): Cell 69: 11-25.
3. Larjava H., Peltonen J., Akiyama S.K., Yamada S.S., Gralnick H.K., Uitto J. and Yamada K.M. (1990): J. Cell Biol. 110: 803-815.
4. Marchisio P.C., Bondanza S., Cremona O., Cancedda R. and De Luca M. (1991): J. Cell Biol. 112: 761-773.
5. Marchisio P.C., and De Luca M. (1994): Trends in Cell Biol., submitted for publication.
6. Rousselle P., Lunstrum G.P., Keene D.R. and Burgeson R.E. (1991): J. Cell Biol. 114 : 567-576.
7. Rouslahti E. (1991): J. Clin. Invest. 87: 1-5.
8. Sonnenberg A., Linders C.J.T., Daams H. and Kennel S.J. (1990): J. Cell Sci. 96: 207-217.
9. Sonnenberg A., Calafat J., Janssen H., Daams H., van der Raaij-Helamer L.M.H., Falcioni R., Kennel S.J., Aplin J.D., Baker J., Loizidou M. and Garrod D. (1991): J. Cell Biol. 113: 907-917.
10. Stepp M.A., Spurr-Michaud S., Tisdale A., Elwell J. and Gipson I.K. (1990): Proc. Natl. Acad. Sci. USA 87: 8970-8974.
11. Takeichi M. (1990): Annu. Rev. Biochem. 59: 224-232.
12. Takeichi M. (1991): Science 251: 1451-1455.
13. Wynford-Thomas D. (1993): Trends Endocrinol. Metab. 4: 224-232.
14. Wollner D.A. and Nelson W.J. (1992): J. Cell Sci. 102: 185-190.

Frontiers in Endocrinology
Volume 9 - 1994

Analysis of ras Mutations in Thyroid Cytologic Smears by Denaturing Gradient Gel Electrophoresis

S. Sciacchitano[1,2], D. Danese[2,3], M. Andreoli[2], A. Di Gregorio[2], A. Sacchi[1] and A. Pontecorvi[1,4]

[1]*Laboratory of Molecular Oncogenesis, Regina Elena Cancer Institute, Via delle Messi D'Oro 156, 00158 Rome;* [2]*Department of Experimental Medicine, University of Rome La Sapienza, Viale Regina Elena 324, 00161 Rome;* [3]*Istituto Medico-Legale, Aeronautica Militare, via P. Gobetti 2, 00185 Rome;* [4]*Institute of Medical Pathology, Catholic University, Largo F. Vito 1, 00168 Rome, Italy*

INTRODUCTION

Cytologic examination of thyroid tissue sampled by fine needle aspiration (FNA) represents a reliable and accurate diagnostic tool in the preoperative identification of thyroid carcinoma (5). The main limit of the technique is that it does not provide reliable information for the correct diagnosis of follicular carcinoma. A smear characterised by a large number of well differentiated thyroid follicular cells, in fact, does not allow the cytopathologist to draw any diagnostic conclusion on the benign or malignant nature of the lesion which is usually referred to as a follicular neoplasm (2). This cytologic picture may be observed in about 7-10% of all cytologic diagnoses (6). Surgical removal of the nodule, with histologic examination to detect signs of blood vessel or capsular invasion, is necessary to distinguish malignant from benign follicular lesions. However, only 15-20% of these cytologically neutral nodules prove to be malignant at final histology (6, 14).

ras mutations and thyroid follicular neoplasms The three *ras* proto-oncogenes (H-*ras*, K-*ras* and N-*ras*) encode proteins ($p21^{ras}$) which share homology with G proteins and play an important role in the transduction of proliferation and differentiation signals (1, 3). Single base substitutions in the guanine nucleotide binding site (codon 12 and 13) or in the intrinsic GTPase domain (codon 61) produce constitutive functional activation of the p21^{ras}. *ras* mutations represent the earliest and most frequent (50-60%) oncogenic alterations in thyroid tumorigenesis (18, 25). However, they are found in all stages of thyroid neoplastic progression (11) and, therefore, lack specificity as molecular markers for the diagnosis of thyroid follicular carcinoma. Recent *in vivo* studies, however, suggest that *ras* alterations may be used as indicators of thyrocyte proliferation. Indeed, transfection of activated *ras* proto-oncogenes into thyroid epithelial cells stimulate their proliferation and extend the proliferative life span of the cell (4, 12). A cooperative effect of other oncogenes (9, 24) or growth factors, such as TSH (17), is required for complete malignant transformation of the thyroid cell. Transgenic mice bearing an activated *K-ras* gene may develop thyroid abnormalities that are mostly benign and appear after a long latency (19). These findings support the hypothesis that thyroid tumorigenesis is a multistep process (4) and that *ras* activation may constitute an early predisposing event that favours the proliferation of the thyroid cell and its subsequent progression toward malignancy. This hypothesis is in agreement with the higher incidence of *ras* mutations reported in microfollicular adenomas, considered more prone to malignant transformation (11).

The identification of *ras* mutations on FNA cytologic specimens may, therefore, represent a valid marker of a pre-neoplastic stage of the thyroid nodule.

Aim of the present study was to preoperatively identify, among the cytological group of follicular neoplasms, those lesions that, due to the presence of *ras* mutations, are to be considered at high risk for progression toward malignancy.

MATERIAL AND METHODS

DNA extraction and amplification DNA was extracted from thyroid cells scraped from stained cytologic smears as previously described (20) and subsequently amplified by the polymerase chain reaction (PCR) in the presence of oligonucleotide primers flanking the first two exons of the *ras* proto-oncogenes (22). Primer sequences were modified by adding a GC-tail to the 5' extremity in order to allow the analysis of the entire DNA fragment by denaturing gradient gel electrophoresis (DGGE) (15).

Denaturing gradient gel electrophoresis analysis DGGE analysis was performed by using a DGGE 2000 system (C.B.S. Scientific Company, Del Mar, CA). Samples were analysed by polyacrylamide gel electrophoresis in the presence of a concentration gradient of denaturants (5.6M Urea and 32% deionized formamide) specific for each DNA fragment to be analysed and parallel to the direction of electrophoresis (16). Denaturant concentration and electrophoretic conditions were previously analysed by using the computer algorithm of Lerman and Silverstain (13) and confirmed in trial gradient gels, perpendicular to the direction of electrophoresis. The electrophoretic separation pattern was visualised by silver staining.

RESULTS

DGGE analysis revealed the presence of a *ras* mutation in 4 (33.3%) out of 12 FNA samples cytologically diagnosed as follicular neoplasms. *ras* mutations were localised in the first exon of *H-ras* in 3 cases and in the second exon of *K-ras* in one case (Table 1). Two DNA fragments showed the presence of four electrophoretic bands, suggesting a heterozygosity of *ras* mutation; in the other two cases, the presence of a single mutated band suggested a homozygous pattern. In these two cases, DGGE allowed also prediction of the type of nucleotide substitution, the altered bands showing a slower migration in comparison to control. This condition, described as B-pattern by Takeda et al. (23), suggests a reduction of the melting temperature of the DNA fragment which is consistent with a nucleotide substitution of a G or C with a T or A residue. The correlation of the results obtained with the final histologic diagnosis indicated that *ras* mutations were detected in 3 out of 6 follicular carcinomas and in 1 of the 6 adenomas. No significant correlation was observed with any clinical parameter considered (Table 1).

Table 1. *Ras gene mutations in thyroid FNA smears from 12 patients with a cytologic pattern of follicular neoplasms*

Patient	Age (yr)	Sex	Tumor size (cm)[a]	Cytology[b]	*ras* gene mutations		Histology[d]
					Localization	Pattern[c]	
1	25	F	6.0	FTN Hürthle cells			FTA Hürthle cells
2	32	M	1.5	FTN			FTA
3	27	F	3.4	FTN Hürthle cells			FTA Hürthle cells
4	50	F	2.3	FTN			FTA
5	16	M	3.0	FTN Hürthle cells			FTA Hürthle cells
6	76	F	3.9	FTN Hürthle cells	H-*ras* exon 1 (codon 12/13)	Het	FTA Hürthle cells
7	36	M	2.5	FTN			FTC
8	40	F	1.5	FTN			FTC
9	53	F	4.2	FTN	H-*ras* exon 1 (codon 12/13)	Hom	FTC
10	34	F	2.5	FTN	H-*ras* exon 1 (codon 12/13)	Het	FTC
11	52	F	1.0	FTN Hürthle cells			FTC Hürthle cells
12	42	F	3.7	FTN	H-*ras* exon 2 (codon 61)	Hom	FTC

[a]Maximum size of tumor nodule; [b]FTN = Follicular Thyroid Neoplasia; [c]Het = Heterozygous, Hom = Homozygous; [d]FTA = Follicular Thyroid Adenoma, FTC = Follicular Thyroid Carcinoma.

DISCUSSION

The preoperative identification of benign and malignant follicular neoplasms is one of the major diagnostic problems in the evaluation of the solitary thyroid nodule by FNA. Several attempts have been made to detect specific markers of malignancy. Clinical characteristics of the nodule (8), morphology of thyroid cells on FNA cell-block sections (10), nuclear morphometry by computerised videophotometry (7) and quantitative analysis of DNA content by flow cytometry (26) have all been evaluated but no conclusive data have been reported.

Results emerging from the present investigation indicate that stained FNA smears are a valid source of DNA for the analysis of early proto-oncogenic alterations associated with neoplastic transformation. *ras* mutations have already been successfully analysed on cytologic samples from pancreatic lesions (21). However, the molecular analysis on thyroid cells obtained by FNA may be cumbersome due to the abundant blood contamination known to interfere with the PCR process and technical advice is therefore necessary to obtain optimal DNA amplification (20). In the small number of follicular neoplasms analysed we have been able to identify a *ras* mutation in about one third of cases, a frequency in agreement with overall data reported in the literature (18). In particular, *ras* mutations were detected in 50% of the follicular carcinomas diagnosed at final histology.

Although *ras* mutations cannot be considered a valid molecular marker of malignancy, they enhance the proliferative behaviour of the thyroid cells, thereby favouring its progression along the tumorigenic pathway. The preoperative identification of these alterations in suspicious thyroid nodules may, therefore, be useful in the surgical selection of those lesions at a higher risk of malignant transformation.

ACKNOWLEDGEMENTS

This work has been supported by research grants from Associazione Italiana per la Ricerca sul Cancro (AIRC) and from Ministero dell'Università e della Ricerca Scientifica e Tecnologica (MURST).

REFERENCES

1. Barbacid M. (1987): Ann. Rev. Biochem. 56: 779-827.
2. Block M.A., Dailey G.E. and Robb J.A. (1983): Am. J. Surg. 146: 72-78.
3. Bos J.L. (1989): Cancer Res. 49: 4682-4689.
4. Burns J.S., Blaydes P., Wright P.A., Lemoine L., Bond J.A., Williams E.D. and Wynford-Thomas D. (1992): Mol. Carcinog. 6: 129-139.
5. Campbell J.P. and Pillsbury III H.C. (1989): Head Neck 11: 414-425.
6. Centanni M., Andreoli M., Sciacchitano S. and Frati L. (1992): Forum. Trends in Experimental and Clinical Medicine 2 (5): 24-37.
7. Crissman J.D., Drozdowicz S., Johnson C. and Kini S.R. (1991): Analyt. Quant. Cytol. Histol. 13: 321-328.

8. Davis N.L., Gordon M., Germann E., Robins R.E. and McGregor G.I. (1991): Am. J. Surg. 161: 567-569.
9. Fusco A., Berlinghieri M.T., Di Fiore P.P., Portella G.G., Grieco M. and Vecchio G. (1987): Mol. Cell. Biol. 7: 3365-3370.
10. Kung I.T.M. and Yuen R.W.S. (1989): Acta Cytol. 33: 53-60.
11. Lemoine N.R., Mayall E.S., Wyllie F.S., Williams E.D., Goyns M., Stringer B. and Wynford-Thomas D. (1989): Oncogene 4: 159-164.
12. Lemoine N.R., Staddon S., Bond J., Wyllie F.S., Shaw J.J. and Wynford-Thomas D. (1990): Oncogene 5: 1833-1837.
13. Lerman L.S. and Silverstain K. (1987): Methods Enzymol. 155: 482-501.
14. Miller J.M., Kini S.R. and Hamburger J.I. (1985): Cancer 55: 2812-2817.
15. Myers R.M., Fisher S.G., Lerman L.S. and Maniatis T. (1985): Nucl. Acid Res. 13: 3111-3129.
16. Myers R.M., Maniatis T. and Lerman L.S. (1987): Methods Enzymol. 155: 501-527.
17. Portella G., Ferulano G., Santoro M., Grieco M., Fusco A. and Vecchio G. (1989): Oncogene 4: 181-188.
18. Said S., Schlumberger M. and Suarez H.G. (1994): J. Endocrinol. Invest. 17: 371-379.
19. Santelli G., de Franciscis V., Portella G., Chiappetta G., D'Alessio A., Califano D., Rosati R., Mineo A., Monaco C., Manzo G., Pozz, L. and Vecchio G. (1993): Cancer Res. 53: 5523-5527.
20. Sciacchitano S., Paliotta S.D., Sacchi A., Nardi F., Andreoli M. and Pontecorvi A. (1994): Diagn. Mol. Pathol. 3(2): 114-121.
21. Shibata D., Almoguera C., Forrester K., Dunitz J., Martin S.L., Cosgrove M.M., Perucho M. and Arnheim N. (1990): Cancer Res. 50: 1279-1283.
22. Tada M., Omata M. and Ohto M. (1990): Cancer Res. 50: 1121-1124.
23. Takeda K., Weiss R.E. and Refetoff S. (1992): J. Clin. Endocrinol. Metab. 74: 712-719.
24. Vecchio G., Di Fiore P.P., Fusco A., Colletta G., Weissman B.E. and Aaronson S.A. (1986): In: Human Genes and Diseases, edited by F. Blasi pp. 415-470. John Wiley & Sons, Ltd. New York.
25. Wynford-Thomas D. (1993): Crit. Rev. Oncog. 4: 1-23.
26. Zedenius J., Auer G., Bäckdahl M., Falkmer U., Grimelius L., Lundell G. and Wallin, G. (1992): World J. Surg. 16: 589-594.

Frontiers in Endocrinology
Volume 9 - 1994

Neutral Amino Acids and Triiodothyronine Transport System in Thymocytes: Effect of Leucine

M. Centanni, A. Bei, A. Casini and S. Migliaccio

II Chair of Endocrinology, Department of Experimental Medicine, University of Rome La Sapienza, Viale Regina Elena, 324, 00161 Rome, Italy

INTRODUCTION

The nuclear receptor represents the target structure to which thyroid hormone binds to exert several biological effects. Due to the intracellular localization of these receptors, thyroid hormone must enter the cells to interact with these structures (7).

Several studies have focused on the triiodothyronine (T3) and thyroxine (T4) entry mechanism into different cell types (1, 4, 5, 11). In mouse thymocytes, cells in which over 4/5 of T3 bound to the nucleus directly derives from plasma (9), a saturable and partly Na-sensitive mechanism mediates T3 entry *in vitro* (2). No evidence of a similar mechanism has been shown for T4 entry. The biochemical characteristics of the above-mentioned T3 entry mechanism into thymocytes resemble the main neutral amino acid transport systems (3). In different tissues, the involvement of systems "L" or "T" has been suggested, based on the tryptophan and leucine effect on the rate of T3 or T4 transport. In particular, it has been reported that aromatic amino acids interfere with specific T3 uptake in erythrocytes (10), suggesting the existence of a countertransport among these substrates. The amino acid leucine represents a typical substrate of "L" transport system for neutral amino acids and has been shown to inhibit T4 uptake in the neuroblastoma cell lines (6).

Therefore, the aim of the present study was to analyse the effect of leucine on cellular and nuclear T3 uptake by mouse thymocytes, as a model of amino acid interference on the T3 internalization process at plasma membrane level.

MATERIAL AND METHODS

Isolation of thymocytes was performed as previously described (8). Whole thymocytes, obtained from young BALB-c mice, were incubated at 25 C at physiological pH, in Krebs-Ringer-Tris buffer containing tracer amounts of labelled T3. Different concentrations of leucine (Leu) were added simultaneously to labelled T3, to the incubation medium. At the end of incubation cell-associated T3 was separated from the free form by means of centrifugation over a sucrose column (30% w/v). The radioactivity in the pellet was measured to determine the labelled T3 associated to cells. The non specific cell-associated radioactivity was measured as the ^{125}I-T3 uptake in the presence of 10μM unlabelled T3.

To determine the nuclear uptake, the cells were centrifuged at 4 C, at the end of each incubation, over a sucrose column and resuspended for 5 minutes in the same medium containing 0.05% BSA, centrifuged again and resuspended in a lysing buffer containing 0.5% Triton X-100. The nuclear pellet was obtained by further centrifugation at 800g. Cell viability, tested before and after the experiments, was greater than 95%.

All experiments were performed in triplicate and the results of at least three independent experiments were plotted.

Statistical analysis was performed using Student t test.

RESULTS

The standard time-course of radioactive T3 uptake by thymocytes at 25 C was investigated. The nonsaturable uptake, measured in each experiment, represented 33±5% of the total at 1 min and 44±6% at 30 min and was subtracted throughout the study to obtain the saturable T3 uptake. The early saturable T3 uptake was linear and represented 1.27±.1% of the total radioactivity/million cells and then approached a plateau. The addition of Leu (1 mM) during the incubation period, reduced the saturable T3 uptake by 29% ($p<0.01$) at 1 min and by 30% ($p<0.01$) at equilibrium.

The above-mentioned effect of Leu was dose-dependent. The incubation of cells in the presence of increasing concentrations of the amino acid (0.1-5 mM) progressively reduced the amount of T3 associated to cells and the half maximal inhibitory concentration (IC_{50}) was 550 μM. Inhibition was not dependent on stereoisomeric configuration of the Leu molecule; in fact, the incubation of thymocytes in the presence of equimolar concentrations of D-leucine reduced the uptake by 27% ($p<0.05$) which was not significantly different from the inhibition obtained using the L-stereoisomer.

The presence of Leu in the incubation buffer also reduced the nuclear T3 uptake in thymus cells. The nuclear T3 uptake represented 8.4% of the cellular uptake (0.080 ± 0.005%/million cells). The presence of 1mM Leu reduced the nuclear associated T3 by 46% ($p<0.01$).

DISCUSSION AND CONCLUSIONS

The results obtained in this *in vitro* study indicate that Leu exerts a dose-dependent inhibition of the saturable cellular and nuclear T3 uptake by mouse thymocytes.

The inhibitory effect of Leu was evident at a concentration (IC_{50}=550 μM) close to the physiological one in the bloodstream (0.1 mM) and was not stereospecific. The effect represented an early event, being maximal after a few minutes incubation, and was not reversed by longer incubation times. It must be noted that the effect, at nuclear level, was greater than that effect at cellular level. This finding would imply that the effect on the availability of T3 for the nuclear interaction is not simply related to the kinetics of transport at the plasma membrane level but more likely to the accumulation of T3 inside the cells. However, the role of other intracellular regulatory events cannot be excluded and further studies are needed.

These findings in thymus cells seem to confirm the hypothesis that, at the plasma membrane level, T3 transport is similar to that of other amino acids, as occurs in erythrocytes (10). However, in these cell lines, the inhibitory effect was exerted by aromatic amino acids and Leu has been shown to inhibit only T4 uptake in neuroblastoma cells (6).

In conclusion, these results indicate that the amino acid Leu, transported by the "L" system into the cells, interferes with cellular and nuclear T3 uptake in thymus cells by a cis-inhibition on the outer surface of the membrane.

REFERENCES

1. Centanni M., Mancini G. and Andreoli M. (1989): Endocrinology 124: 2443-2448.
2. Centanni M., Sapone A., Taglienti A. and Andreoli M. (1991): Endocrinology 129: 2175-2179.
3. Christensen H.N. (1990): Physiol. Rev. 70: 43-77.
4. Docter R,, Krenning E., Bernard H. and Hennemann G. (1987): J. Clin. Endocrinol. Metab. 65: 624-628.
5. Everts M.E., Docter R., van Buuren J.C., van Koetsveld J., Hofland L.J., De Jong M., Krenning E.P. and Hennemann G. (1993): Endocrinology 132 (3): 1278-1285.
6. Lakshmanan M., Goncalves E., Lessly G., Foti D. and Robbins J. (1990): Endocrinology 126: 3245-3250.
7. Oppenheimer J.H. (1983): In: Molecular Basis of Thyroid Hormone Action, J. Oppenheimer and H. Samuels (eds): Academic Press. Orlando, Florida 1-35.

8. Segal J. and Ingbar S.H. (1979): J. Clin. Invest. 63 : 507- 515.
9. Van Doorn J., Roelfsema F. and van der Heide D. (1985): Endocrinology 117: 1201-1208.
10. Zhou Y., Samson M., Osty J., Francon J. and Blondeau J.P. (1990): J. Biol. Chem. 265: 17000 -17004.
11. Zhou Y., Samson M., Francon J. and Blondeau J.P. (1992): Biochem. J. 281: 81-86.

Frontiers in Endocrinology
Volume 9 - 1994

Role of Forebrain VIP in the Neuroendocrine Pathophysiology of SIADH in Hypothyroidism

R. Toni[1], S. Mosca[1], R.M. Lechan[2] and P. Vezzadini[3]

[1]Institute of Human Anatomy, [3]Division of Medicine and Endocrinology at Bellaria Hospital, University of Bologna, Italy; [2]Division of Endocrinology, NEMCH-Tufts University, Boston, MA, USA

INTRODUCTION

Impaired water excretion and/or hyponatremia can occur during severe hypothyroidism as a part of the syndrome of inappropriate secretion of antidiuretic hormone (ADH or AVP) release (SIADH) (14). As increased levels of AVP have been found in the magnocellular nuclei of the hypothalamus in congenitally hypothyroid rats (2) but thyroid hormone does not appear to directly regulate AVP biosynthesis either *in vitro* (1) or *in vivo* in magnocellullar-neurohypophysial nuclei of the rat hypothalamus (5), it is presumed that other factors may be responsible for increased secretion of AVP in hypothyroidism.

MORPHOFUNCTIONAL CORRELATIONS

Effect of hypothyroidism on VIP content in forebrain-neurohypophysial centers We have recently reported that hypothyroidism stimulates the biosynthesis of vasoactive intestinal polypeptide (VIP) in both parvocellular and magnocellular neurons of the paraventricular nucleus (PVN) of the adult, male, rat hypothalamus (15) (Fig. 1). Since VIP potently stimulates AVP release (3, 6, 12) and VIP has been found in magnocellular nuclei of the rat hypothalamus and in the posterior pituitary (10, 11), we have hypothesized that increased VIP in the magnocellular PVN might stimulate AVP secretion in hypothyroidism and thus contribute to SIADH of the hypothyroid rat.

To determine whether the effect of hypothyroidism on VIP biosynthesis in the PVN implies the existence of a VIPergic system capable of controlling AVP neurons, we conducted immunocytochemical studies on the distribution of immunoreactive (IR)-VIP neurons in forebrain centers known to regulate AVP

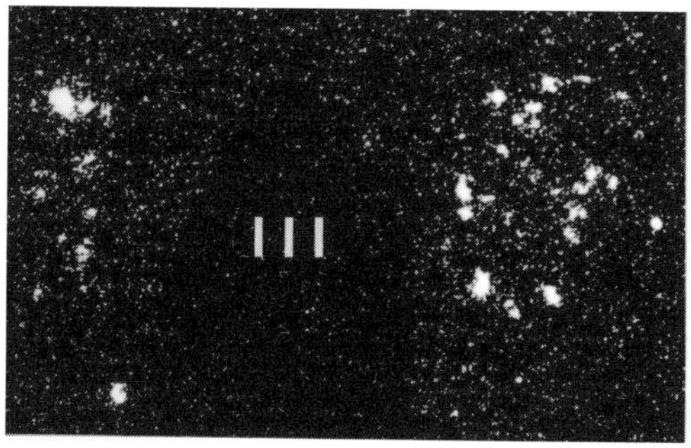

FIG. 1. Darkfield photomicrograph of hybridized VIP mRNA in the PVN of the hypothyroid rat. III = third ventricle.

neurons in the hypothalamic supraoptic nucleus (SON) and PVN (Fig. 2), both in controls and rats made hypothyroid by thionamide treatment.

Hypothyroidism promptly induced the appearance of IR-VIP in perikarya and fibers in regions of the diencephalon and telencephalon (Table 1) that stimulate AVP release, increase thirst, activate drinking behavior, inhibit baroreceptor reflexes and decrease heart rate and blood pressure (4).

Table 1. *Effect of hypothyroidism of IR-VIP in forebrain-neurohypophysial nuclei of the male rat*

Nuclei	Control		Hypothyroid	
	perikarya	fibers	perikarya	fibers
Hypothalamus				
MPOA	-	-	+	+
PVpo	-	+	+	+
PVNp	-	-	+	+
PVNmp	-	-	+	+
PVNpm	-	-	+	+
SON	+	+	++	++
SCN	+	+	+	+
APv	-	-	+	+
Thalamus				
Re	-	+	+	+
PVA	+	+	+	+
Circumventricular region				
SFO	-	+	+	++
Olfactory system				
NLOT	+	+	++	++

- = absence of IR-VIP perikarya or fibers; + = presence of IR-VIP perikarya or fibers; ++ = increase in number of IR-VIP perikarya or fibers with respect to control. MPOA = medial preoptic area; PVpo = periventricular preoptic nucleus; PVN = hypothalamic paraventricular nucleus, p = periventricular parvocellular subdivision, mp = medial parvocellular subdivision; pm = posterior magnocellular subdivision; SON = supraoptic nucleus; SCN = suprachiasmatic nucleus; APv = anterior periventricular nucleus; Re = nucleus reuniens; PVA = thalamic paraventricular nucleus; SFO = subfornical organ; NLOT = nucleus of the lateral olfactory tract.

It is conceivable, therefore, that VIP may be involved in the neuroendocrine mechanism to enhance endocrine, autonomic and behavioral responses associated with hypothyroidism-induced SIADH.

Distribution of thyroid hormone receptor beta 2 in forebrain-neurohypophysial centers As VIP-producing neurons in the forebrain can be regulated by

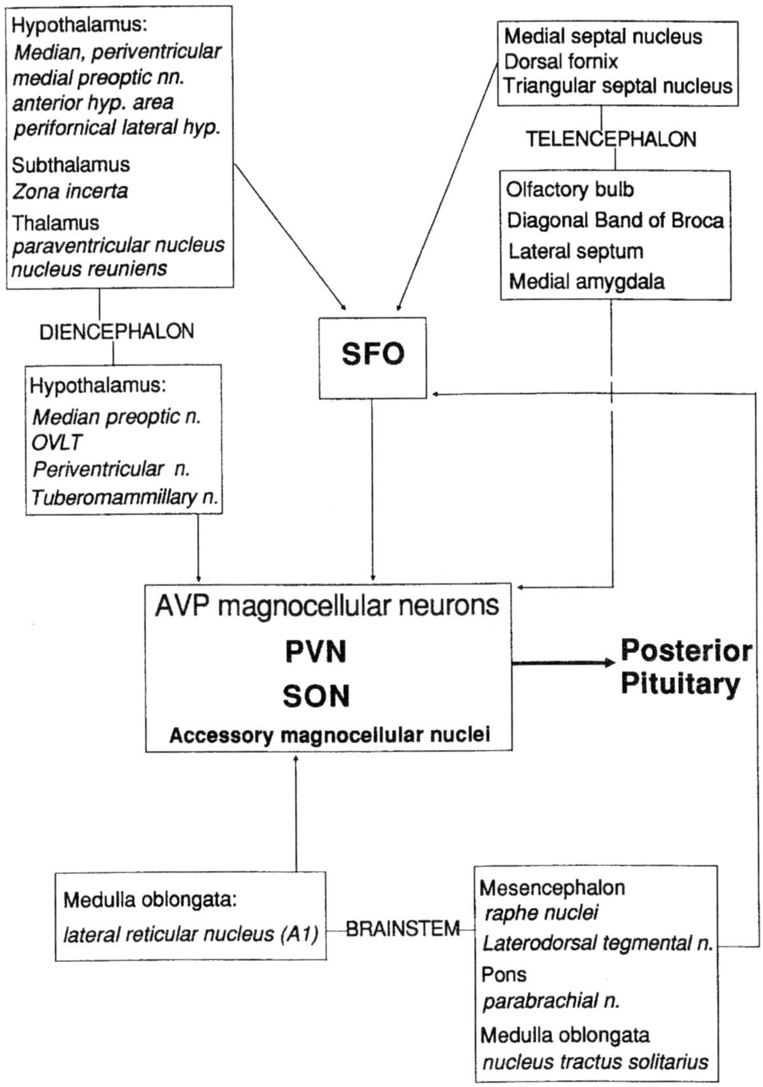

FIG. 2. Organization of projections from different regions of the central nervous system to the vasopressinergic neurons of the magnocellular neurohypophysial system in the rat. OVLT = *Organum Vasculosum* of the *Lamina Terminalis*. For other abbreviations see Table 1.

thyroid hormone, we have begun a study of thyroid hormone receptors (TR) in these cells. Several thyroid hormone receptors are present in the brain including TR alpha and TR beta isoforms that differ entirely at their amino terminal end (7). To begin these studies, we used a highly specific antiserum raised against the N-terminal sequence 131-145 of TR beta 2 (provided by Dr. M.A. Lazar). This antiserum has been shown in previous studies from our laboratories to immunostain the nucleus of neurons distributed throughout the brain (8). When used on immunoprecipitated nuclear extracts from whole brain, total T3 binding capacity was reduced 20% suggesting that immunoreactive TR beta 2 comprises a substantial portion of the total content of nuclear thyroid hormone binding proteins in the central nervous system (8). Preliminary observations indicate that IR-TR beta 2 is present in the nucleus of neurons of many diencephalic and telencephalic regions containing IR-VIP cells and its immunostaining is particularly intense in the SON and NLOT (Table 2). This evidence suggests that T3 may have direct effects on VIP-synthesizing forebrain neurons that control fluid and electrolyte balance and support a role for VIP in these regions as a neuroendocrine mediator of SIADH in hypothyroidism.

Table 2. *Distribution of IR-thyroid hormone receptor beta 2 in forebrain-neurohypophysial nuclei of the male rat*

Nuclei	Intensity of immunolabeling
Hypothalamus	
MPOA	++
PvPo	+
PVNp	+
PVNmp	++
PVNpm	++
SON	+++
SCN	+
APv	+
Thalamus	
Re	+
PVA	++
Olfactory system	
NLOT	+++

+ = low intensity, ++ = medium intensity, +++ = high intensity with respect to background staining. For abbreviations see Table 1.

Effect of hypothyroidism on the size of IR-VIP neurons in forebrain-neurohypophysial centers Hypothyroidism did not cause any statistically significant change in the size of VIP neurons in the SON with respect to controls (Fig. 3). Instead, hypothyroidism may produce a reduction in the number of axons afferent to target neurons in the SON as well as in the number of dendrites available for postsynaptic reception, thereby leading to impoverishment of afferent neural information (9). This reduction in neuropil might set into motion compensatory mechanisms that stimulate AVP secretion by inducing an autocrine and/or paracrine release of VIP (6). VIP was also increased in parvocellular PVN neurons, as demonstrated by the small size of these cells (Fig. 3), and this could indicate that thyroid hormone influences VIP neurons involved in the control of anterior pituitary function and as a result, contributes to its role in the coordination of fluid and electrolyte balance. The absence of statistically significant differences in the size of VIP neurons in the SCN between control and hypothyroid rats (Fig. 3) is in keeping with the results of Paula-Barbosa et al. (13) and raises the possibility that hypothyroidism alters the neuropil of SCN VIP neurons, thereby leading to the derangement in drinking rhythm that occurs in SIADH.

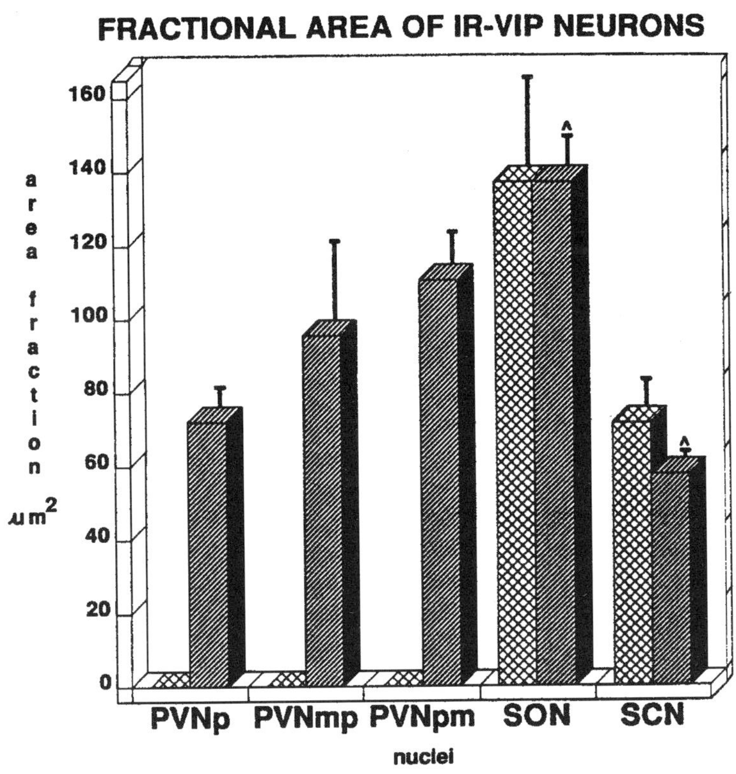

FIG. 3. Distribution of mean cell area fraction of IR-VIP perikarya in hypothalamic nuclei of control (bar by network) and hypothyroid (bar by oblique lines) rats, as determined by the morphometric principle of grid area fraction. ^ = $p > 0.05$ respect to controls. For abbreviations see Table 1.

CONCLUSIONS

These results indicate that hypothyroidism increases IR-VIP in neurohypophysial nuclei and other forebrain regions known to regulate AVP release, body fluid and electrolyte balance and blood pressure. The presence of thyroid hormone receptors in these regions suggests that the effects of thyroid hormone on the expression, distribution and morphological features of VIP neurons may be direct and specific to VIP cells. We conclude that increased VIP in forebrain-neurohypophysial neurons may contribute to the neuroendocrine pathohysiology of the hypothyroidism-induced SIADH.

ACKNOWLEDGEMENTS

This study was supported by Grants CNR 9300434CT04, 9303603CT11, 9400809CT11, 9402500CT04, ACRO, MURST 40% and 60% 1993-1994, Cassa di Risparmio di Imola, NIH DK 37021.

REFERENCES

1. Adan R.A.H. and Burbach. J.P.H. (1992): In: Progress in Brain Research, vol. 92., edited by J. Joosse, R.M. Bujis, F.J.H. Tilders, pp.127-136. Elsevier. Amsterdam.
2. Ali M. and Clos J. (1987): J. Physiol. (Paris) 82: 25-35.
3. Bardrum B., Ottensen B. and Fahrenkrug J., Fuchs A-R (1988): Endocrinology 123: 2249-2254.
4. Bourque C.W. and Renaud L.P. (1990): Frontiers in Neuroendocrinology 11: 183-212.
5. Ceccatelli S., Giardino L. and Calzà L. (1992): Neuroendocrinology 56: 694-703.
6. Falke N. (1991): Neuropeptides 18: 143-147.
7. Lazar M.A. and Chin W.W. (1990): J. Clin. Invest. 86: 1777-1782.
8. Lechan R.M., Qi Y., Berrodin T.J., Davis K.D., Schwartz H.L., Strait K.A., Oppenheimer J.H. and Lazar M.A. (1993): Endocrinology 132: 2461-2469.
9. Madeira M.D., Cadete-Leite A., Sousa N. and Paula-Barbosa M.M. (1991): Neuroscience 41: 827-839.
10. Meister B., Villar M.J., Ceccatelli S. and Hokfelt T. (1990): Neuroscience 37: 603-633.
11. Mikkelsen J.D. (1989): Cell Tissue Res. 255: 307-313.
12. Ottensen B., Pedersen B.L., Vangsted A., Rogowsky P., Nielsen J., Dalgaard D., Bardrum B., Fahrenkrug J. and Fuchs A-R. (1988): J. Obstet. Gynaecol. 9: 83-86.
13. Paula-Barbosa M.M., Sousa N. and Madeira M.D. (1990): Neuroendocrinology 52 supp 1: 59.
14. Skowsky W.R. and Kikuchi T.A. (1978): Am. J. Med. 64: 613-621.
15. Toni R., Kakuscka I., Mosca S., Marrama P. and Lechan R.M. (1992): Endocrinology 131: 976-978.

Frontiers in Endocrinology
Volume 9 - 1994

Variant Thyroid Hormone Receptor (THR) Isoforms in Developing Rat Testis

E.A. Jannini, S. Ulisse, E. Carosa, F.M. Graziano, D. Piersanti and M. D'Armiento

Department of Experimental Medicine, University of L'Aquila, Coppito, Bldg 2, Room A2/54, 67100 L'Aquila, Italy

INTRODUCTION

Although the importance of thyroid hormone in the development of vertebrates and invertebrates is well recognized, it is unclear how the two major THR_s, α and β, their variants (V) and Rev contribute to this process (4). While most tissues are thyroid hormone-responsive at all times concomitant with expression of both THR_{α} and THR_{β}, the adult rat testis appears to be unresponsive because of a lack of increase in oxygen consumption upon treatment with thyroxine (1), the absence of nuclear binding sites for thyroid hormone (12) and of the two major THR mRNAs (15). However, we demonstrated that Sertoli cells from prenatal, neonatal and prepuberal, but not adult, rat testes possess a T_3 nuclear binding activity (7) that is exclusively due to the expression of THR_{α} mRNA (10). These findings suggest a *critical window* of thyroid hormone responsiveness coinciding with the prepuberal period.

In this study, we evaluated the ontogenetic expression of THR_{α}-V_s and of their anti-sense Rev, and their regulation by exogenous thyroid hormone treatment and experimental hypothyroidism.

RESULTS

*Ontogenesis of the c-*erbA_{α} *genomic locus expression* Northern analysis of total RNA from whole testes of various ages showed the presence of THR_{α} mRNA in fetuses, in perinatal and prepuberal periods, but not in adulthood.

The 5.4 and 6.8 kb bands corresponding to the THR_{α} mRNA paralelled the ontogenetic profile of thyroid hormone nuclear receptor previously demonstrated in rat testis (7). The THR_{α} was maximally expressed in fetal and perinatal age, then declined to be virtually absent in adult testis. On the contrary, the 2.6 kb band corresponding to the variant mRNA was present at all ages, but adult rat testis showed a significantly lower amount with respect to prepuberal ages ($p < 0.05$). To define possible differential expression of THR_{α}-V_1 and THR_{α}-V_2, RNase protection assays were performed using a new specific riboprobe. Densitometric scanning of the 98 b fragment corresponding to THR_{α} expression in testis from 15-day-old rats showed a significant decrease of the mRNA expression with respect to younger ages ($p < 0.05$). In adult testis, the protected fragment was undetectable also in longer exposures of autoradiograms. The expression of THR_{α}-V_1 was predominant at all ages studied and was detectable at all ages, but adult testes showed a lower expression level than that of prepuberal ages ($p < 0.001$). The expression of Rev mRNA was then studied using RNase protection assay by hybridizing the specific riboprobe with samples previously checked for integrity in a denaturing agarose gel. Unlike the expression of the other mRNAs encoded by the c-*erb*A_{α} genomic *locus*, the Rev mRNA was barely detectable in the fetal period, but it was expressed at high levels in the adult gonad.

Regulation by thyroid hormone of c-erbA_{α} *mRNA*$_s$ The effect of T_3 administration and of experimental hypothyroidism on the expression of the c-*erb*A_{α} genomic locus products in testis was studied. THR_{α} in prepuberal, THR_{α}-V_1 in prepuberal and adult, and Rev mRNA levels in adult rats were unaffected by thyroid hormone treatment (T_3, 1µg/g/BW/day for 3 days). Short term neonatal hypothyroidism (methimazole, 0.05% from birth to day 21), a treatment able to increase the size of adult testis (3) and sperm number (2), apparently increased the expression of THR_{α} and THR_{α}-V. In fact, at day 60 after birth, when in coeval euthyroid animals THR_{α} is absent, it is still expressed in animals hypothyroid from birth to day 21. T_3 replacement during MMI treatment reverses the effects of hypothyroidism.

DISCUSSION AND CONCLUSIONS

Spermatogenesis represents a developmental system which has been the subject of intense scrutiny in recent years, with particular emphasis on the study of proto-oncogene expression throughout its various stages. The transition from the observation that a proto-oncogene is transcribed in a population of germ or somatic cells to the elucidation of its relevance to their developmental program has been generally difficult. However, c-*erb*A_{α} may be regarded as a notable exception, together with a few others, like c-*mos* and c-*kit*. In fact, the localization of THR_α mRNA (10) and its nuclear binding activity (7) in prenatal, neonatal and prepuberal Sertoli cell, the main regulator of seminiferous epithelium development, is coupled with the dramatic effects of thyroid hormone on testis differentiation (9). Here we show that rat testes express THR_α from fetal life to the prepuberal period. We previously demonstrated by RNase protection assay the absence of THR_β and the ontogenetic profile of THR_α and its variant in rat testis (10). The Northern analysis shows that the TRH $mRNA_s$ are expressed at high levels in testis before puberty and that transcripts have the canonical size. The presence of THR_α and T_3 nuclear binding activity in prepuberal Sertoli cells accounts for the thyroid hormone responsivity of these cells both *in vivo* and *in vitro*. T_3 administration during the neonatal period increases the number of germ cells and stimulates their maturation from gonocytes to spermatogonia (9), probably by stimulating Sertoli cell metabolism (16). Longer *in vivo* exposure to T_3 reduces the period of Sertoli cell proliferation and accelerates tubular lumen formation (19). Furthermore, these treatments are able to increase the testis size, as well as the diameter of the seminiferous tubule. In addition, T_3 stimulates IGF-I synthesis (13), glucose uptake and GLUT1 mRNA accumulation (16), while it decreases the production of androgen binding protein (6) and its mRNA (10) and the aromatase activity induced by FSH (17).

Since the Rev sequence overlaps that of THR_α-V, the possibility that a sense-antisense hybrid might exist *in vivo* has been raised and demonstrated *in vitro* (11). This mechanism should modulate the levels of THR_α-V mRNA with concomitant increase in production of THR_α, if temporal expression patterns of both mRNAs are coordinated. Our data partially suggest that this mechanism is operating in the testis, contrary to findings in other tissues (brain, liver, muscle, spleen, lung, and kidney) (8). In fact, the time-dependent dramatic increase in Rev mRNA coincides with the decrease in THR_α-V expression, but also with the loss of THR_α expression demonstrated in the adult testis. Localization studies of Rev mRNA in the testis are currently under way to determine this possibility. However, the expression pattern of Rev in the testis as well as in other tissues (8) suggests that this receptor-like protein may be involved in the establishment of the differentiated phenotype of postpuberal tissues.

Chronic hypothyroidism from birth to adulthood reduces testis size, the diameter of the seminiferous tubules and germ cell number, on account of a delay in Sertoli cell maturation (5). On the contrary, it has been shown that short-term prepuberal hypothyroidism increases adult testis size (3), doubles germ cell number (2) and extends the period of Sertoli cell maturation, delaying their maturation (18). Since these effects were observed only in adult animals, at the time when THR_α is absent, we hypothesized that prepuberal hypothyroidism may affect the levels of THR_s. Furthermore, it has been shown that T_3 nuclear binding activity is higher in testes from 35-day-old-animals treated with MMI from day 1 to day 21 after birth, with respect to control (14). Hypothyroidism delays the maturation of Sertoli cells, as demonstrated by the prolongation of the proliferation of these cells in hypothyroid animals (18). Thus, the presence of detectable levels of THR_{α} mRNA in adult rats made hypothyroid in the prepuberal period may be due to the delayed differentiation of Sertoli cells. The apparent responsivity of adult testis to hypothyroidism may be referred to the resumption of thyroid hormone secretion after the goitrogen withdrawal. The re-circulating thyroid hormone can bind to a receptor still expressed in a seminiferous epithelium functionally younger with respect to its chronological age. This is also suggested by the lack of any acute effects of thyroid hormone on the expression of THR $mRNA_{s}$.

In summary, the testis should be regarded now as a unique model for the study of developmental expression of THR_{s} and their variant isoforms, and the seminiferous epithelium as a target for thyroid hormone action.

REFERENCES

1. Barker S.B. and Klitgard H.M. (1952): Am. J. Physiol. 170: 81-86.
2. Cooke P.S., Hess R.A., Porcelli J. and Meisami E. (1991): Endocrinology 129: 244-248.
3. Cooke P.S. and Meisami E. (1991): Endocrinology 129: 237-243.
4. D'Armiento M. and Jannini E.A. (1993): In: Thyroid Diseases: Basic Science, Pathology, Clinical and Laboratory Diagnoses. pp 145-154. edited by L. Troncone, B. Shapiro, M.A. Satta, F. Monaco. CRC Press. Boca Raton.
5. Francavilla S., Cordeschi G., Properzi G., Di Cicco L., Jannini E.A., Palmero S., Fugassa E., Loras B. and D'Armiento M. (1991): J. Endocrinol. 129: 35-42.
6. Fugassa E., Palmero S. and Gallo G. (1987): Biochem. Biophys. Res. Comm. 143: 241-247.
7. Jannini E.A., Olivieri M., Francavilla S., Gulino A., Ziparo E. and D'Armiento M. (1990): Endocrinology 12: 2521-2526.
8. Jannini E.A., Mitsuhashi T. and Nikodem V.M. (1992): Biochem. Biophys. Res. Comm. 184: 739-745.
9. Jannini E.A., Ulisse S., Piersanti D., Carosa E., Muzi P., Lazar J. and D'Armiento M. (1993): Endocrinology 132: 2726-2728.
10. Jannini E.A., Dolci S., Ulisse S, and Nikodem V.M. (1994): Mol. Endocrinol. 8: 89-96.
11. Munroe S.H. and Lazar M.A. (1991): J. Biol. Chem. 266: 22083-22086.
12. Oppenheimer J.H., Schwartz H.L. and Suks M.I. (1974): Endocrinology 95: 897-903.
13. Palmero S., Prati M., Barreca A., Minuto F., Giordano G. and Fugassa E. (1990): Mol. Cell. Endocrinol. 68: 61-65.
14. Palmero S., Prati M., De Marco P. and Fugassa E. (1993): J. Endocrinol. 136: 277-282.
15. Strait K.A., Schwartz H.L., Perez-Castillo A. and Oppenheimer J.H. (1990): J. Biol. Chem. 265: 10514-10521.
16. Ulisse S., Jannini E.A., Pepe M., De Matteis S. and D'Armiento M. (1992): Mol. Cell. Endocrinol. 87: 131-137
17. Ulisse S, Jannini EA, Carosa E, Piersanti D, Graziano F.M. and D'Armiento M (1994): J. Endocrinol. 140: 431-436.
18. Van Haaster L.H., De Jong F.H., Docter R. and De Rooij D.G. (1992): Endocrinology 131: 1574-1576.
19. Van Haaster L.H., De Jong F.H., Docter R. and De Rooij D.G. (1993): Endocrinology 133: 755-760.

Frontiers in Endocrinology
Volume 9 - 1994

Effects of TRH and Thyroid Hormones on Circulating TSH Bioactivity in Various Clinical Conditions

L. Persani[1,2], E. Giammona[2], C. Asteria[1], G. Pivano[3] and P. Beck-Peccoz[1]

[1]*Institute of Endocrine Sciences, University of Milan, Ospedale Maggiore IRCCS, Via F. Sforza 35, 20122 Milan;*
[2]*Centro Auxologico Italiano IRCCS, Via L. Ariosto 13, 20145 Milan;*
[3]*Department of Clinical and Biological Sciences, University of Turin, Italy*

INTRODUCTION

Intrapituitary and serum TSH, like the other pituitary glycoprotein hormones, are constituted by several isoforms characterized by different oligosaccharide structure and possessing different bioactivity (3, 9). When TSH, in a given sample, is simultaneously quantified by immunometric and biological assay, the ratio between bioactivity (B) and immunoreactivity (I) may serve as an index of its overall potency (2, 3, 5, 8).

Variations of circulating TSH B/I have been documented in both physiological and pathological conditions associated with an alteration in the two most important mechanisms controlling TSH synthesis and secretion, i.e., TRH release and thyroid hormone feedback system (2, 3, 5). In fact, TRH and thyroid hormones are known to modulate the quantity, but also the bioactivity of TSH molecules produced by rat pituitary cells *in vitro* (4). Moreover, TSH forms with impaired thyroid receptor binding and reduced biological activity circulate in patients with hypothalamic hypothyroidism (HH). Chronic TRH treatment in these patients restores normal thyroid receptor binding and bioactivity of endogenous TSH, as demonstrated *in vivo* by the normalization of thyroid hormone circulating levels (1).

The aim of the present work was to study how these two principal factors regulating TSH secretion, TRH and thyroid hormones, may affect the biological activity of TSH molecules secreted in humans *in vivo*.

MATERIAL AND METHODS

Circulating TSH B/I was assessed before and after TRH and/or thyroid hormone administration in various clinical conditions, as reported in Table 1.

Table 1. *Study groups and treatment*

Condition (n, baseline studies)	Treatment (n)
Normal Controls (n. 14)	TRH (200 μg, iv) (n. 6)
Primary Hypothyroidism (PH, n. 20)	TRH (200 μg, iv) (n. 2) L-T4 (0.9 μg/kg/day) (n. 4)
Resistance to Thyroid Hormones (RTH, n. 13)	TRH (200 μg, iv) (n. 7) L-T3 (100 μg/day) (n. 3)
TSH-Secreting Adenomas (TSHoma, n. 10)	TRH (200 μg, iv) (n. 2)

Blood was collected 120-180 min after TRH injection, and after 1 month of L-T4 or 10 days of L-T3 administration.

TSH immunoreactivity was measured using a third generation IFMA method (Delfia®).

For bioactivity studies, circulating TSH was partially purified from serum by an immuno-concentration method resulting in constant recovery, as previously described (7). Immuno-concentrated TSH bioactivity was assessed using either FRTL-5 cells or CHO cells transfected with recombinant human TSH receptor (kindly provided by Dr. G. Vassart, Belgium). Both cell types were cultured under well standardized conditions. Both bioassays were based on the measurement of cAMP accumulation in the hypotonic extracellular fluid collected after incubation, displaying good analytical characteristics (7). A highly significant correlation between results obtained with the two bioassays has been described (7). As dilution curves of immuno-concentrated TSH samples and TSH standard (WHO, 80/558) were parallel in both biological and immunological assays, results were expressed as TSH B/I ratios.

RESULTS

In normal controls, basal circulating TSH B/I ranged between 0.6-2.1 (1.4±0.4). No significant changes in the average mean of TSH B/I were observed 120-180 min after TRH injection. However, a significant reduction in TSH B/I was observed when only paired data (obtained in the same subject before and after TRH) were considered.

In patients with PH, TSH B/I largely overlapped the normal range (0.3-1.5), but the average mean of TSH B/I was significantly lower than in controls (0.7 ± 0.3, $p<0.001$). TRH injection did not cause variations of TSH B/I. During low-dose L-T4 administration mean TSH B/I returned to normal in all cases.

In patients with an altered feedback mechanism due to thyroid hormone resistance, TSH B/I was always enhanced (2.2-11.9). TRH injection induced a normal response of TSH immunoreactive levels, but did not significantly modify its bioactivity. High doses of L-T3, partially overcoming the dominant negative effects of mutated thyroid hormone receptor β, induced a return to normal of the circulating TSH bioactivity.

TSH secreted from TSHoma is characterized by highly variable B/I ratios (0.3-5.0), which were unchanged after TRH injection.

DISCUSSION

Reduced TSH biological activity may be recorded when the circulating levels of thyroid hormones are low, as in PH patients, or TRH release is impaired, as in HH patients (1-3). Enhanced TSH bioactivity may be found in conditions where the negative feedback mechanism is intrinsically altered, as in TSHomas and patients with RTH (7). The administration of TRH to normal subjects is followed by secretion of TSH molecules with reduced bioactivity, while no modification of TSH B/I is observed in patients with PH, or RTH, or TSHoma. Only in patients with HH, did chronic TRH treatment induce a return to normal of TSH receptor-binding and bioactivity.

The above findings do not support the general assumption that TRH administration is invariably followed by the secretion of TSH molecules with enhanced bioactivity. Specific treatments, such as L-T4 in PH or high doses of L-T3 in RTH, can restore the secretion of TSH molecules with normal bioactivity.

The present data show that both TRH and thyroid hormones play an important role in the *in vivo* regulation of TSH bioactivity in humans.

REFERENCES

1. Beck-Peccoz P., Amr S., Menezes-Ferreira M., Faglia G. and Weintraub B.D. (1985): N. Engl. J. Med. 312: 1085-1090.
2. Beck-Peccoz P. and Persani L. (1994): Eur. J. Endocrinol. 1 (in press).
3. Magner J.A. (1990): Endocr. Rev. 11: 354-385.
4. Menezes-Ferreira M.M., Petrick P.A. and Weintraub B.D. (1986): Endocrinology 118: 2125-2130.
5. Persani L., Asteria C. and Beck-Peccoz P. (1994): Exp. Clin. Endocrinol. (in press).
6. Persani L., Asteria C., Tonacchera M., Vitti P., Chatterjee V.K.K. and Beck-Peccoz P. (1994): J. Clin. Endocrinol. Metab. 78 (in press).

7. Persani L., Tonacchera M., Beck-Peccoz P., Vitti P., Mammoli C. Chiovato L., Elisei R., Faglia G., Ludgate M., Vassart G. and Pinchera A. (1993): J. Endocrinol. Invest. 16: 511-519.
8. Robertson W.R., Lambert A. and Loveridge N. (1987): Clin. Endocrinol. 27: 259-278.
9. Weintraub B.D., Stannard B.S., Magner J.A., Ronin C., Taylor T., Joshi L., Constant R.B., Menezes-Ferreira M.M., Petrick P. and Gesundheit N. (1985): Recent Prog. Horm. Res. 41: 577-606.

Frontiers in Endocrinology
Volume 9 - 1994

Impairment of Intellectual Capacities in Children as a Consequence of Neonatal Transient Hypothyroidism

F. Calaciura, R.M. Motta, M. Distefano, L. Barbagallo, G. Mendorla[1], S. Castorina[1], L. Sava and R. Vigneri

Chair of Endocrinology, Ospedale Garibaldi, University of Catania;
[1]Chair of Psychology, University of Catania, Italy

INTRODUCTION

Transient congenital hypothyroidism (TCH) is characterized by a variable degree of thyroid failure that is present at birth but spontaneously remits during the post-natal period. The alterations of thyroid function at birth are much more frequent in newborns from endemic goiter areas (3) since an inadequate iodine intake is the most frequent cause of TCH.

Hypothyroidism, when occurring during the critical period of brain development, even if transient, may theoretically cause partial mental retardation and be the cause of the intellectual impairment reported in clinically and biochemically euthyroid subjects from endemic areas (2). The neuropsychointellectual outcome of newborns with TCH, however, is not known.

MATERIAL AND METHODS

Investigations were here carried out on thyroid function, auxometric parameters and neuropsychological evaluation in a series of 16 children born in an endemic goiter area with documented short-term transient congenital hypothyroidism. Two control groups were also studied: a)

children born in the same area at the same time and having normal thyroid function at birth and, b) children with late treated (over 2 months of age) sporadic congenital hypothyroidism.

Subjects A) Sixteen *transient congenital hypothyroid* newborns with elevated (above 50 mU/ml) cord serum TSH had either low or normal T4 and were, therefore, classified as having either transient hypothyroidism (high TSH and low T4) or transient hyperthyrotropinemia (high TSH and normal T4), a more attenuated form of congenital hypothyroidism. Both TSH and T4 spontaneously returned to normal a few weeks after birth, at the time of recall examination (at age 38-91 days, median=57) indicating that their hypothyroidism had been of short, although indeterminate, duration. They were examined at age 4.5-10.4 years (median=7.8). None had ever been treated with thyroid hormones.

B) Sixteen *euthyroid controls* with documented normal TSH and T4 at birth were selected as a control group because of being born in the same area, matching the birth date (within a 90-day interval) and having similar socio-economic conditions for each patient with transient congenital hypothyroidism. Their evaluation was carried out at 5.1-10.6 years (median = 8.0). None had ever been treated with thyroid hormone.

C) *Sporadic congenital hypothyroid patients* The psychological examination was carried out also in 9 children aged 7.2-11.9 years (median = 9.7) with congenital hypothyroidism diagnosed and treated late, when hypothyroidism was clinically evident. They were evaluated as a control group for impaired mental function due to congenital hypothyroidism.

Methods Thyroid function studies included the measurements of total thyroid hormone, TSH and thyroglobulin (Tg) in serum. A TRH test (TRH 100 µg iv, TSH at time 0' and 20' min) was performed in all TCH patients and euthyroid controls. In these two groups, an ultrasound scan examination was performed in order to assess their thyroid volume. Statural (Tanner's centile charts of height) and bone age (TW2 method) were also calculated.

In 27 children (9 TCH, 9 controls and 9 congenital hypothyroid), the Full scale IQ, Verbal IQ and Performance IQ was assessed by the Wechsler Intelligence Scale for Children - Revised (WISC) (4) in order to evaluate their cognitive ability. Because of the transversal characteristics of our study, care was taken to have paired children from different groups examined at a similar age (less than 1 year difference).

RESULTS

Auxonomic and thyroid function data (m ± SD) in children with TCH and in controls are shown in Table 1.

Table 1. *Auxonomic and thyroid function data (m±SD) in TCH and controls*

Variables	Controls n = 16	Transient hypothyroidism n = 16
At birth		
Gestational age	39.9 ± 1.6	39.6 ± 1.7 NS
Weight (g)	3240 ± 490	2920 ± 740 NS
Cord serum TSH (μU/ml)	8.8 ± 3.6	100.5 ± 70.5**
T4 (μg/dl)	9.4 ± 2.1	5.3 ± 2.5*
Late evaluation		
Chronological age (years)	7.9 ± 1.5	7.2 ± 1.7 NS
Statural age (years)	7.5 ± 1.9	6.6 ± 1.7 NS
Bone age (years)	8.5 ± 7.4	7.4 ± 1.9 NS
Thyroid volume (ml)	5.6 ± 3.0	5.7 ± 2.2 NS
Serum TSH 0' (μU/ml)	2.3 ± 1.2	3.5 ± 2.8 NS
20'	17.6 ± 9.1	23.6 ± 17.5 NS
T4 (μg/dl)	9.0 ± 1.6	8.8 ± 2.0 NS
T3 (ng/ml)	1.7 ± 0.2	1.6 ± 0.3 NS
Tg (ng/ml)	102.4 ± 110.2	215.9 ± 331.2 NS

NS = non significant; * p < 0. 05; ** p < 0.001.

Values in the two groups are very similar and when small differences are present (basal and TRH induced serum TSH, serum Tg) they are not statistically significant.

Values for performance, verbal and global intellectual quotients (IQ) in the three groups under investigation are shown in Table 2.

Table 2. *Performance, verbal and global IQ in the series under study*

	Controls	Congenital hypothyroidism	
		Transient	Permanent
	n = 9	n = 9	n = 9
Performance IQ	89.2 ± 12.5	75.0 ± 8.5**a	71.7 ± 8.0 NSb
Verbal IQ	96.2 ± 14.8	84.4 ± 15.4NSa	69.7 ± 9.7*b
Global IQ	90.9 ± 14.2	78.3 ± 11.1*a	69.1 ± 7.8*b

a) TCH vs controls b) permanent vs TCH; NS = non significant, * = p < 0.05, ** = p < 0.01.

The IQ values progressively decreased from the controls through the children with TCH to the children with permanent congenital hypothyroidism. The difference between the group with TCH and the controls was significant for global as well as performance IQ. No difference was observed in the results obtained for Performance, Verbal and Global IQ in the infants of the TCH group with either normal or slightly altered thyroid function (TSH > 4.0 μU/ml) at the time of IQ tests.

DISCUSSION

Infants born and living in an endemic iodine deficient area and who exhibited biochemical signs of TCH at birth, at the age of 7-8 years had an intelligence quotient (IQ) lower than matched controls living in the same environmental conditions but with normal thyroid function at birth.

At school age, physical and bone maturation in the hypothyroid and control groups were not significantly different. No patient exhibited signs or symptoms of hypothyroidism. The results obtained for thyroid function tests were within the limits of normal in most subjects from both groups. However, as a likely consequence of the iodine deficiency, there were 9 children (6 in the TCH and 3 in the control group) with basal TSH levels higher than normal.

The intellectual outcome was lower in infants with transient congenital hypothyroidism than in controls. The observation that IQ values were not different in TCH patients with or without signs of subclinical thyroid impairment at the time of late reevaluation precludes the possibility that IQ difference between TCH and controls is a consequence of the moderate thyroid insufficiency at the time of IQ testing observed in some children. Consequently, the difference in the intellectual ability between TCH and control groups can reasonably be attributed to the presence of thyroid impairment occurring during the critical period of brain development during fetal and early postnatal life in TCH infants.

Moderate but definite impairment of the mental ability in clinically and biochemically euthyroid schoolchildren born and living in conditions of iodine deficiency is well established both in severe and moderate iodine deficiency (1).

Since transient congenital hypothyroidism is frequent in these conditions and may cause intellectual impairment (2), our results strongly support the view that this type of neonatal hypothyroidism has long-term consequences on intellectual development.

REFERENCES

1. Bleichrodt N., Escobar del Rey F., Morreale de Escobar G., Garcia I. and Rubio C. (1989): In: Iodine and the Brain. edited by De Long G.R., Robbins J. and Condliffe P.G. pp 269-287. Plenum Press. New York.
2. Delange F. (1991): In: The Thyroid. A Fundamental and Clinical Text. Braverman L.E., Utiger R.D. eds. pp 942-955. J.B. Lippincott publ. Philadelphia.
3. Sava L., Delange F., Belfiore A., Purrello F. and Vigneri R. (1984): J. Clin. Endocrinol. Metab. 59: 90-95.
4. Wechsler D. (1974): WISC-R Manual of the Wechsler Intelligence Scale for Children - Revised Psychological Corporation. New York.

Frontiers in Endocrinology
Volume 9 - 1994

Anti-Thyroid Autoantibodies and Aging: Influence of Overall Health Status

G. Barbesino, L. Bartalena, R. Bechi[1], P. Sansoni[2], A. Mancato, F. Fagnoni[2], A. Cossarizza[3], D. Monti[3], U. Fagiolo[4], C. Franceschi[3] and A. Pinchera

Institute of Endocrinology, University of Pisa, Viale del Tirreno 64, 56018 Pisa;
[1]Department of Medicine, Viareggio;
[2]Institute of Internal Medicine, University of Parma;
[3]Institute of General Pathology, University of Modena;
[4]Internal Medicine, University of Padova, Italy

INTRODUCTION

The age-dependent increase in the prevalence of positive serum thyroid peroxidase (anti-TPO) and thyroglobulin (anti-TG) autoantibodies in subjects without overt thyroid disease is a well established phenomenon, recognized since the early sixties (1). The biological and clinical significance of this finding is still unknown (2). In particular, it is not clear whether it represents the lower end of the clinical spectrum of thyroid autoimmune disease or it is one of the consequences of the aging process on the immune system, without direct involvement of the target gland. The prevalence of clinically overt thyroid autoimmune disease is generally not increased in the elderly (6), these observations suggesting that age-associated thyroid autoimmune phenomena and fully expressed thyroid autoimmune disease are separate entities.

We recently reported (4) that neither anti-TG nor anti-TPO prevalence are increased in healthy centenarians. It is still unknown whether this phenomenon is due to the disappearance of autoantibodies present in "younger" elderly or to the extreme selection of centenarians, who may indeed include subjects with an unusually efficient immune system (5).

To clarify the relationship between aging, thyroid autoimmune phenomena and health status in the present study the prevalence of circulating anti-thyroid antibodies was assessed in an apparently normal population with a wide age range and in three groups of aged individuals, strictly selected according to their age and general health status.

MATERIAL AND METHODS

Group A consisted of 54 elderly hospitalized patients (aged 61-95 years), affected by various acute or chronic diseases.

Group B included a larger number (n = 54) of apparently healthy subjects over 100 years of age. All centenarians were in good health, without relevant acute or chronic disorders and standard hematochemical parameters were normal in all of them.

Group C included sera from 33 healthy elderly subjects (aged 65-80 years) selected according to the restrictive criteria Eurage-Senieur protocol (3). The observed prevalence of anti-TG and anti-TPO were compared to those found in two groups of unselected subjects without clinical evidence of thyroid disease aged 7-49 years (n = 436) and 70-95 years (n = 40), respectively.

Serum thyroid autoantibodies were assayed in all subjects using several independent techniques including passive hemaglutination for both anti-TG and anti-TPO, a solid-phase ELISA technique for anti-TG and a monoclonal antibody assisted radioimmunoassay (RIA) for anti-TPO. Antibody titres ≥ 1/100 by passive agglutination were considered as positive results; using ELISA and RIA techniques, antibody levels were expressed in International Units (IU/ml); values >120 IU/ml were considered positive anti-Tg and >10 U/ml positive anti-TPO assays. Statistical analysis was performed by the X^2 method.

RESULTS

The results obtained in the assay of anti-TG showed a significant increase in the prevalence of positive tests in control subjects aged >69 years, when compared to younger individuals (aged <50 years) of the same group (Table 1).

Table 1. *Anti-TPO and Anti-TG prevalence in the study groups*

Groups	n.	Anti-TG positive (%)	Anti-TPO positive (%)
A	54	7 (12.9)[1]	12 (22.2)[2,3]
B	54	2 (3.7)	3 (5.5)
C	33	2 (6.0)	3 (9.1)
Controls aged 7-49	436	14 (3.2)	22 (5.0)
Controls aged 70-95	40	5 (12.5)[1]	12 (30.0)[2]

[2]p<0.0001 vs controls <50; [1]p<0.01 vs controls <50; [3]p<0.05 vs B.

As also shown in Table 1, when the selected elderly populations were considered, a significant increase in the prevalence of positive anti-TG when compared to unselected normal subjects aged <50 years was only observed in old hospitalized patients of group A. The prevalence of positive anti-TG tests found in group C patients and in unselected group D subjects aged >69 years were higher when compared to groups A and B, but the difference did not reach the level of statistical significance.

The results obtained in the assay of anti-TPO are also reported in Table 1. The trend was very similar to that observed for anti-TG, but the differences between the various study groups were more evident. A highly significant difference was found in the prevalence of positive anti-TPO in unselected control subjects aged >69 years when compared to younger individuals of the same group. When the other three selected elderly groups were considered, only group C patients showed a significant increase of anti-TPO prevalence, when compared to control subjects aged <50 years. Moreover, the prevalence of anti-TPO found in group D subjects aged >69 years and in group C patients was significantly higher than that found in centenarians ($p<0.05$), but did not reach the level of statistical significance when compared to elderly subjects of group B. Finally, no significant difference in the prevalence of both anti-TG and anti-TPO was found between unselected controls aged >69 and elderly hospitalized patients.

DISCUSSION AND CONCLUSIONS

The results of this study confirm and extend our previous report (4) on a relatively low thyroid autoantibody prevalence in healthy centenarians. Interestingly, no significant increase in the thyroid autoantibody prevalence was found even in healthy elderly subjects aged 65-80 years. This finding is in apparent contrast with several other studies, including our own (4), showing increased thyroid autoantibody prevalence in apparently healthy general population over the sixth decade. A significant increase in the prevalence of anti-TPO and, to a lesser degree, anti-TG, was actually confirmed in the present investigation only in the unselected general population but was found only in hospitalized patients when carefully selected elderly groups were examined. As previously hypothesized by us for centenarians, it is conceivable that old subjects fulfilling the Eurage criteria represent a highly selected healthy population with an unusually efficient immune system. We are tempted to speculate that these may actually represent a cohort of individuals with high potential for longevity and may include future centenarians.

These results are in keeping with the hypothesis discussed above that the association between anti-thyroid autoantibodies and aging is not an effect of the aging process per se, but is maybe related to age-associated disease. If an unusually efficient immune system is an important pre-requisite for longevity, the question may be raised as to whether the appearance of organ-specific autoantibodies at the beginning of senescence is a risk factor for a shorter life-expectancy.

Longitudinal cohort studies, although very difficult to perform, are needed to clarify this point.

ACKNOWLEDGEMENTS

This work was partially supported by National Research Council (CNR, Rome, Italy), Target Project Aging, Subproject Gerontobiology, Grants 92.00355.PF40 and 92.00293.PF40.

REFERENCES

1. Hackett E. and Beech M. (1960): Lancet 2: 402-404.
2. Hawkins B.R., Cheah P.S., Dawkins R.L., Whittingham S., Burger H.G., Patel Y., Mackay I.R. and Welborn T.A. (1980): Lancet 2: 1369-1370.
3. Lighart G.J., Corber J.X., Geertzen H.G., Meinders A.E., Knook D.L. and Hijmans W. (1990): Mech. Ageing Dev. 55: 89-105.
4. Mariotti S., Sansoni P., Barbesino G., Caturegli P., Monti D., Cossarizza A., Giacomelli T., Passeri G., Fagiolo U., Pinchera A. and Franceschi C. (1992): Lancet 339; 1506-8
5. Thompson J.S., Wekstein D.R., Rhoades J.L., Kirkpatrick C., Brown S.A., Roszman T., Straus R. and Tietz N. (1984): J. Am. Geriatr. Soc. 32: 274-281.
6. Volpé R., Clarke P.V. and Row V.V. (1973): CMA Journal 109: 898-901.

Frontiers in Endocrinology
Volume 9 - 1994

Human PTH/PTHrP Receptor: its Role in Pseudohypoparathyroidism Type Ib

E. Schipani, C. Bergwitz, H.M. Kronenberg, G.V. Segre and H. Jüppner

Endocrine Unit, Medical and Children's Services, Massachusetts General Hospital and Harvard Medical School, Boston, MA 02114, USA

INTRODUCTION

Parathyroid hormone (PTH) is the most important regulator of mineral ion metabolism in mammals (10). PTH-related peptide (PTHrP), discovered initially as the cause of the syndrome of malignancy-associated humoral hypercalcemia, is now known to be of importance for normal embryonic development and may act as a paracrine factor throughout life (3, 8, 22).

PTH and PTHrP bind and activate a common G protein-coupled receptor with seven putative membrane-spanning helices which has dual signaling properties (1, 7, 17). The PTH/PTHrP receptor belongs to a newly discovered receptor family (6): the members of this novel receptor family share many common motifs including a relatively long amino-terminal extracellular region, at least two potential glycosylation sites, eight conserved extracellular cysteine residues, and multiple conserved amino acids that are scattered throughout the extracellular domains, the membrane spanning helices, and the intracellular loops.

This pattern of amino acid conservation suggests a structural and functional organization that is shared among all members of this novel receptor family.

The organization of the PTH/PTHrP receptor gene is highly homologous in the three mammalian species, rat, human and mouse (9). It extends over 22 kb and contains at least 15 exons and 14 introns.

For many G protein-coupled receptors, interesting information about important functional domains has been derived from the molecular analysis of human diseases or animal models, i.e. ACTH-resistance (21), nephrogenic diabetes insipidus (5, 13, 15), murine congenital hypothyroidism (20), and the little mouse phenotype (12). These disorders are due to mutations in the gene's coding exons that resulted in non-functioning receptors. Mutations that are the cause of constitutively activated or hypersensitive receptor have been described as well, i.e. retinitis pigmentosa (4), thyroid adenomas (14), gonadotropin-independent male precocious puberty (18).

METHODS AND RESULTS

To determine the molecular basis of a human disease, and to extend our understanding of the functional properties of the PTH/PTHrP receptor, we searched for receptor mutations in patients with pseudohypoparathyroidism type Ib.

The classical form of pseudohypoparathyroidism (PHP), PHP type Ia, was described by Fuller Albright almost 50 years ago (2). This disease is usually characterized by end-organ resistance to PTH, typical skeletal abnormalities, so-called Albright's Hereditary Osteodystrophy, and additional associated endocrine abnormalities. Patients with pseudo pseudohypoparathyroidism have the same skeletal findings but no abnormalities of their mineral ion metabolism. Both diseases can occur in members of the same family, and they have been attributed to a defect or deficiency of the alpha subunit of the Gs protein (11). Patients with PHP type Ib present with a selective end-organ resistance to PTH, but no other abnormalities are usually observed. Based on *in vivo* and *in vitro* findings, the pathogenesis of PHP type Ib is thought to involve a defect in the PTH/PTHrP receptor (19).

The isolation of genomic DNA clones encoding the human PTH/PTHrP receptor allowed us to investigate whether PHP type Ib is caused by a defect involving its coding exons or adjacent introns.

Each exon was amplified by polymerase chain reaction (PCR) from the patients' genomic DNA. Nucleotide primers were based on DNA sequences adjacent to each exon, modified by the addition of GC-rich high melting oligomers to either the forward or the reverse primer. Each PCR product was then analyzed by temperature gradient gel electrophoresis (TGGE) (18) or by sequencing alone.

PCR products representing all 14 coding exons from 18 patients with this syndrome were of the predicted size. Only one heterozygotic base substitution resulted in a missense mutation in the intracellular tail of the receptor (3/18). Infrequent heterozygotic polymorphisms were identified in two coding exons (1/18 and 1/18, respectively) and in two intronic sequences

(1/18 and 2/18, respectively). A frequent polymorphism in exon M7 which was recently described for the normal population (16), was also identified in this group of patients.

It is possible that TGGE failed to detect abnormalities in the patients' DNA. However, since 6 independent base-changes were detected in this study with a large number of patients, it seems unlikely that functionally important mutations in the coding exons or in adjacent intronic sequences occur frequently in PHP-Ib.

We must, therefore, conclude that PHP-Ib is only rarely, if at all, caused by mutations in the coding region of the PTH/PTHrP receptor gene or the intron/exon junctions.

REFERENCES

1. Abou-Samra A.B., Jüppner H., Force T., Freeman M.W., Kong X.F., Schipani E., Urena P., Richards J., Bonventre J.V., Potts J.T., jr., Kronenberg H.M. and Segre G.V. (1992): Proc. Natl. Acad. Sci. USA 89: 2732-2736.
2. Albright F., Burnett C.H., Smith P.H. and Parson W. (1942): Endocrinology 30: 922-932.
3. Broadus A. E. and Stewart A.F. (1994): In: The Parathyroids. Basic and Clinical Concepts. edited by J.P. Bilzikian, M.A. Levine and R. Marcus. Raven Press. New York. 259-294.
4. Dryja T.P., Hahn L.B., Cowley G.S., McGee T.L. and Berson E.L. (1991): Proc. Natl. Acad. Sci. USA 88: 9370-9374.
5. Holtzman E., Harris H. Kolakowski L.F., jr., Guay-Woodford L., Botelho B. and Ausiello D. (1993): New Engl. J. Med. 328: 1534-1537.
6. Jüppner H. (1994): Current Opinion in Nephrology and Hypertension 3: 371-378.
7. Jüppner H., Abou-Samra A.B., Freeman M.W., Kong X.F., Schipani S., Richards J., Kolakowski L.F., Jr., Hock J., Potts J.T., Jr., Kronenberg H.M. and Segre G.V. (1991): Science 254: 1024-1026.
8. Karaplis A.C., Luz A., Glowacki J., Bronson R., Tybulewicz V., Kronenberg H.M. and Mulligan R.C. (1994): Genes Develop. 8: 277-289.
9. Kong X.F., Schipani E., Lanske B., Joun H., Karperien M., Defize L.H.K., Jüppner H., Potts J.T., Segre G.V., Kronenberg H.M. and Abou-Samra A.B. (1994): Biochem. Biophys. Res. Comm. 200: 1290-1299.
10. Kronenberg H.M., Bringhurst F.R., Nussbaum S., Jüppner H., Abou-Samra A.B., Segre G.V. and Potts J.T., jr. (1993): In: Handbook of Experimental Pharmacology: Physiology and Pharmacology of Bone. G.R. Mundy, and T.J. Martin (ed.). Springer-Verlag. Heidelberg. 185-201.
11. Levine M.A. and Aurbach G.D. (1989): In: Endocrinology. L.J. DeGroot (ed.). Saunders. Philadelphia. 1065-1079.
12. Lin S.C., Lin C.R., Gukovsky I., Lusis A.J., Sawchenko P.E. and Rosenfeld M.G. (1993): Nature 364: 208-213.
13. Merendino J.J., jr., Spiegel A.M., Crawford J.D., O'Carroll A.M., Brownstein M.J. and Lolait S.J. (1993): New Engl. J. Med. 328: 1538-1541.
14. Parma J., Duprez L., Van Sande J., Cochaux P., Gervy C., Mockel J., Dumont J. and Vassart G. (1993): Nature 365: 649-651.
15. Rosenthal W., Seibold A., Antaramian A., Lonergan M., Arthus M.F., Hendy G.N., Birnbaumer M. and Bichet D.G. (1992): Nature 359: 233-235.
16. Schipani E., Hustmyer F.G., Bergwitz C. and Jüppner H. (1994): Hum. Mol. Genet. 3: 1210.
17. Schipani E., Karga H., Karaplis A.C., Potts J.T., jr., Kronenberg H.M., Segre G.V., Abou-Samra A.B. and Jüppner H. (1993): Endocrinology 132: 2157-2165.
18. Shenker A., Laue L., Kosugi S., Merendino J.J., jr., Minegishi T. and Cutler G.B. (1993): Nature 365: 652-654.

19. Silve C., Santora A., Breslau N., Moses A. and Spiegel A. (1986): J. Clin. Endocrinol. Metab. 62: 640-644.
20. Stein S.A., Oates E.L., Hall C.R., Grumbles R.M., Fernandez L.M., Taylor N.A., Puett D. and Jin S. (1994): Mol. Endocrinol. 8: 129-138.
21. Tsigos C., Arai K., Hung W. and Chrousos G. P. (1993): J. Clin. Invest. 92: 2458-2461.
22. van de Stolpe A., Karperien M., Löwik C.W.G.M., Jüppner H., Abou-Samra A.B., Segre G.V., de Laat S. W. and Defize L.H.K. (1993): J. Cell. Biol. 120: 235-243.

Frontiers in Endocrinology
Volume 9 - 1994

INTRODUCTORY REMARKS

Thyroid Autoimmunity: Controversies and Future Developments

L. Chiovato, S. Filetti[1] and A. Pinchera

Institute of Endocrinology, University of Pisa;[1]Chair of Endocrinology, University of Reggio Calabria in Catanzaro, Italy

Autoimmune reactions against the thyroid gland result in a wide spectrum of disorders ranging from hyperthyroid Graves' disease to atrophic autoimmune thyroiditis with hypothyroidism. Goitrous Hashimoto's thyroiditis, either euthyroid or hypothyroid, is the central disease in this spectrum. Despite this heterogeneity of clinical manifestations, thyroid autoimmune diseases share a common feature: the presence of autoreactive lymphocytes and of antibodies against specific thyroid antigens. Although much is known about the nature and consequences of thyroid autoimmune reactions, the underlying abnormalities leading to the development and progress of thyroid autoimmunity are still a matter of active research.

During the last two decades, extensive research has focused mainly on two goals: 1) definition of the etiologic factors and mechanisms leading to the breakdown of immune tolerance to thyroid antigens; 2) assessment of the role of humoral and cellular effectors in the pathogenesis of the clinical manifestations of thyroid autoimmune diseases. These studies led to new developments in our understanding of the generation and expansion of autoreactive immune cells, of the effects of lymphocytes and cytokines on the thyroid and of the interactions between thyroid autoantigens and antibodies at molecular level.

With the identification of thyroperoxidase (TPO) as the main component of the so-called microsomal antigen, and the elucidation of the biological properties of different TSH-receptor antibodies, it has been possible to carry out much new basic and clinical work.

The application of recombinant DNA technology provided a further key to the research in thyroid autoimmunity. Indeed, the cloning of TPO and

TSH receptor, and the elucidation of their primary aminoacid sequence provided a refined approach to the identification of the epitopes recognized by autoreactive lymphocytes and antibodies.

In the first part of this Workshop, the role of immunogloubin genes in the development of thyroid autoimmunity, the effects of lymphocytes and cytokines on thyroid cells, and the clinical importance of TPO and TSH-receptor antibodies are reviewed by scientists actively engaged in these fields of thyroid research.

In the second section, specific clinical aspects of autoimmune thyroidits (AT), the archetype of autoimmune thyroid diseases, are discussed. The topics of this debate include; epidemiology of AT; techniques for measuring thyroid autoantibodies; diagnostic relevance of ultrasound examination of the gland, fine needle aspiration biopsy and detection of thyroid antibodies; of therapeutic approach to AT, and complications. Attention is also focused on several controversial aspects such as: the role of iodine intake in the development of AT, pregnancy and AT, post-partum thyroiditis, the association of AT with other organ-specific and nonorgan-specific diseases, the effects of interferon therapy on AT development and progress.

Research in thyroid autoimmunity is moving rapidly, and this will probably have a great clinical impact in the near future. In particular, the identification and the definition at the molecular level of the mechanisms responsible for the breakdown of immune tolerance to thyroid antigens might result in new strategies of intervention for a specific immune therapy.

In the effort to bring together, and to discuss, basic and clinical experiences, the topics of this Workshop were chosen on the basis of their implications for clinical practice and of their relevance for future research.

From: JEI, Vol. 17, Suppl. 2 to n. 3, 1994, p. 15.
Abstracts of the XXV National Congress of the Italian Endocrine Society

Frontiers in Endocrinology
Volume 9 - 1994

Immunoglobulin Genes and Autoimmune Thyroid Disease

S. McLachlan, S. Portolano, G. Chazenbalk, J.C. Jaume, M. Prummel and B. Rapoport

Thyroid Molecular Biology Unit, V.A. Medical Center and the University of California San Francisco, California, 4150 Clement Street, San Francisco, CA 94121, USA

Graves' disease and Hashimoto's thyroiditis have long been known to have a familial basis. Autoantibodies to thyroid peroxidase (TPO) and thyroglobulin (Tg) also cluster in families. The genes responsible for overt clinical disease or thyroid autoantibody production are unknown at present. Recent studies of families with Graves' and Hashimoto's disease demonstrated a lack of linkage between Major Histo-Compatibility antigens (MHC) and either thyroid autoantibody production or disease (12, 17). Consequently, it is unlikely that MHC gene polymorphism plays a major role in the inheritance of autoimmune thyroid disease.

Inheritance of the ability to produce TPO and Tg autoantibodies is in agreement with other observations. Thus, the ability to make pemphigus vulgaris cadherin autoantibodies (1) is inherited and the response involves MHC genes. Production of antibodies to malarial antigens is also genetically controlled but MHC genes are *not* involved (19).

IMMUNOGLOBULIN GENES AND THYROID AUTOANTIBODY INHERITANCE

A role for immunoglobulin genes in human antibody responses was first suggested by the association between antibodies to a bacterial pathogen and polymorphisms of the immunoglobulin heavy chain constant region, Gm allotypes (reviewed in 21). Such an association could arise because the genes encoding the immunoglobulin heavy chain constant regions lie on the same chromosome as the set of genes encoding the antigen-binding regions, the immunoglobulin *variable* region genes. To investigate whether immunoglobulin gene polymorphism is involved in the development of thyroid autoimmunity, *human* monoclonal thyroid autoantibodies derived from patients' B cells are required.

MONOCLONAL ANTIBODY PRODUCTION USING COMBINATORIAL LIBRARIES

Immortalization of *human* antibody-producing cells for monoclonal antibody generation is more difficult than conventional hybridoma technology in mice (reviewed in 7). However, many of these problems are overcome by a new technique, which involves cloning and expressing immunoglobulin heavy (H) and light (L) chain genes in bacteria (5). In this "combinatorial library" approach, cDNA is reverse transcribed from lymphocyte mRNA. The cDNA is used as template in the polymerase chain reaction with oligonucleotide primers to generate separate immunoglobulin H and L chain cDNA libraries in a bacteriophage vector. The H and L chain libraries are then combined and the random H and L chain combinations are screened with purified antigen to identify antigen-specific antibodies.

Using the combinatorial library approach, we have generated a panel of human IgG class antibodies, in the form of F(ab), to thyroid peroxidase (TPO) from thyroid-infiltrating B cell cDNA (13-15, 4). This panel of TPO F(ab) resembles TPO auto-antibodies in patients' sera in terms of IgG subclass, specificity and affinity for TPO. Further, the F(ab) interact with epitopes on TPO recognized by >80% of serum TPO autoantibodies (4).

GENES ENCODING H AND L CHAINS OF TPO F(AB)

The variable regions of TPO F(ab) H and L chain nucleotide sequences can be described in terms of their homology to the germline minigenes which generate the antigen binding site. An H chain antigen-binding region is encoded by the combination of 1 of ~100 variable (VH) genes, 1 of ~20 diversity (D) genes, 1 of 6 joining (JH) genes. The variable region of human kappa L chain is formed from 1 of ~100 VK genes and 1 of 6 JK genes.

Analysis of the putative germline genes used by our TPO F(ab), derived from 4 Graves' patients, demonstrated a relatively restricted number and combinations of H and L chain genes: 5 different H and L chain combinations involving 4 H chains and 3 L chains (Table 1) (4). In addition, one combination of H and L chains (HV1L1 and KL012) was obtained from combinatorial libraries prepared from 3 patients. Another H and L chain combination (V1-3b and KL012) was found in libraries prepared from 2 patients.

Information from this panel of TPO F(ab) may provide insight into the question of thyroid autoantibody V region gene inheritance. Thus, TPO

F(ab) TR1.8 is encoded by a VH gene 91% homologous to germline gene hv1263 (4). hv1263 is closely related to 51p1, a member of a highly polymorphic group of VH1 genes (18). Some variants of 51p1 were detected in up to 58% of individuals studied. In contrast, the two hv1263 variants were *only* observed in 4% and 8% of the study group (18). These findings raise the possibility that the ability to produce autoantibodies to the TR1.8 epitope on TPO may be determined by the inheritance of a particular hv1263 variant.

Table 1. *TPO-specific human F(ab)*

Library	No. clones	H Chain Germline	VH	JH	L Chain Germline	VK	JK
SP	1 clone	HV1L1	1	6	KL012	1	2
	2 clones	HV1L1	1	6	KL012	1	1
	1 clone	HV1L1	1	4	KL012	1	2
WR	20 clones	HV1L1	1	4	KL012	1	2
JA	1 clone	HV1L1	1	6	KL012	1	4
TR	2 clones	V1-3b	1	4	A'	1	4
	1 clone	V1-3b	1	4	KL012	1	1
WR	2 clones	V1-3b	1	4	KL012	1	1
TR	2 clones	8-1b	3	4	KL012	1	2
TR	2 clones	HV1263	1	3	A3	2	2

PHAGE DISPLAY SYSTEM

Screening for antibody binding with a bacteriophage lambda vector requires a source of purified antigen. A modification of the combinatorial library approach, the "phage display system" (2, 9), permits combinatorial library screening with either purified or *unpurified* antigen.

The ability to screen with unpurified antigen is potentially useful in the case of antigens (like the TSH receptor) which are difficult to purify. However, there had been no comparison of F(ab) obtained from the same cDNA by screening plaques in a bacteriophage library with *purified* antigen and by panning a phage display library with *impure* antigen. We, therefore, performed such a study for TPO F(ab) by transferring the H and L chain cDNA combinations from one bacteriophage library (TR) into a phage display vector, pComb3. This library was screened by panning on live, stably-transfected Chinese hamster ovary (CHO) cells expressing human TPO on their surface (8). We obtained 6 new TPO-specific F(ab), all with high affinities (Kd ~10^{-10} M) for TPO, comparable with those for F(ab) generated by screening bacteriophage plaques with purified TPO (16).

A second important feature of the phage display system is the ability to screen very large numbers of recombinant phage, >10^{11} compared with 10^5 - 10^6 by the lytic plaque method. Consequently, the phage display system permits screening for rare antibodies, and screening may be performed using antigens on living cells.

COMBINATORIAL LIBRARIES AND GRAVES' OPHTHALMOPATHY

The evidence for autoantibodies to orbital specific antigens in Graves' ophthalmopathy is controversial (reviewed in 20). A major problem in screening sera for antibody binding to relatively crude antigen extracts or cultured cells is distinguishing a specific signal from the background.

Lymphocytic infiltrates present in Graves' orbital muscle and, to a lesser extent in fat/connective tissue, contain predominantly T cells, although plasma cells have been observed (3, 20). It is a reasonable assumption that some of these B cells are synthesising autoantibodies to orbital specific antigens. Monoclonal antibodies, derived from infiltrating orbital B cells, might overcome the difficulties in using polyclonal serum antibodies in screening for orbital autoantigens.

As a first step to cloning orbital antibodies, we established that immunoglobulin H and L chain products could be obtained by PCR from Graves' orbital connective tissue/fat and muscle cDNA (10, 11). Subsequently, we constructed immunoglobulin H chain and kappa L chain cDNA libraries from the orbital fat/connective tissue of a patient with active ophthalmopathy. We then analyzed the V regions of 15 H chains and 15 kappa L chains, randomly selected without regard to antigen specificity (6). We observed a restricted spectrum of both H and kappa genes. In addition, there was a similarity between some H and L chain genes expressed in the orbital fat/connective tissue of patient n. 7 and those used to code for other autoantibodies.

We are currently constructing combinatorial libraries from Graves' orbital tissue B cells. These orbital phage display libraries will be potentially powerful probes for identifying the autoantigens responsible for Graves' ophthalmopathy.

REFERENCES

1. Ahmed A.R. Mohimen A., Yunis E.J., Mirza M., Kumar V., Beutner E.H. and Alper C.A. (1993): J. Exp. Med. 177, 419-424.
2. Barbas III, C.F., Kang A.S., Lerner R.A. and Benkovic S.J. (1991): Proc. Natl. Acad. Sci. USA 88: 7978-7982.

3. Campbell R.J. (1989): Acta Endocrinol. 121 (Suppl. 2), 9-16.
4. Chazenbalk G.D., Portolano S., Russo D., Hutchison J.S., Rapoport B. and McLachlan S.M. (1993): J Clin. Invest. 92: 62-74.
5. Huse W.D. Sastry L., Iverson S.A., Kang A.S., Alting-Mees M., Burton D.R., Benkovic S.J. and Lerner R.A. (1989): Science 246: 1275-1281.
6. Jaume J.C., Portolano S., Prummel M.F., McLachlan S.M. and Rapoport B. (1994): J. Clin. Endocrinol. Metab. 378: 348-352.
7. Kalsi J.K. and Isenberg D.A. (1992): Autoimmunity 13: 249-258.
8. Kaufman K.D., Rapoport B., Seto P., Chazenbalk G.D. and Magnusson R.P. (1989): J. Clin. Invest. 8: 394-403.
9. McCafferty J., Griffiths A.D., Winter G. and Chiswell D.J. (1990): Nature 348: 552-554.
10. McLachlan S.M., Prummel M.F., Dallow R.L., Wiersinga W.M. and Rapoport B. (1993): Autoimmunity 16: 149-152.
11. McLachlan S.M., Prummel M.F., Jaume J.C . and Rapoport B. (1994): J. Endocrinol. Invest. 17: 247-252.
12. Phillips D., McLachlan S., Stephenson A., Roberts D., Moffitt S., McDonald D., Ad'Hiah A., Strattton S., Young E., Clark F. Beever K., Bradbury J. and Rees Smith B. (1990): J. Clin. Endocrinol. Metab. 70: 742-746.
13. Portolano S., Seto P., Chazenbalk G.D., Nagayama Y., McLachlan S. and Rapoport B. (1991): Biochem. Biophys. Res. Comm. 179: 372-379.
14. Portolano S., Chazenbalk G.D., Seto P., Hutchison J.S. Rapoport B. and McLachlan S.M. (1992): J. Clin. Invest. 90: 720-726.
15. Portolano S., Chazenbalk G.D., Hutchison J.S., McLachlan S.M. and Rapoport B. (1993): J. Immunol. 150: 880-887.
16. Portolano S., McLachlan S.M. and Rapoport B. (1993): J. Immunol. 151: 2839-2851.
17. Roman S.H., Greenberg D., Rubinstein P., Wallenstein S. and Davies T.F. (1992): J. Clin. Endocrinol. Metab. 74: 496-503.
18. Sasso E.H., van Dijk K.W., Bull A.P. and Milner E.C.B. (1993): J. Clin Invest. 91: 2358-2367.
19. Sjoberg K., Lepers J.P., Raharimalala L. et al. (1992): Proc. Natl. Acad. Sci. USA 89: 2101-2104.
20. Weetman A.P. (1992): Autoimmunity 12: 215-222.
21. Whittingham S. and Propert D.N. (1986): Monogr. Allergy 19: 52-70.

Frontiers in Endocrinology
Volume 9 - 1994

Pathogenetic Role of Lymphocytes and Cytokines in Autoimmune Thyroid Disease

S. Mariotti, G. Barbesino, L. Chiovato, M. De Carli[1] and G.F. Del Prete[1]

Endocrinology, University of Pisa, Viale del Tirreno 64, I-56018 Tirrenia Pisa;
[1]Clinical Immunology, University of Florence, Florence, Italy

INTRODUCTION

Graves' disease, Hashimoto's thyroiditis and idiopathic myxedema are regarded as typical organ-specific autoimmune disorders (autoimmune thyroid disease, AITD) (11, 20, 21). Independently of the precise etiologic factor involved, dysregulation of the immune system leads to ongoing expansion of autoreactive T cells and to the activation of several effector systems responsible for thyroid damage and/or dysfunction (5, 14, 20, 21). Destructive processes may be mediated by complement-fixing antibodies, by *in situ* formation of immune complexes, by nonspecific mononuclear (killer) cells through antibody-dependent cellular cytotoxicity and by specific cytotoxic T lymphocytes. Autoantibodies directed against thyrotropin (TSH) receptor and able to stimulate or block thyroid function are responsible for hyperthyroidism of Graves' disease and thyroid atrophy of primary adult myxedema, respectively. In this framework, cytokines could exert important modulatory effects in triggering and/or maintaining the autoimmune reaction, as well as in the effector system activation.

Attention will be focused here on recent progress in our understanding the pathogenetic role of cellular mechanisms and cytokines in AITD, with emphasis on experimental work carried out in our laboratories.

T-LYMPHOCYTES AND THYROID AUTOIMMUNITY

Although the initial event of thyroid autoimmunity remains elusive, the ongoing expansion of thyroid antigen-specific autoreactive T-lymphocytes plays a central role in the development and maintainence of effector mechanisms leading to thyroid damage. In the past few years, the development of high efficiency T-cell cloning methods allowed detailed characterization of T-lymphocytes of thyroid autoimmune infiltrates.

Antigen-specificity of infiltrating T-lymphocytes in AITD The study of T-cell clones (TCC) derived from infiltrates led to the unequivocal demonstration of the specific sensitization to thyroid antigen(s) at cell level (5). This was obtained by the demonstration of TCC proliferating when co-cultured with autologous thyroid cells, but not reacting with autologous monuclear cells or heterologous thyrocytes (13). These thyroid-specific TCC are both CD4+ and CD8+ and appear to represent <10% of the total TCC obtained from thyroid infiltrating cells (14). Further characterization of thyroid-specific TCC showed that they were able to recognize at least two of the major thyroid antigens (i.e. thyroglobulin -Tg, and thyroid peroxidase -TPO), while evidence for TCC specific for TSH (TSHr) is only indirect. The fine specificity of thyroid-specific TCC appears to be complex, as shown by the existence of clones reacting with distinct aminoacid sequences of TPO (6).

Quite recently, a peculiar resistance to *in vitro* induced anergy has been described from thyroid-specific TCC from the thyroid infiltrate of a patient with Graves' disease; in contrast, TCC derived from the peripheral blood of the same patient were easily anergized (5). Although it is difficult to generalize on the basis of data obtained from a single patient, this finding could be relevant in the understanding of the mechanisms leading to loss of tolerance to thyroid autoantigens.

Studies on T-cell receptor (TCR) of thyroid-infiltrating lymphocytes The antigen-specificity of T-lymphocytes involved in thyroid autoimmunity has recently been studied from a different point of view, by attempting to define the molecular characteristics of TCR of lymphocytes involved in thyroid autoimmunity. Briefly, T-lymphocytes recognize antigenic fragments bound to major histocompatibility complex (MHC) molecules through TCR, a surface heterodimer formed by an a and a b chain (19). TCR is encoded by random rearrangements of discontinuous DNA segments during T-cell maturation: this phenomenon provides the "generation of diversity" needed to the immune system to recognize a vast array of antigen-MHC complexes (4). It is believed that the random nature of this process may result in T-lymphocytes recognizing self-antigens potentially able to initiate an autoimmune response, when immunolgical tolerance is circumvented. In this regard, several studies have recently been carried out to investigate whether and to what extent there is a restricted TCR usage in autoimmune diseases (19). Limiting the present discussion to thyroid autoimmunity, mRNA analsyis by polymerase chain reaction has been carried out on total lymphoid cell populations obtained from surgical samples or thin needle aspiration biopsies from Graves' or Hashimoto's glands. The results obtained are contradictory, with some degree of restriction being observed for Vα gene by some investigators (1-3), but not confirmed by others (1-3, 17, 18); in contrast, the Vβ rearrangement appears to be mostly polyclonal (19). The apparent lack of a TCR restriction in AITD could be due to technical problems such as the prevalence in thyroid infiltrates of T-lymphocytes non-specifically sensitized to thyroid antigens and to different disease stages of the patients studied so far. It is conceivable that the study of TCR gene rearrangements in thyroid antigen-specific TCC and/or in very early phases of AITD might provide different results. It should be noted, however, that the heterogeneity in autoantigen recognition found in thyroid-specific TCC strongly argues against a very restricted TCR gene usage in AITD.

Phenotypical and functional characterization of thyroid-derived TCC in AITD In the past few years, we have analysed phenotypic and functional characteristics of TCC derived from thyroid infiltrating lymphocytes of patients with Hashimoto's thyroiditis (HT) or Graves' disease (GD). To this purpose, T lymphocytes from surgical specimens were cloned at limiting dilutions in the presence of irradiated feeder cells, phytohemagglutinin (PHA) and interleukin-2 (IL-2). Most T-cell clones (TCC) obtained appeared to be a progeny of CD4+ and CD8+ *in vivo* activated lymphocytes with natural killer (NK)-like activity (9, 12). When stimulated by PHA, most TCC were able to secrete high amounts of interferon-gamma (IFN-γ), whereas the ability to co-secrete tumor necrosis factor-alpha (TNF-α) was peculiar of most HT derived TCC (10, 11). In agreement with other reports, a minority of thyroid derived TCC were able to proliferate *in vitro* in response to autologous thyroid epithelial cells (TEC) under MHC restricted conditions. The pattern of cytokine secretion by thyroid-specific TCC after co-culture with autologous TEC was very similar to that observed in total TCC population. It is interesting to note that, according to the profile of cytokine secretion, most CD4+ TCC from HT and GD infiltrates could be assigned to the subpopulations of Th1-type "inflammatory" T cells able to produce high amounts of IFN-γ and IL-2, but not IL-4 (8, 15).

ROLE OF CYTOKINES ON THYROID AUTOIMMUNITY AND FUNCTION

IFN-γ, TNF-α and other cytokines exert several immunological activities which may be important in triggering and maintaining thyroid autoimmune reaction. Cytokines could also modulate the clinical expression of AITD by exerting direct functional effects on thyroid epithelial cells. Recent *in vitro* studies indicate that IFN-γ, IL-1, IL-6 and TNF-α exhibit a potent action, mostly inhibitory, on thyroid cell growth and differentiated functions (16).

The role of IL-1 and IL-6 in thyroid autoimmune reaction may be more complex. It has been shown that thyroid cells are not only target, but also produce these cytokines (16, 20). This phenomenon could be particularly relevant, since a DR^+ thyroid cell producing IL-1 and IL-6 could be considered a functioning antigen-presenting cell, able to trigger autoimmune reactions without the involvement of macrophages. The precise *in vivo* relevance of these observations still remains to be established. It may be speculated that the enhanced local generation of TNF-α suggested by our studies on HT TCC might play an important and specific role in the mechanisms leading to thyroid hypofunction and damage characteristic of this disease.

To address this question, we assessed the effects of culture supernatants of thyroid derived Th1 clones rich in IFN-γ and TNF-α on TSH induced proliferation and ^{131}I uptake in FRTL-5 cells (8). FRTL-5 cells were pre-incubated for 48 hours with culture supernatants of HT or GD TCC stimulated with autologous TEC, and then stimulated with TSH. Supernatants from autoreactive HT derived TCC containing both TNF-α and IFN-γ were found to inhibit, in a dose-dependent fashion, TSH-induced growth of FRTL-5 cells. Similar results were found for ^{131}I uptake. In contrast, supernatants of GD derived autoreactive TCC, containing IFN-γ but not TNF-α, were ineffective. Furthermore, the inhibitory effect of TNF-α containing supernatants of HT TCC was specifically abrogated by addition of neutralising antibodies to TNF-α.

In a subsequent series of experiments (8) we investigated whether the different mixture of cytokines secreted by autoreactive thyroid derived TCC were able to induce human TEC to develop *in vitro* functions peculiar to professional antigen presenting cells (i.e. expression of HLA class II molecules and secretion of IL-1 and/or IL-6). To this purpose autoreactive HT and GD TCC were stimulated with autologous TEC and their supernatants were incubated with primary cultures of normal TEC. When incubated for 4 days with either HT- or GD-supernatants the majority of DR-negative normal TEC were induced to express DR molecules (63-78%, as assessed by FACS analysis). This effect was due to IFN-γ since it was observed also in IFN containing GD-TCC devoid of TNF-α and, more importantly, it was specifically prevented by the addition of neutralising anti-IFN-γ antibodies.

Finally, we assessed whether thyroid specific TCC were able to induce human cloned TEC (8) to secrete co-stimulatory cytokines, such as IL-6 and IL-1β. A spontaneous secretion of IL-6, but not of IL-1β, was found in TEC supernatants. The addition of supernatants from autoreactive TCC resulted in increased IL-6 production, without any change in IL-1β production. This effect was inhibited by addition of anti-IFN-γ antibody, while anti-IL-2 antibody was ineffective. An even greater reduction of IL-6 secretion was obtained with anti-TNF-α antibody. These data provide evidence for an up-regulation of IL-6 production by TEC exerted by IFN-γ and TNF-α.

T-LYMPHOCYTES AND CYTOKINES IN GRAVES OPHTHALMOPATHY

It is widely accepted that Graves' ophthalmopathy is an autoimmune condition, although its pathogenesis remains elusive. We recently characterized phenotypic and functional features of TCC derived from orbital infiltrates of Graves' patients (7). Retrobulbar tissue and peripheral blood lymphocytes (PBL) were obtained from 4 patients with severe ophthalmopathy during surgical decompression. Four healthy donors provided control PBL. Orbital lymphocyte (OL) suspensions were obtained by seeding surgical material in RPMI medium supplemented with rIL-2. PBL and OL were then cloned by limiting dilution on feeder irradiated splenocytes, in the presence of rIL-2 and PHA. Surface phenotype analysis of freshly isolated PBL from both controls and patients showed a predominance of CD4+ cells with CD4+/CD8+ ratios ranging from 1.9-2.5. In contrast, OL displayed equal proportions of CD4+ and CD8+ cells, with CD4+/CD8+ ratios ranging from 0.9-1.2. Further analysis was carried out on a total of 153 TCC from OL, 166 from patients and 236 from control PBL. Assessment of lectin-dependent cytolytic activity showed similar percentages of cytolytic cells in TCC derived from PBL of both patients and controls (37.3% and 38%, respectively), most of cytolytic TCC being CD8+. In contrast, cytolytic TCC from OL were markedly increased (106/153, 69.2%) and also included a high proportion (53/79, 67%) of CD4+ TCC. Analysis of PHA-induced cytokine secretion by TCC showed increased proportion of CD8+ and CD4+ OL TCC able to produce IL-2, IFN-γ and TNF-α when compared to patient and control PBL clones. Only rare CD4+ TCC from ROL produced IL-4 and IL-5, while these cytokines were secreted by 27-32% of CD4+ TCC from patient and control PBL. This finding is consistent with a quite homogeneous (90%) pattern of Th1 T-cell phenotype in OL. Thus, cytolytic lymphocytes predominate in the orbital infiltrate of Graves' ophthalmopathy. Furthermore, the prevalence of Th1 phenotype in orbital CD4+ infiltrating T-cells is a pattern quite similar to that previously found in thyroid infiltrate of Hashimoto's thyroiditis and possibly plays an important role in the tissue damage and in the fibrogenic process of Graves' ophthalmopathy.

CONCLUSIONS

Taken together, tha data discussed above suggest a model by which infiltrating T cells may cross-talk with thyroid cells in thyroid autoimmunity. Upon interaction with autologous class II-positive TEC, autoreactive T cells can release different cytokines which can not only trigger a number of immune effector mechanisms, but also affect the function of TEC. *In situ* secreted IFN-γ seems to be mainly responsible for the up regulation of HLA class II molecules, whereas TNF-α (possibly enhanced by IFN-γ) would be mainly responsible for functional damage and up regulation of IL-6 production by TEC. These data also suggest that in thyroid autoimmunity TEC may be induced by locally secreted cytokines to increase their aberrant capacity to function as antigen presenting cells, thus actively contributing to maintain and amplify the autoimmune reaction.

ACKNOWLEDGEMENTS

This paper was partially supported by grants from the National Research Council (CNR, Rome, Italy), Target Project: "Ageing" (Grants #91.00418.PF40 and #92.00355.PF40), and by MURST (40%).

REFERENCES

1. Davies T.F., Concepcion E.S., Ben N.A., Graves P.N. and Tarjan G. (1993): J. Clin. Endocrinol. Metab. 76: 660-6.
2. Davies T.F., Martin A., Concepcion E.S., Graves P., Cohen L. and Ben N.A. (1991): N. Engl. J. Med. 325: 238-44.
3. Davies T.F., Martin A., Concepcion E.S., Graves P., Lahat N., Cohen W.L. and Ben N.A. (1992): J. Clin. Invest. 89: 157-62.
4. Davis M.M. (1990): Annu. Rev. Biochem., 59: 475-96.
5. Dayan C.M., Chu N.R., Londei M., Rapoport B. and Feldmann M. (1993): J. Immunol. 151: 1606-13.
6. Dayan C.M., Londei M., Corcoran A.E., Grubeck L.B., James R.F., Rapoport B. and Feldmann M. (1991): Proc. Natl. Acad. Sci. USA 88: 7415-9.
7. De Carli M., D'Elios M.M., Mariotti S., Marcocci C., Pinchera A., Ricci M., Romagnani S. and Del Prete G.F. (1993): J. Clin. Endocrinol. Metab. 77: 1120-24.
8. Del Prete G.F., De Carli M.C.M., Mavilia C., Romagnani S., Ricci M., Mariotti S., Marcocci C., Chiovato C. and Pinchera A. (1991): In: Progress in Thyroid Research, edited by A. Gordon, J. Gross and G. Hennemann, pp 415-417. A.A. Balkema. Rotterdam.
9. Del Prete G.F., Maggi E., Mariotti S., Tiri A., Vercelli D., Parronchi P., Macchia D., Pinchera A., Ricci M. and Romagnani S. (1986): J. Clin. Endocrinol. Metab. 62: 52-7.
10. Del Prete G. F., Tiri A., De C.M., Mariotti S., Pinchera A., Chretien I., Romagnani S. and Ricci M. (1989): Autoimmunity 4: 267-76.
11. Del Prete G.F., Tiri A., Mariotti S., Pinchera A., Ricci M. and Romagnani S. (1987): Clin. Exp. Immunol. 69: 323-31.
12. Del Prete G.F., Vercelli D., Tiri A., Maggi E., Mariotti S., Pinchera A., Ricci M. and Romagnani S. (1986): Clin. Exp. Immunol. 65: 140-7.
13. Londei M., Lamb J.R., Bottazzo G.F. and Feldmann M. (1984): Nature , 312: 639-41.
14. Mariotti S., Chiovato L., Vitti P., Marcocci C., Fenzi G.F., Del P.G., Tiri A., Romagnani S., Ricci M. and Pinchera A. (1989): Clin. Immunol. Immunopathol. 50: s73-s84.
15. Mariotti S., Del Prete G.F., Caturegli,P., Barbesino G., Marinò M., Manetti L., Chiovato L., Marcocci C., Iacconi P., Miccoli P., Romagnani S. and Pinchera A. (1993): In: 80 Years of Hashimoto Disease, edited by S. Nagataki, T. Mori, and K. Torizuka, pp 307-312. Excerpta Medica. Amsterdam.
16. Mariotti S. and Pinchera A. (1990): In: The Thyroid Gland. edited by M.A. Greer, pp 147-219. Raven Press. New York.
17. McIntosh R.S., Tandon N., Pickerill A.P., Davies R., Barnett D. and Weetman A.P. (1993): J. Immunol. 151: 3884-93.
18. McIntosh R.S., Watson P.F., Pickerill A.P., Davies R. and Weetman A.P. (1993): Clin. Exp. Immunol. 91: 147-52.
19. Navarrete C. and Bottazzo G.F. (1993): Clin. Exp. Immunol. 91: 189-92.
20. Weetman A.P. (1992): Clin. Endocrinol. (Oxf.) 36: 307-23.
21. Weetman A.P. and McGregor A.M. (1984): Endocr. Rev. 5: 309-55.

Frontiers in Endocrinology
Volume 9 - 1994

Autoantibody Epitopes in Autoimmune Thyroid Disease: Potential Clinical Importance

B. Rapoport, T. Nishikawa, G. Chazenbalk, S. Portolano and S. McLachlan

Thyroid Molecular Biology Unit, V.A. Medical Center and the University of California, San Francisco, California, 4150 Clement Street, San Francisco, CA 94121, USA

The most common organ-specific autoimmune disease in man involves the thyroid. Autoantibodies against thyroid peroxidase (TPO) are present in the sera of virtually all patients with active disease. However, many normal individuals also have TPO autoantibodies. Serum TPO autoantibodies are polyclonal. An important question, therefore, is whether or not epitopes recognized by TPO autoantibodies in patients with disease differ from the epitopes recognized by autoantibodies in euthyroid individuals. Such an association would be of diagnostic, prognostic and (potentially) of therapeutic importance.

Monoclonal antibodies are essential tools for defining B cell epitopes. However, monoclonal human autoantibodies would define epitopes on autoantingens more precisely than mouse monoclonal antibodies. We have used the heavy and light chain gene combinatorial library approach to clone the genes for a repertoire of ~40 high affinity, IgG-class human autoantibodies to TPO from thyroid-infiltrating B cells (1, 8-10). Selected genes have been expressed in bacteria to generate, as F(ab), recombinant, TPO-specific human autoantibodies. All F(ab) bind with specificity and high affinity (~10^{-10} M) to TPO, comparable to autoantibodies in patients' sera.

Competition between pairs of F(ab)s for binding to recombinant human TPO was used to define their respective binding domains. In this approach, increasing concentrations of one Fab were pre-incubated with radiolabeled TPO and then, added to a second, immobilized Fab. These competition studies, covering all permutations of immobilized and free F(ab)s, suggest that these autoantibodies recognize two closely associated domains, A and B, on TPO (1).

A number of epitopes for TPO autoantibodies have been defined previously using polyclonal autoantibodies in patients' sera. These studies all used peptide or polypeptide fragments of TPO. By definition, these epitopes are linear, i.e. they comprise a small, continuous sequence of amino acid residues. In particular, the region between TPO amino acids 590 and 767 contains a "hotspot" within which two linear epitopes have been defined; the first between amino acids 713-721 (3, 5) and the second between amino acids 590-622 (5). However, it is known that most antibodies to complex globular proteins interact with conformational epitopes (4). These epitopes are created by the apposition of different segments of the linear polypeptide chain during molecular folding. Unlike linear epitopes, recognition of conformational epitopes is destroyed by protein denaturation because of disruption of the three-dimensional structure of the antigen.

Testing of the monoclonal, human autoantibodies revealed that they interact with conformational, not linear epitopes (9, 2). Consistent with this finding, the well-defined Mab47/C21 linear epitope was found to lie outside the conformational epitopes in the A and B domains (2). The relationship between the A and B domains and the C2 linear epitope cannot be evaluated because of the absence of a specific Mab to this segment.

An important issue, that is frequently not appreciated, is the difference between the prevalence in the patient population of autoantibodies to a particular epitope and epitopic dominance of an antibody component in an individual serum containing polyclonal autoantibodies. All studies on linear epitopes have examined only the prevalence. For example, autoantibodies to the C2 epitope appear to occur in ~63% of TPO autoantibody positive sera (6). However, there is no information on what proportion of the TPO autoantibodies in a particular serum are to the linear C2 epitope. Such information cannot be obtained from a study using polyclonal serum and TPO fragments.

The availability of monoclonal human autoantibody F(ab) allowed us to perform competition studies between these F(ab) and polyclonal TPO autoantibodies, in patients' sera. In this way, it was possible to determine both the prevalence of TPO autoantibodies to the A and B domains as well as the proportion of TPO autoantibodies to these regions in individual sera. The prevalence was 100%. Even more striking, we found that the A and B domains contain the binding sites of most of the IgG-class TPO autoantibodies in the sera of patients with autoimmune thyroid disease. This conclusion is based on experiments in which we used a pool of 4 human monoclonal TPO autoantibodies (Fab SP1.4, WR1.7, TR1.8 and TR1.9) that define the immunodominant region to map the binding sites for TPO autoantibodies in the sera of 32 patients. The F(ab) pool inhibited TPO binding by 32 patients' sera by 82 ± 14% (mean ± SD), with a range from 51% to 100%. The closely associated A and B domains are, therefore, truly an epitopic dominant region on the antigen. A corollary of these data is that the majority of TPO autoantibodies in patients' sera interact with the antigen in its native, undenatured, state. It seems likely, therefore, that autoantibodies to linear epitopes comprise only a minority of TPO autoantibodies and that at least some of these linear epitopes lie outside the immunodominant region

When the monoclonal human autoantibodies to TPO were used individually to compete for binding of serum autoantibodies to radiolabeled TPO, it was possible to define an epitopic "fingerprint" of the polyclonal TPO autoantibodies present in the sera of individual patients (7). Serum autoantibodies to the TR1.8 F(ab) region were strongly represented among the autoantibodies to the immunodominant region. There was a close association between the proportions of TPO autoantibodies to the TR1.8 and TR1.9 epitopes, as well as between those to the SP1.4 and WR1.7 epitopes. These associations correspond to the previously described A and B epitopic domains in the TPO immunodominant region. No TPO epitope was seen to be associated with clinically apparent ophthalmopathy of Graves' disease, nor was there an association between TPO epitopes and patient age or sex.

As mentioned above, it is an enigma why only some individuals with TPO autoantibodies develop hypothyroidism. In an attempt to address this question, we determined the TPO epitopic fingerprint in a selected, very well controlled group of hypothyroid patients and euthyroid individuals. Because of the latency in developing hypothyroidism, the selected patients and controls were all elderly (61-70 years old). All were female, of similar genetic and environmental background and all had similar titers of TPO autoantibodies. In studies to be reported elsewhere, we did not observe a statistically significant qualitative, epitopic difference between TPO autoantibodies in elderly women who do and do not develop hypothyroidism, additional studies will be needed to clarify this issue.

It should be appreciated that an association between an epitopic fingerprint and the development of hypothyroidism would not imply that autoantibodies to a certain segment of TPO are directly responsible for induction of disease. More likely, in our opinion, is that autoantibodies to a particular domain would be markers for an underlying predisposition to the disease. As described elsewhere in this Volume, TPO autoantibodies with particular epitopic domains are coded for by a specific group of immunoglobulin genes. It is the inheritance of these genes that may be linked to the development of hypothyroidism. Future studies of TPO epitopic fingerprinting in families with autoimmune thyroid disease will be important to address this issue.

In summary, the cloning and expression of human autoantibodies, to TPO provide powerful tools to study the pathogenesis of autoimmune thyroid disease.

REFERENCES

1. Chazenbalk G.D., Portolano S., Russo D., Hutchison J.S., Rapoport B. and McLachlan S.M. (1993): J. Clin. Invest. 92: 62-74.
2. Chazenbalk G.D., Costante G., Portolano S., McLachlan S.M. and Rapoport B. (1993): J. Clin. Endocrinol. Metab. 77: 1715-1718.
3. Finke R., Seto P., Ruf J., Carayon P. and Rapoport B. (1991): J. Clin. Endocrinol. Metab. 73: 919-921.
4. Laver W.G., Air G.M., Webster R.G. and Smith-Gill S.J. (1990): Cell. 61: 553-556.
5. Libert F., Ludgate M., Dinsart C. and Vassart G. (1991): J. Clin. Endocrinol. Metab. 73: 857-860.
6. Ludgate M., Mariotti S., Libert F., Dinsart C., Piccolo P., Santini F., Ruf J., Pinchera A. and Vassart G. (1989): J. Clin. Endocrinol. Metab. 68: 1091-1096.
7. Nishikawa T., Costante G., Prummel M.F., McLachlan S.M. and Rapoport B. (1994): J. Clin. Endocrinol. Metab. 78: 944-949.
8. Portolano S., Seto P., Chazenbalk G.D., Nagayama,Y., McLachlan S. and Rapoport B (1991): Biochem Biophys. Res. Comm. 179: 372-379.
9. Portolano S., Chazenbalk G.D., Seto P., Hutchison J.S., Rapoport B. and McLachlan S.M. (1992): J. Clin. Invest. 90: 720-726.
10. Portolano S., Chazenbalk G.D., Hutchison J.S., McLachlan S.M. and Rapoport B. (1993): J. Immunol. 150: 880-887.

Frontiers in Endocrinology
Volume 9 - 1994

Pathogenetic Role of TSH-Receptor Antibodies in Autoimmune Thyroid Diseases

L. Chiovato, P. Vitti, F. Santini, G. Bendinelli, P. Lapi, E. Fiore and A. Pinchera

Institute of Endocrinology, University of Pisa, V.le del Tirreno 64, 56018 Tirrenia, Pisa, Italy

Autoantibodies to the TSH-receptor may either directly stimulate thyroid function or inhibit the biological effects of TSH (15). Thyroid stimulating antibodies (TSAb) are typically found in sera of hyperthyroid patients with Graves' disease and in a minority of those with other thyroid autoimmune disorders. TSH-receptor antibodies with blocking activity (TSH-BAb) are present in variable percentages of patients with autoimmune thyroiditis, and contribute to the development of thyroid failure.

The clinical relevance of TSH-receptor antibodies will be discussed in the following paragraphs.

THYROID STIMULATING ANTIBODIES

The pivotal observation by Adams and Purves (1) of a long-acting thyroid stimulator in sera of hyperthyroid patients with Graves' disease provided the basis for the subsequent demonstration that the stimulator was an antibody directed to the TSH-receptor (15).

Biological Activity of TSAb The biological effects of TSAb have been investigated in primary cultures of human thyroid cells and in the differentiated strain of rat thyroid cells, FRTL-5. Similar to TSH, TSAb stimulate thyroid adenylate cyclase, iodide, uptake and T3 production (15, 18). Thyroid cell growth, as assessed by 3H-thymidine incorporation, DNA accumulation, and mitotic activity in rat thyroid cells, in also stimulated by TSAb of Graves' disease (15, 18). Like TSA, TSAb produce their biological effects by increasing intracellular cAMP, the main regulator of differentiation and growth in thyroid cells (8).

The ability of TSAb to stimulate the phosphatidylinositol (PI) pathway was also investigated. While TSAb increase PI levels in non-thyroid cells transfected with the TSH-receptor cDNA (22), other studies failed to demonstrate an effect of TSAb on PI cascade in human thyroid slices (8) or a stimulation of protein kinase C in porcine thyroid cells (10). Graves' IgG can increase arachidonic acid release in FRTL-5 cells, but the latter effect could be mediated by an activation of phospholipase-A2 (7).

The question of whether these discrepancies are due to variations in the structure of TSH receptors in different species, concentrations of TSAb insufficient to stimulate the PI cascade, or insensitivity of *in vitro* assays, is a matter of future investigations. This is, however, an important point since TSH-receptor antibodies, active through the PI or other growth pathways unrelated to cAMP, could stimulate thyroid growth but not function. To explore this possibility we simultaneously evaluated the effect of Graves' IgGs on thyroid cell function (iodide uptake) and growth (3H-thymidine incorporation) in FRTL-5 cells. Most IgGs had a similar potency in the two assays and a significant positive correlation was found (18). Thus, our data strongly support the concept that TSAb can be regarded as a sufficient pathogenetic agent for thyroid enlargement of hyperfunction in Graves' disease.

Assays for TSAb Two major types of assays for TSAb are currently available (15, 17): 1) bioassays that assess the effect of TSAb on thyroid cell function, 2) radioreceptor assays that assess the inhibition of binding of radioactive TSH to its receptor (TBIAb). Radioreceptor assays use either porcine solubilized receptor or cells transfected with the recombinant human TSH-receptor (9), but are not specific for TSAb since they also detect antibodies that bind to the TSH-receptor, but do not activate adenylate cyclase. Specific *in vitro* bioassays for TSAb are based on the stimulation of cAMP production in human thyroid slices or cells, in FRTL-5 cells (15, 18), or in CHO cells transfected with the human TSH-receptor (23). The latter assay is both extremely sensitive and has the advantage of employing a species-specific receptor of TSAb.

Pathogenetic role of TSAb The crucial role of TSAb in the pathogenesis of hyperthyroidism and thyroid enlargement in Graves' disease is supported by an array of clinical observations. Using sensitive *in vitro* bioassays. TSAb can be demonstrated in sera of more than 90% of thyrotoxic patients with Graves' disease (15-18). In these patients there is a relationship between TSAb levels and thyroid radioiodine uptake, serum T3 levels, or goiter size (15, 17, 18).

The occurrence of TSAb in euthyroid patients with goiter or a family history of thyroid autoimmune disorders forecasts the development of hyperthyroidism (12). In Graves' patients treated with thionamides, there is a correlation between TSAb levels and relapse or remission of hyperthyroidism after discontinuation of therapy (15, 17, 18).

The proportion of patients with Graves' disease who relapse after initial treatment with anti-thyroid drugs ranges from over 80% to less than 50% (15, 17, 18). The measurement of TBIAb or TSAb at the end of therapy has been used to predict post-treatment outcome. The abundant literature on this topic suggests that the presence of high levels of TSAb at the end of anti-thyroid drug therapy is a good indicator of relapse (15, 17, 18). The absence of detectable antibody in the bioassay at the time of drug withdrawal, however, does not necessarily predict remission.

Neonatal thyrotoxicosis, due to the transplacental transfer of TSAb from a mother with Graves' disease, is a rare condition (15, 17). In most instances of congenital hyperthyroidism, the onset of clinical thyrotoxicosis is delayed until the neonatal period, due to ongoing therapy with thionamides in the mother.

In rare infants, the onset of clinical thyrotoxicosis may be delayed 1 to 2 months because of the coexistence of TSAb and TSH-BAb in the mother's serum (15). The rare case of a neonate with delayed and prolonged hyperthyroidism was also described in whom TSAb, TSH-BAb and an antibody enhancer of TSAb action coexisted in variable concentrations during time (15).

TSH-BLOCKING ANTIBODIES

TSH-receptor antibodies have been described in patients with autoimmune hypothyroidism that compete with TSH for its receptor and block the biological effects of thyrotropin on thyroid cells (TSHBAb) (15, 18).

Biological activity of TSH-BAb TSH-BAb inhibit the binding of thyrotropin to its receptor, and block TSH-induced cAMP production, iodide uptake, T3 secretion and thyroid cell growth (15, 18). In most cases, this blocking effect occurs at the receptor level, but an antibody producing a post-receptorial inhibition of iodide organification has been described (19).

Assays for TSH-BAb The radioreceptor assay does not discriminate between TSAb of Graves' disease and TSH-BAb. *in vitro* bioassays for blocking antibodies are based on the ability of TSH-BAb to inhibit the stimulation of adenylate cyclase induced by TSH in human or porcine thyroid cells, in FRTL-5 cells (15, 17, 18), and recently in CHO cells transfected with the human TSH receptor (CHO-R cells) (5). The sensitivity of this assay is slightly greater than that obtained in FRTL-5 cells. CHO-R cells also have the advantage of expressing the human TSH-receptor and of requiring easier culture conditions than FRTL-5 cells.

Pathogenetic role of TSH-BAb TSH-BAb are mainly found in patients with atrophic thyroiditis (AT) (idiopathic myxedema), and to a lesser extent in hypothyroid patients with goitrous Hashimoto's thyroiditis (3). In a different series of patients with AT, the prevalence of TSH-BAb ranges from 14% to nearly 80% (20). In our experience, the prevalence of TSH-BAb in AT ranges from 34% to 46%. Genetic differences in the populations studied do not completely explain these discrepancies, since both extremely low or high prevalence (20) has been reported in Japan. Differences in assays for TSH-BAb, selection of patients, inclusion of samples drawn before or after therapy with L-thyroxine may account for the wide range of positive results reported in the literature.

Several lines of evidence support the role of TSH-BAb in the development of hypothyroidism and thyroid atrophy: i) TSH-BAb are not detectable in euthryoid patients with autoimmune thyroiditis; ii) their prevalence is higher in overt hypothyroidism than in subclinical thyroid failure; iii) the prevalence and levels of TSH-BAb are greater in AT than in goitrous Hashimoto's (3).

Finally, recovery of thyroid function has been reported upon disappearance of TSH-BAb in patients with autoimmune thyroiditis (19).

TSH-BAb, on crossing the placenta, induce transient neonatal hypothyroidism (15, 17). Most cases of transient neonatal hypothyroidism due to TSH-BAb have been described in the offspring of women with euthyroid or hypothyroid Hashimoto's thyroiditis, but TSH-BAb may also occur in Graves' mothers (15). Although TSAb usually predominate in Graves' mothers, transient hypothyroidism may be possible in the neonate when TSH-BAb titers are very high and concentrations of TSAb are relatively low (15).

TSH-RECEPTOR ANTIBODIES IN NON-AUTOIMMUNE THYROID DISORDERS

Sporadic and endemic goiter Early reports indicating that TSAb could be involved in the pathogenesis of toxic nodular goiter were not confirmed by studies from our (18) and other (15) laboratories. The development of Graves' disease on a preexisting nodular goiter in iodine-deficient populations, may explain some conflicting reports.

In the last 10 years, evidence was also accumulated for the existence of a category of IgG that specifically stimulates growth of thyroid cells (TGI), but does not affect adenylate cyclase. TGI might cause simple diffuse or nodular goiter, toxic adenoma, and even endemic iodine-deficiency goiters (15, 18). While initial reports were based on intriguing cytochemical bioassays, subsequent studies were performed by 3H-thymidine incorporation or a mitotic arrest assay in FRTL-5 cells (15, 18). Using the same culture system we were unable to confirm these results. Indeed, no IgG from 37 patients with endemic goiter living in Italy or Peru produced a stimulation of 3H-thymidine incorporation in FRTL-5 cells different from that obtained with IgGs of normal nongoitrous subjects residing in endemic or nonendemic areas (13). Moreover, IgGs of patients with endemic goiter did not promote DNA accumulation in FRTL-5 cells, nor stimulate adenylate cyclase.

Thus, our data show that sera of endemic goiter patients are devoid of TGI and TSAb activities, and argue against a direct role of thyroid autoimmunity in the development of goiter in iodine-deficient areas. Similar results indicating the absence of TGI or TSAb in patients with sporadic non-toxic goiter were reported by McKenzie and Zakarija (15).

Sporadic and endemic cretinism Permanent sporadic congenital hypothyroidism (CH) is mainly due to thyroid dysgenesis, but its etiology remains obscure. Autoimmune thyroid processes have been suggested as a possible pathophysiological mechanism for CH, but conventional thyroid antibodies, such as anti-thyroperoxidase antibodies are usually absent (4, 15). However, Van Der Gaag et al. (21) reported that 44% of mothers of children with sporadic CH had thyroid growth blocking antibodies (TGBI), despite being euthyroid themselves. Fifty per cent of affected children also had TGBI. In subsequent studies, the same authors reported that 85% of athyreotic myxedematous cretins from an endemic area in China had TGBI as opposed to the negative results found in euthyroid goitrous neurologic cretins (2).

These intriguing findings have not been confirmed in other studies. In our laboratory, 84 children with sporadic CH and their mothers were examined for the presence of TSH-blocking antibodies. Autoantibodies blocking TSH-dependent adenylate cyclase or thyroid cell growth were found in only 2 neonates born to mothers with Hashimoto's thyroiditis, who were hypothyroid and had the blocking antibody in their serum.

In a subsequent study, we examined for TSH-BAb and TGBI IgGs from 18 euthyroid-neurologic and from 21 myxedematous endemic cretins living in areas of severe iodine deficiency in Italy and Peru. TGBI were assessed by measuring the effect of IgGs on TSH-stimulated 3H-thymidine incorporation and DNA accumulation in FRTL-5 cells.

In the same cell culture system, the effect of IgGs on the TSH-dependent adenylate cyclase was evaluated. None of the IgGs of myxedematous cretins without goiter produced a significant inhibition of TSH-stimulated FRTL-5 cell growth, and the results obtained did not differ from those produced by IgGs of euthryoid neurologic cretins. Negative results were also obtained in the adenylate cyclase inhibition assay (4).

Therefore, our studies do not support the view that antibodies blocking thyroid growth or function play a major role in the pathogenesis of sporadic permanent congenital hypothyroidism or endemic myxedematous cretinism.

TOWARDS A UNIFYING CONCEPT OF AUTOIMMUNE TSH-RECEPTOR DISEASES

An interesting subgroup of patients that have attracted much attention recently are those who demonstrate clinical evidence of hypothyroidism followed by overt hyperthyroidism (14). The contrasting situation, hypothyroidism following hyperthyroid Graves' disease, has also been described. In both instances, evidence was provided for the contribution of TSH-receptor antibodies with opposite biological activities in changes of thyroid function Thus, the disappearance of TSAb producing hyperthyroidism may be accompanied by the appearance of TSH-BAb and the development of hypothyroidism, or vice versa.

The occurrence of spontaneous changes of thyroid function, due to the appearance or disappearance of TSAb or TSH-BAb, the observation that TSH-BAb are present in only a minority of hypothyroid patients with AT, and the possible recovery of thyroid function upon disappearance of blocking antibodies, all suggest that in these disorders the accompanying lymphocytic destruction of the thyroid plays a minor role.

By going further in this argument we could hypothesize that there is a subgroup of thyroid autoimmune disorders in which immunity to the TSH-receptor has a preponderant role, while destructive cellular reactions are only marginally involved. These autoimmune TSH-receptor diseases could comprise most cases of Graves' disease, TSH-BAb, positive AT, and intermediate disorders characterized by changes of thyroid function conditioned by TSH-receptor antibodies with different biological activities. Support to this hypothesis comes from genetic studies.

Analysis of HLA types in Japanese patients with primary hypothyroidism revealed that TSH-BAb positive patients with AT have decreased frequency of DPw2 and are genetically similar to Graves' disease, whereas TSH-BAb negative patients with AT are characterized by high frequency of DPw2 and are genetically similar to classical goitrous Hashimoto's thyroiditis (11). A similar genetic clustering was reported in a Korean series of patients with thyroid autoimmune disorders (6).

REFERENCES

1. Adams D.D. and Purves H.D. (1956): Proc. Univ. Otago Med. Sch. 34: 11-15.
2. Boyages S.C. Halpner J.P., Maberly G.F., Eastman C.J., Chen J., Zhen-Hua W., van Der Gaag, R.D. and Drexhage H.A. (1989): Lancet 2: 529-32.
3. Chiovato L., Vitti P., Santini F., Lopez G., Mammoli C., Bassi P., Giusti L., Tonacchera M., Fenzi G.F. and Pinchera A. (1990): J. Clin. Endocrinol. Metab. 71: 40-45.
4. Chiovato L., Tonacchera M., Lapi P., Fiore E., Vitti P. and Pinchera A. (1992): Acta Med. Austr. 19: 91-95.

5. Chiovato L., Pinchera A., Ludgate M., Tonacchera M., Bendinelli G., Fiore E., Mammoli C., Capaccioli A., Lapi P. and Vitti P. (1993): J. Endocrinol. Invest. 16: 23 (abstract).
6. Cho B.Y., Chung J.H., Shong Y.K. Chang Y.B., Han H., Lee J.-B., Lee H.K. and Koh C.-S. (1993): J. Clin. Endocrinol. Metab. 77: 611-615.
7. Di Cerbo A., Di Girolamo M., Guardabasso V., De Filippis V. and Corda D. (1992): J. Clin. Endocrinol. Metab. 74: 585-592.
8. Dumont J.E., Lamy F., Roger P. and Maenhaut C. (1992): Physiol. Rev. 72: 667-697.
9. Filetti S., Foti D., Costante G. and Rapoport B. (1991): J. Clin. Endocrinol. Metab. 72: 1096-1101.
10. Ginsberg J. and Murray P.G. (1993): Clin. Endocrinol. (Oxf.) 38: 45-48.
11. Inoue D., Sato K., Sugawa H., Akamizu T., Maeda M., Inoko H., Tsuji K. and Mori T. (1993): J. Clin. Endocrinol. Metab. 77: 606-610.
12. Kasagi K., Tamai H., Morita T., Hidaka A., Hatabu H., Misaki T., Iida Y., Ishihara T., Ikekubo K., Kuma K. and Konishi J. (1989): J. Clin. Endocrinol. Metab. 68: 1189-1194.
13. Mammoli C., Tonacchera M., Giachetti M., Bendinell, G., Santin, F., Rago T., Cianciosi C., Lapi P., Fenzi G.F., Vitti P. and Chiovato L. (1991): In: Progress in Thyroid Research, edited by A. Gordono, J. Gross and G. Hennemann, pp. 663-666. A.A. Balkema. Rotterdam.
14. McGrego, A.M. (1990): Clin. Endocrinol. (Oxf) 33: 683-685.
15. McKenzie M.J. and Zakarija M. (1991): In: The Thyroid, edited by L.E. Braverman and R.D. Utiger, pp. 506-524. J.B. Lippincott Co. Philadelphia.
16. Rapoport B., Greenspan F.S., Filetti S. and Pepitone M. (1984): J. Clin. Endocrinol. Metab. 58: 332-338.
17. Rees-Smith B., McLachlan S.M. and Furmaniak J. (1988): Endocr. Rev. 9: 106-121.
18. Pinchera A., Mariotti S., Vitti P., Marcocci C., Chiovato L., Fenzi G.F. and Santini F. (1989): Biochimie 71: 237-245.
19. Takasu N., Yamada T., Takasu M., Komiya I., Nagasawa Y., Asawa T., Shinoda T., Aizawa T. and Koizumi Y. (1992): N. Engl. J. Med. 326: 513-563.
20. Tamaki H., Amino N., Kimura M., Hidaka Y., Takeoka K. and Miyai K. (1990): J. Clin Endocrinol. Metab. 71: 1382-1386.
21. Van Der Gaag R.D., Drexhage H.A. and Dussault,J.H. (1985): Lancet 2: 246-250.
22. Van Sande J., Lejeune C., Ludgate M. et al. (1992): Mol. Cell. Endocrinol. 88: R1-R5.
23. Vitti P., Elisei R., Tonacchera M., Chiovato L., Mancusi F., Rago T., Mammoli C., Ludgate M., Vassart G. and Pinchera A. (1993): J. Clin. Endocrinol. Metab. 76: 499-503.

Frontiers in Endocrinology
Volume 9 - 1994

Clinical Aspects of Autoimmune Thyroiditis

L. Chiovato, S. Filetti[1] and A. Pinchera

Institute of Endocrinology, University of Pisa; [1]Chair of Endocrinology, University of Reggio Calabria in Catanzaro, Italy

This paper is an edited summary of the *Clinical Panel* held 24 May 1994 in Rome during the XXV National Congress of the Italian Endocrine Society.

Moderators:
L. Chiovato, S. Filetti, A. Pinchera

Discussants:
M. Bagnasco (Department of Internal Medicine, University of Genoa)
P. Beck-Peccoz (Institute of Endocrine Sciences, University of Milan)
S. Benvenga (Chair of Endocrinology, University of Messina)
C. Betterle (Chair of Endocrinology, University of Padua)
G. Costante (Chair of Endocrinology, University of Reggio Calabria in Catanzaro)
A. De Bellis (Institute of Endocrinology, University of Naples)
G.F. Fenzi (Chair of Endocrinology, University of Naples)
D. Giuffrida (Chair of Endocrinology, University of Catania)
S. Mariotti (Institute of Endocrinology, University of Pisa)
E. Martino (Institute of Endocrinology, University of Pisa)
E. Roti (Chair of Endocrinology, University of Parma)
F. Vermiglio (Chair of Endocrinology, University of Messina)
P. Vitti (Institute of Endocrinology, University of Pisa)
G.A. Zampa (Division of Endocrinology and Metabolic Diseases, Ospedale Maggiore Pizzardi, Bologna).

CLINICAL PRESENTATION - EPIDEMIOLOGY

The prototype of autoimmune thyroiditis, Hashimoto's thyroiditis, is a chronic disorder of the thyroid gland that is characterized histologically by diffuse lymphocytic infiltration, and clinically by goiter, with or without hypothyroidism (27, 32). Although thyroid enlargement is generally diffuse, it can be asymmetric or nodular. The gland is usually quite firm, but occasionally rock-hard. Hashimoto's thyroiditis can present with hypothyroidism, or as euthyroid goiter, rarely with transient hyperthyroidism (Hashitoxicosis). In addition to the classical disorder, several variants have been recognized: fibrous, focal, adolescent, and atrophic (27, 32). These conditions may represent different stages of a common disorder, or more probably, distinct entities with common pathogenetic mechanisms. Most cases of silent (painless) thyroiditis and postpartum thyroiditis also recognize an autoimmune origin, but their clinical course is typically transient.

Autoimmune thyroiditis is a common clinical disorder, and its incidence appears to be increasing, even in geographic areas of iodine sufficiency (32). Autoimmune thyroiditis shows a higher prevalence in women, and is most often diagnosed between the ages of 30 and 50 years. An autopsy study in the mid 1960s showed that 2% of women had histologic features of autoimmune thyroiditis (26). A survey from Wickham, England, demonstrated positive thyroid antibodies (a hallmark of the disease) in sera of nearly 10% of unselected individuals, with 2% having hypothyroidism (10). A population study in Italy reported positive thyroid antibodies ranging from 6% in the first 3 decades of life to as high as 28% in women over 60 years of age (24). The rate of progression to overt hypothyroidism may be as high as 2% per year among patients who have both thyroid antibodies and elevated serum TSH at the time of diagnosis (10). Conversely, when untreated adult patients present with complaints of hypothyroidism, autoimmune thyroiditis is nearly always the cause.

DIAGNOSTIC TOOLS

Thyroid autoantibodies Autoimmune thyroiditis is nearly always associated with positive thyroid peroxidase antibodies (TPO-Ab) that can be detected in sera of approximately 90% or more of cases (23). Thyroglobulin antibodies (Tg-Ab) are less frequently positive, being present in up to 50% of patients.

Several techniques are presently available to measure thyroid antibodies, including passive hemagglutination (PH), immunoenzymatic (ELISA) and radioimmunological (RIA) techniques. In general, PH provides satisfactory results, but ELISA and RIA techniques are both more sensitive and specific, provided that purified autoantigens (thyroglobulin and thyroid peroxidase) are used (14, 23). With the ELISA and RIA methods the assay design is also important, since sporadic false negative results may be found in competitive assays for TPO-Ab employing monoclonal antibodies. High titers of TPO-Ab and/or Tg-Ab are observed, almost exclusively, in clinically overt thyroid autoimmune diseases, but low or undetectable serum thyroid antibody may be encountered in a minority of patients with Hashimoto's thyroiditis. On the other hand, low to medium titers of thyroid antibodies are found in a minority of apparently normal subjects or patients with nonautoimmune thyroid diseases (24). Thus, it must be stressed that, irrespective of the assay employed for the measurement of thyroid antibodies, the specificity of thyroid antibody tests will never be absolute.

Measurement of TSH-receptor antibodies, either by radioreceptor or *in vitro* bioassay (13), is not usually necessary for the diagnosis of autoimmune thyroiditis, but their presence in the serum of a pregnant woman with autoimmune thyroiditis may forecast the occurrence of transient congenital hypothyroidism in her neonate (11, 17).

Antibodies against thyroid hormones (TH-Ab) are not useful in the diagnosis of autoimmune thyroiditis, but their presence in serum may interfere with the measurement of thyroid hormones resulting in falsely high or low thyroid hormone levels, depending on the particular assay used (7). For example, in assays using the analog or the solid phase design, thyroid hormone levels will be overestimated. The prevalence of TH-Ab in the general population is around 0.04%, but these antibodies are more frequently encountered in autoimmune thyroiditis (7). TH-Ab are directed to T3 alone, T4 alone or both thyroid hormones in approximately 50%, 25%, and 25% of positive cases, respectively. Demonstration of TH-Ab requires evaluation of nonspecific binding of thyroid hormones in serum (PEG precipitation) or specific radioimmunoprecipitation with a human anti-IgG antibody. TH-Ab do not affect thyroid function, since circulating thyroid hormones are in equilibrium with their plasma transport proteins (and with TH-Ab, when present) and their biologically active moiety is the free form.

Echography An abnormal ultrasound pattern of the thyroid, characterized by a diffusely reduced echogenicity, has been found in autoimmune thyroid disorders. This observation established the role of thyroid ultrasound examination in the diagnosis of autoimmune thyroiditis. In particular, thyroid hypoechogenicity by ultrasound is associated with overt hypothyroidism or may predict the development of hypothyroidism in goitrous patients who, while having thyroid autoantibodies in serum, are still euthyroid (22).

In patients with Hashimoto's thyroiditis, submitted to thyroidectomy for tracheal decompression, it was shown that the hypoechogenic pattern is associated with a diffuse lymphocytic infiltrate disrupting the normal follicular structure. This observation explains the correlation between thyroid hypoechogenicity and the development of hypothyroidism.

Fine needle aspiration cytology (FNAC) provides an important tool in the diagnostic work-up of autoimmune thyroiditis, particularly if the patient presents with a single (or multiple) thyroid nodule (32). Cytological smears of Hashimoto's thyroiditis are rich in cells, including moderate to large numbers of lymphoid cells and thyroid follicular cells. Transformed follicular cells, referred to as Askanazy cells (Hurthle cells, oncocytes, or oxyphilc cells), follicular cells with a granular cytoplasm, giant multinucleated cells, and vacuolized follicular cells containing colloid, may be observed (20). A low epithelial to lymphoid ratio, and lymphocytic cells in various stages of differentiation are characteristic features of the disease. Cytological aspects resembling a papillary structure may also be observed. In this instance, the differential diagnosis between Hashimoto's thyroiditis and papillary thyroid cancer is mainly based on the epithelial to lymphoid ratio, since in Hashimoto's thyroiditis the number of lymphoid cells is at least five-fold greater than that of epithelial cells. In this regard, it should also be mentioned that primary thyroid lymphoma may be associated with Hashimoto's thyroiditis, and requires differentiation on clinical and cytological grounds (18).

In vitro evaluation of thyroid function Nowadays, sensitive TSH measurements provide the most accurate assessment of thyroid function (5, 6, 25). According to their sensitivity, ultrasensitive TSH assays have been subdivided into 2nd, 3rd and 4th generation methods (30). The major advantage of the more recent ultrasensitive TSH assays is their reduced (<10%) intra- and inter-assay coefficient of variation for extremely low concentrations of serum TSH (0.03-0.06 mU/L and 0.003-0.006 mU/L for 3rd and 4th generation methods, respectively). Using these sensitive assays, hyperthyroid patients with reduced or undetectable serum TSH levels can be differentiated from normal euthyroid subjects. On the other hand, the first and most sensitive indicator of thyroid deficiency is an increase in serum TSH concentrations, that may occur before any decline in serum thyroid hormone levels (subclinical hypothyroidism). Rare cases of central hyper- or hypothyroidism represent an exception to this rule. Because of this, free T4 and free T3 measurements are needed as second key tests. The specificity and sensitivity of combined measurement of TSH and free T4 is over 90% (6).

In the management of patients on L-thyroxine replacement therapy, free T4 is the best test to monitor the initial response to treatment while ultrasensitive TSH is most effective for the fine tuning of treatment toward biochemical euthyroidism. During suppressive therapy with L-thyroxine, assessment of free T3 is mandatory since high levels of this hormone invariably indicate excessive treatment (3). In the latter condition, assessment of sex hormone binding globulin, angiotensin converting enzyme, soluble IL-2 receptor, and osteocalcin has also been used to avoid overtreatment with L-thyroxine.

TREATMENT

Although autoimmune thyroiditis is an immune process, any type of immunosuppressive treatment is unwarranted in this condition. Indeed, the serious side effects of immunosuppressive agents, including corticosteroids, are not justified in a benign disease that can be safely and economically managed with L-thyroxine (32).

When hypothyroidism, either overt or subclinical, is present, chronic replacement therapy with L-thyroxine is indicated. Spontaneous recovery of thyroid function rarely occurs, and may be expected when hypothyroidism has been precipitated by an iodine overload or when TSH-blocking antibodies present in serum before starting treatment disappear in the subsequent follow-up (32). The goal of L-thyroxine replacement therapy is the return to normal of serum TSH levels. Successful L-thyroxine therapy is often accompanied by a decrease in thyroid antibody titers, mainly in patients with extremely elevated serum TSH levels before treatment (12).

The indication of suppressive L-thyroxine therapy in euthyroid patients with thyroid enlargement due to Hashimoto's thyroiditis is still debated. Although shrinkage of goiter occurs less often than in patients in whom TSH levels are elevated, suppressive L-thyroxine therapy appears a reasonable approach in areas of iodine deficiency where a background of endemic goiter may contribute to thyroid enlargement.

Surgery is only rarely necessary in huge Hashimoto's goiters producing symptoms of compression, or when an associated thyroid malignancy is suspected.

AUTOIMMUNE THYROIDITIS DURING PREGNANCY AND IN THE POSTPARTUM PERIOD

Untreated autoimmune hypothyroidism during pregnancy may adversely affect the outcome of gestation, producing a higher incidence of miscarriages, maternal complications, and congenital malformations (11). Maternal hypothyroidism also impairs the neurological development of the fetus due to reduced availability of maternal thyroxine during early gestation. Carefully monitored L-thyroxine replacement therapy is, therefore, mandatory in hypothyroid pregnant women with autoimmune thyroiditis. The physiological immunosuppression of pregnancy may favorably influence the clinical course of autoimmune thyroiditis, so that serum levels of TSH may spontaneously decrease in late pregnancy, while FT4 has a tendency to increase (11). This transient improvement does not justify discontinuation of replacement therapy, since it is followed by a rebound exacerbation of thyroid autoimmunity in the postpartum period.

TSH-receptor antibodies present in sera of patients with autoimmune thyroiditis cross the placenta. Therefore, infants born to mothers with autoimmune thyroid diseases may present with transient neonatal hypo- or more rarely hyperthyroidism, depending on whether the maternal antibody to the TSH receptor is stimulating or inhibiting in nature (17).

Postpartum thyroiditis (PPT) is a syndrome of thyroid dysfunction that occurs during the first year after parturition (28, 31). The prevalence of the syndrome varies widely between the different populations screened; the lowest prevalence being reported in Thailand (1.1%) and the highest in the United Kingdom (16.7%). This wide variability in prevalence of PPT can be attributed to environmental and genetic factors, as well as to different methods of screening. PPT is characterized by a transient thyrotoxic phase occurring 1 to 3 months postpartum, followed by a hypothyroid phase developing 3 to 6 months after delivery. Afterwards, complete recovery may occur. A thyrotoxic phase followed by hypothyroidism occurs in 26% of cases, while thyrotoxicosis alone or hypothyroidism alone occur in 38% and 36% of cases, respectively.

Thyroid dysfunction is usually followed by recovery of euthyroidism, but long-term follow-up studies have revealed that 10.3% to 29% of women presenting PPT will develop permanent hypothyroidism (28, 31). Furthermore, 64% of women with PPT will develop a functional condition characterized by impaired hormone synthesis as revealed by a positive thiocyanate discharge test, and 72% will be prone to develop iodine-induced hypothyroidism (29). PPT is, nowadays, regarded as an autoimmune thyroid disease. Lymphocytic infiltration of the gland, and circulating TPO-Ab are present in approximately 75% of patients. PPT occurs more frequently in women with a previous history of Hashimoto's thyroiditis, Graves' disease, or type I diabetes mellitus. Diagnosis may be difficult, but the disease should be suspected in women with a previous episode of PPT or other thyroid autoimmune disorders. Palpitation, fatigue, depression and goiter in the postpartum period should alert the physician. Positive TPO-Ab tests during the first trimester of pregnancy may also forecast the development of PPT since approximately 30% of pregnant women with high TPO-Ab levels will develop PPT in the post partum period. Administration of beta-blocker drugs is indicated to improve symptoms of thyrotoxicosis. L-thyroxine treatment is required during the hypothyroid phase, and should be maintained for the first year after parturition. Thereafter, an attempt should be made to withdraw replacement therapy to check whether the hypothyroidism was transient or, indeed, is permanent.

ASSOCIATED AUTOIMMUNE DISEASES

Thyroid-associated (autoimmune) ophthalmopathy In the large majority of cases (nearly 85%), thyroid-associated ophthalmopathy (TAO) occurs in patients with hyperthyroid Graves' disease. The remaining 10% of patients with TAO are euthyroid (euthyroid Graves' disease), and 5% have

Hashimoto's thyroiditis with hypothyroidism (27, 32). As in Graves' disease, an antigen shared by both the thyroid gland and the retroorbital tissue is believed to be involved in the pathogenesis of TAO in Hashimoto's thyroiditis. Recent evidence indicates that the TSH receptor is expressed in the retroorbital fat and might, therefore, function as a common target of thyroid and retroorbital autoimmunity (16). The diagnosis of TAO in patients with autoimmune thyroiditis is based on common clinical criteria, and is confirmed by examining the orbit with ultrasounds, computed tomography and/or magnetic resonance. Specific treatment does not differ from that of TAO in Graves' disease.

Autoimmune polyendocrine syndrome (APS) Patients with thyroid autoimmune disorders, and, in particular, with autoimmune thyroiditis, are prone to develop other autoimmune conditions. Four types of APS have been described so far, and of these two (type 2 and 3) are associated with thyroid autoimmunity (15, 33).

Type 2 APS (also known as Schmidt or Carpenter syndrome) is a condition characterized by the coexistence of autoimmune thyroiditis and Addison's disease. Some of these patients may also develop insulin dependent diabetes mellitus (IDDM). The syndrome predominates in young females, and is associated with DR3 and/or DR4 genotypes. In most cases, Addison's disease or IDDM appears first, and is then followed by the manifestations of autoimmune thyroiditis. Other autoimmune conditions that may be associated with Type 2 APS include: atrophic gastritis with or without pernicious anemia, hypergonadotropic hypogonadism, vitiligo, alopecia, myasthenia gravis, and hypophysitis (15, 33).

Type 3 APS is characterized by the association of thyroid autoimmune diseases with the above-mentioned autoimmune conditions except Addison's disease and hypoparathyroidism. It is more frequent than type 2 APS and prevails in middle-aged females. The syndrome can be further classified into 3 subgroups depending on the diseases associated with thyroid autoimmunity. APS type 3A includes IDDM (this condition occurs in 1-5% of patients with Graves' disease and in 3-8% of those with Hashimoto's thyroiditis); type 3B is characterized by atrophic gastritis (10-15%) or pernicious anemia (0.5-3%); type 3C involves vitiligo, alopecia, myasthenia gravis, or other organ-specific autoimmune diseases not included in the previous subgroups (2-6%). A further subgroup, type 3D, has been proposed for patients with the coexistence of thyroid autoimmune diseases and non-organ specific or intermediate autoimmune diseases (1-3%) (15, 33).

Rarely, do all the diseases involved in a given APS appear simultaneously. In general, a latency of months or years is observed from the clinical onset of the first to the last disease. However, the clinical manifestations of each autoimmune disease are preceded by the appearance of the specific antibody in the serum. Therefore, the concept of APS could be extended to those incomplete forms characterized by only one clinical disease associated with the serological evidence of other autoimmune conditions. In these cases, APS will be only potential if specific function tests are normal, or subclinical if the impairment of the endocrine function is only partial. Therefore, an incomplete type 2 APS is characterized by the association of a clinical thyroid autoimmune disease with adrenal cortex antibodies (1-2%), or of Addison's disease with circulating thyroid antibodies (30%). Incomplete type 3A APS is defined as a clinical thyroid autoimmune disease associated with the presence of pancreatic islet-cell antibodies (1-3%), or with IDDM and thyroid autoantibodies (8-18%). The association of clinical thyroid autoimmune disease with gastric parietal cell (10-30%) or intrinsic factor antibodies (1%), or the coexistence of atrophic gastritis (and/or pernicious anemia) with thyroid antibodies (10-40%) identify incomplete type 3B APS. An incomplete type 3C APS is defined as thyroid autoimmune disease having anti-ss or anti-ds DNA, anti-mitochondrial, anti-extractable nuclear antigen, anti-phospholipid or anti-IgG antibodies (5-15%). The same applies to patients with LES, rheumatoid arthritis, Sjogren syndrome, primary biliary cirrhosis or other collagen diseases and thyroid antibodies (5-15%). Since these patients with incomplete APS have a greater chance to develop the complete syndrome, they must be examined periodically to promptly diagnose and treat these conditions when are only subclinical (8, 9).

AUTOIMMUNE THYROIDITIS AND THYROID MALIGNANCY

Thyroid carcinoma An association between differentiated thyroid cancer (mainly of the papillary type) and autoimmune thyroiditis has been hypothesized already for several years (4). This assumption derived from the serological evidence of a high prevalence of Tg-Ab and/or TPO-Ab (20% to 50%) in patients with thyroid cancer, and from the histological observation that lymphocytic infiltrates were frequent (30% to 50%) in these glands. Thus, several questions were raised: 1) is autoimmune thyroiditis a risk factor for thyroid carcinoma? 2) Is the infiltrate of thyroid cancer patients similar to that of autoimmune thyroiditis, as evaluated by phenotypic and functional analysis? 3) Do autoimmune and neoplastic thyroid cells share any immunologically relevant feature? 4) Do cancer patients with thyroid antibodies and/or lymphocytic infiltrate differ from other cancer patients as far as clinical course or prognosis of the disease are concerned?

Experimental and epidemiological data published in the last 2-3 decades provide an answer to most of these questions. First of all, there is no convincing evidence for an increased prevalence of thyroid cancer in patients correctly diagnosed as having Hashimoto's thyroiditis (4, 21). In many studies reporting an association between the two diseases the diagnosis of Hashimoto's thyroiditis was based mainly on the observation of lymphocytic infiltrates (without differentiation between focal or diffuse areas of infiltration) at histology, and of circulating thyroid antibodies. A clear histological diagnosis of Hashimoto's thyroiditis was lacking. Indeed most lymphocytic infiltrates associated with thyroid cancer are focal, while a diffuse autoimmune thyroiditis pattern is unusual. Phenotypic and functional analysis of lymphocytes present in focal infiltrates around thyroid papillary cancer demonstrated major differences with respect to autoimmune thyroiditis (2). Once again this supports the view that those patients should not be considered as having Hashimoto's thyroiditis, and that the latter condition should not be considered as a precarcinomatous lesion. On the other hand, it is worth noting that thyroid epithelial cells of some differentiated thyroid cancers may express HLA Class II antigens, as commonly found in autoimmune thyroiditis (1). Despite the fact that no relationship exists between the presence of circulating thyroid antibodies and the clinical course of thyroid cancer, a more favorable outcome has been reported in patients with thyroid malignancy and diffuse thyroiditis-like infiltrates. This observation led to the hypothesis that the autoimmune reaction could have a protective role, and to the speculation that induction of thyroid autoimmunity could serve as a therapeutic tool in patients with thyroid cancer. A better knowledge of the role of immunity against thyroid cancer appears necessary to confirm this hypothesis.

Thyroid lymphoma The relative risk of developing primary non-Hodgkin lymphoma of the thyroid is nearly 67 times higher in patients with Hashimoto's thyroiditis with respect to matched controls (18). On the other hand, virtually all patients with lymphoma of the thyroid have Hashimoto's thyroiditis. Despite this increased incidence, lymphomas of the thyroid are still rare tumors. The histological pattern of primary lymphoma of the thyroid is similar to that of B-cell lymphomas of the Mucosa Associated Lymphoid Tissues (MALT) that may be found in the stomach, small intestine, salivary glands and lung (19). Both low-grade and high-grade B-cell lymphomas may occur in the thyroid gland.

REFERENCES

1. Bagnasco M., Caretto A., Olive D., Pedini B., Canonica G.W. and Betterle C. (1991): Clin. Exp. Immunol. 83: 309-313.
2. Bagnasco M., Venuti D., Paolieri F., Torre G., Ferrini S. and Canonica G.W. (1989): J. Clin. Endocrinol. Metab. 69: 832-836.
3. Bartalena L., Martino E., Pacchiarotti A., Grasso L., Aghini-Lombardi F., Buratti L., Bambini G., Breccia M. and Pinchera A. (1987): J. Clin. Endocrinol. Metab. 64: 849-855.
4. Baker J.R. and Fosso C.K. (1993): Endocr. Rev. 14: 729-746.
5. Bayer M.F. (1991): Med. Clin. North Am. 75: 1-26.
6. Beck-Peccoz P. (1991): Ligand Quarterly 10: 547-553.
7. Benvenga S., Trimarchi F. and Robbins J. (1987): J. Endocrinol. Invest. 10: 605-619.
8. Betterle C., Presotto F., Magrin L., Pedini B., Moro L., Caretto A. and Zanchetta R. (1994): Diabetologia 37: 95-103.

9. Betterle C., Scalici C., Presotto F., Pedini B., Moro L., Rigon F. and Mantero F. (1988): J. Endocrinol. 117: 467-475.
10. Bilous R.W. and Tunbridge W.M.G. (1988): Bailliere's Clin. Endocrinol. Metabol. 2: 531-540.
11. Chiovato L., Lapi P., Fiore E., Tonacchera M. and Pinchera A. (1993): J. Endocrinol. Invest. 16: 384-391.
12. Chiovato L., Marcocci C., Mariotti S., Mori A. and Pinchera A. (1986): J. Endocrinol. Invest. 9: 299-305.
13. Chiovato L., Vitti P., Santini F., Lopez G., Mammoli C., Bassi P., Giusti L., Tonacchera M., Fenzi G.F. and Pinchera A. (1990): J. Clin. Endocrinol. Metab. 71: 40-45.
14. Di Mario U., Betterle C., Dondero F., Fenzi G.F., Mariotti S. and Trimarchi F. (1994): J. Endocrinol. Invest. 17: 355-365.
15. Doniach D. and Bottazzo G.F. (1981): In: Clinical Immunology Update, edited by E.C. Franklin, pp. 95-121, Elsevier. Amsterdam.
16. Feliciello A., Porcellini A., Ciullo I., Bonavolonta G., Avvedimento E.V. and Fenzi G.F. (1993): Lancet 342: 337-338.
17. Filetti S., Costante G., Foti D. and Sava L. (1993): In: Thyroid Disease. Clinical Fundamentals and Therapy, edited by F. Monaco, M.A. Satta, B. Shapiro and L. Troncone, pp. 507-516, CRC Press. Boca Raton.
18. Holm L.-E., Blomgren H. and Lowhagen T. (1985): N. Engl. J. Med. 312: 601-604.
19. Hyjek E. and Isaacson P.G. (1988): Hum. Pathol. 19: 1315-1320.
20. Jayram G., Marwaha K.R., Gupta R.K. and Sharma, S.K. (1987): Acta Cytol. 31: 687-693.
21. Marceri D.R., Sullivan M.J. and McClatchney K.D. (1986): Laryngoscope 96: 82-86.
22. Marcocci C., Vitti P., Cetani F., Catalano F., Concetti R. and Pinchera A. (1991): J. Clin. Endocrinol. Metab. 72: 209-213.
23. Mariotti S., Caturegli P., Piccolo P., Barbesino G. and Pinchera A. (1990): J. Clin. Endocrinol. Metab. 71: 661-669.
24. Mariotti S., Sansoni P., Barbesino G., Caturegli P., Momti D., Cossarizza A., Giacomelli T., Passeri G., Fagiolo U. and Pinchera A. (1992): Lancet 339: 1506-1508.
25. Martino E., Bambini G., Bartalena L., Mammoli C., Aghini-Lombardi F., Baschieri L. and Pinchera A. (1986): Clin. Endocrinol. 24: 141-148.
26. Masi A.T. (1965): J. Chronic Dis. 18: 35-57.
27. Pinchera A., Fenzi G.F., Bartalena L., Chiovato L. and Marcocci C. (1980): In: The Thyroid Gland, edited by M. De Visscher, pp. 413-439. Raven Press. New York.
28. Roti E. and Emerson C.H. (1992): J. Clin. Endocrinol. Metab. 74: 3-5.
29. Roti E., Minelli R., Gardini E., Bianconi L., Neri T.M., Gavaruzzi G., Ugolotti G., Salso D. and Braverman L.E. (1991): J. Clin. Endocrinol. Metab. 73: 958-963.
30. Spenser C.A., Schwarzbein D., Guttler R.B., LoPresti J.S. and Nicoloff J.T. (1993): J. Clin. Endocrinol. Metab. 76: 494-498.
31. Stagnaro-Green A. (1993): Thyroid Today 16: 1-9.
32. Volpè R. (1991): In: The Thyroid, edited by Braverman L.E. and Utiger R.D., pp. 921-933. Lippincott Co. Philadelphia.
33. Weetman A.P., editor (1991): Autoimmune Endocrine Disease. Cambridge University Press. Cambridge.

NEUROENDOCRINOLOGY - HYPOPHYSIS

SOCIETA'
ITALIANA
DI ENDOCRINOLOGIA

Frontiers in Endocrinology
Volume 9 - 1994

Tianeptine, an Antiserotoninergic Drug, increases GHRH Release into the Hypophysial Portal Blood of the Sheep

M. Cataldi[1,2], E. Magnan[1], V. Guillaume[1], F. Héry[1], A. Dutour[1], M.-C. Rettori[3], A. Kamoun[3], F. Orio[2], G. Lombardi[2] and C. Oliver[1]

[1]Laboratoire de Neuroendocrinologie Experimentale, INSERM U297, Institut Federatif Jean Roche, Faculté de Medecine Nord, Bd Pierre Dramard, 13396 Marseille, France; [2]Chair of Endocrinology, II[a] Facoltà di Medicina, University Federico II°, Via Sergio Pansini 5, 80131 Naples, Italy; [3]Institut de Recherches Internationales Servier, 6 Places des Pléiades, Curbevoie, France

INTRODUCTION

The effect of serotoninergic neural pathways on GH secretion shows a great interspecies variability. Even though the reports on this subject are confusing, serotonin (5HT), its precursors and 5HT-releasing drugs and/or agonists are believed to induce GH release in the rat and to inhibit the secretion of this hormone in the dog and in the chicken (5). The icv injection of 5HT in the sheep induces a brisk reduction in GH concentration in peripheral plasma and this effect is not abolished by the concomitant icv injection of anti-somatostatin serum (6).

To clarify the effect of 5HT on GH secretion in the sheep and to establish the mechanism of the non-SRIH dependent GH inhibition reported by Spencer, we studied the modification in GHRH and SRIH release into hypophysial portal blood (HPB) induced by the "antiserotoninergic" drug Tianeptine in sheep bearing perihypophysial twin cannulae.

Tianeptine is a newly developed antidepressive drug. It was chosen because of its unique pharmacological properties. Indeed, studies using ^{3}H-5HT showed that this drug increases 5HT uptake in rat synaptosomes (4). So, Tianeptine acutely induces a brisk decrease in 5HT concentration in the synaptic cleft and the administration of this drug can be used as a tool to generally inhibit endogenous "tonic" serotoninergic neurotransmission.

MATERIAL AND METHODS

Seven Merinos rams (9-11 months old, weighing 35-45 kg) were prepared for HPB collection as previously described (2). Briefly, the animals were deeply anesthetized and a tunnel was drilled into the sphenoidal bone as far as the pituitary stalk. A twin cannula was embedded in this tunnel using dental rubber. Ten days after, lesions were created in some long portal vessels by pushing a stainless needle into the lower cannula and HPB collection was started. HPB was collected in discrete fractions of 15 min. At the end of each fraction, a

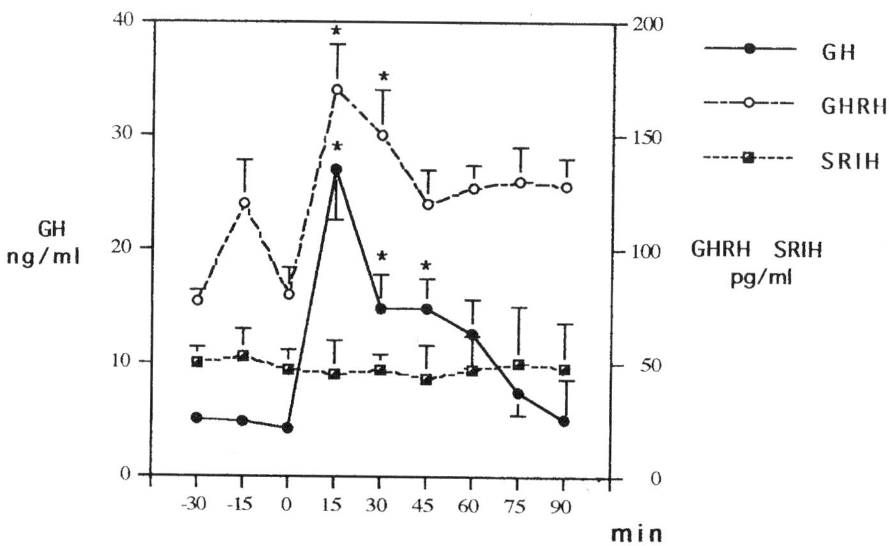

FIG. 1. Tianeptine: iv injection. Effect on GH portal GHRH and somatostatin levels.

sample of peripheral blood was collected from a jugular catheter. After 5 hours of baseline collection, Tianeptine was injected as an iv bolus at the dose of 10 mg/kg. GH was assayed in peripheral blood by RIA using the reagents kindly provided by Dr. Parlow (NIADDK). oGHRH and SRIH-1-14 were assayed in portal plasma after HCl-Acetone extraction, using RIA method as described elsewhere (3).

RESULTS

Tianeptine administration induced marked behavioral changes. The animals actively ruminated and tried to gnaw the catheters. Then, they appeared deeply sedated. GH concentrations rapidly increased after the injection and 15 min after the bolus were 7.5-fold higher than basal levels. In portal blood, GHRH concentrations rose 1.8-fold over the baseline while SRIH levels were unchanged.

DISCUSSION AND CONCLUSIONS

As the acute inhibition of the serotoninergic system in sheep brain is followed by GHRH release, these results suggest that serotoninergic pathways tonically inhibit GHRH secretion into the HPB. We (3) and others (8) have reported that the immunoneutralization of SRIH fails to increase basal GH concentration and to affect spontaneous GH secretion in the sheep. Similarly, in our hands, it is extremely difficult to detect pharmacologically induced changes in SRIH concentrations into the HPB. Up to now, the only stimulus able to induce an increase in portal SRIH concentration in our sheep is exogenous GHRH (1).

Therefore, a great problem, waiting for a solution, is the role effectively played by SRIH in ovine GH neuroregulation. Similarly, it is to be established how GH release in the interpeak periods can be inhibited if the SRIH dogma is not verified in this animal. The data reported here possibly suggest that GHRH neurons are tonically inhibited by serotoninergic neurons: a non SRIH-dependent mechanism to keep GH secretion low.

The chemical neuroanatomy of sheep brain is only partially known, so the pathways involved in the serotoninergic control of GHRH neurons remain to be defined. Tillet (7) showed that the hypothalamus is innervated by the ventral serotoninergic bundle originating from the serotoninergic nucleus B7 in periacqueductal gray. These fibers reach the arcuate nucleus and many of them terminate in the external layer of median eminence.

On the other hand, the effect on GHRH neurons could be indirect, being mediated by other neurotransmitters. Indeed, 5HT inhibits both dopamine and acetylcholine neurons while tianeptine has the opposite effect. Acetylcholine stimulates GH release in the sheep and we have demonstrated that this effect is dependent upon GHRH secretion (2).

In conclusion, we report some evidence that GHRH neurons in the sheep are tonically inhibited by a serotoninergic mechanism. Possibly, this mechanism represents a non-SRIH dependent way to keep the concentrations of GH low during the interpeak periods of spontaneous GH secretion.

REFERENCES

1. Cataldi M., Magnan E., Guillaume V., Mazzocchi L., Dutour A., Conte-Devolx B. and Oliver C. Endocr. J. (in press).
2. Magnan E., Cataldi M., Guillaume V., Mazzocchi L., Dutour A., Conte-Devolx B. and Oliver C. (1993): Endocrinology 132: 1247.
3. Magnan E., Mazzocchi L., Cataldi M., Guillaume V., Dutour A., Dadoun F., Le Bouc Y., Sauze N., Renard M., Conte-Devolx B. and Oliver C. (submitted to J. Endocr.).
4. Mennini T., Mocaer E. and Garattini S. (1987): Naunyn-Schmiedeberg Arch. Pharmacol. 336: 478.
5. Müller E.E. (1987): Physiol. Rev. 67: 962.
6. Spencer G.S.G., Dobbie P. and Bass J.J. (1991): Domest. Anim. Endocr. 8: 383.
7. Tillet Y. (1987): Neuroscience 23: 501.
8. Van Kessel A.G. and Laarveld B. (1993): J. Endocr. 136: 261.

Frontiers in Endocrinology
Volume 9 - 1994

Endothelin Expression in Pituitary Adenomas

U. Pagotto[1,3], M. Lange[1,2], U. Hopfner[1], C.J. Newton[1], J. Sauer[1], U. Renner[1] and G.K. Stalla[1]

[1]*Max-Planck-Institut of Psychiatry, Clinical Institute, 80804 Munich, Germany;* [2]*Department of Neurosurgery, Städt. Klinikum, 68167 Mannheim, Germany;* [3]*Division of Endocrinology, University of Padova, 35128 Padova, Italy*

INTRODUCTION

Endothelins (ET-1, ET-2 and ET-3), a family of potent vasoconstrictor peptides synthesized by the endothelium, have a variety of biological actions, including mitogenic effects (see Review 1).

ET-1 stimulates proliferation of vascular cells, fibroblasts and mesangial cells, moreover several cancer cell lines express ET-1 suggesting its potential role as a growth factor (7). Futhermore ETs are important regulators of function and growth in many endocrine tissues including pituitary. ET-3 appears to be highly expressed in both rat (4) and human (8) pituitary. Both ET-1 and ET-3 have been shown to influence pituitary hormone secretion (3).

The relevant role in pituitary and the potential involvement of ETs in tumor pathogenesis prompted us to examine the expression of ETs in pituitary adenomas in comparison to human normal anterior pituitary by using immunohistochemical techniques and the polymerase chain reaction on reverse transcribed RNA (RT-PCR).

MATERIAL AND METHODS

13 normal human anterior pituitary and 58 pituitary adenomas (33 non-functioning, 16 somatotrophic, 5 corticotrophic and 4 lactotrophic adenomas)

were examined. ET-1 and ET-3 rabbit polyclonal antisera (1:800-1:3000) were from Peninsula Inc. (Heidelberg, Germany), rabbit anti-human ACTH (1:500), PRL (1:400), TSH (1:800) antibodies were from Dako Inc. (Hamburg, Germany) and FSH (1:800), LH (1:1000), GH (1:1000) rabbit antisera were a generous gift from Dr. Raiti (N.H.P.P., Baltimore, Maryland, USA).

Immunohistochemical staining using anti-ET or anti-pituitary hormone serum was carried out in deparaffined and rehydrated tissue sections (5 μm), after preincubation with swine serum. Then biotinylated swine anti-rabbit serum was used(1:300, Dako), followed by avidin-biotinylated horseradish peroxidase. 3,3-diamino-benzidine-tetrahydrochloride was then added, followed by haemalaun counterstaining.

For the characterization of pituitary cells expressing ETs, a double-staining method (6) was used (Figs. 1, 2). For RT-PCR 1 μg of total RNA was isolated from 4 of the 13 normal pituitaries and 28 of the 58 pituitary adenomas, reverse transcribed and subjected to 45-cycle PCR amplification (1 min at 94 C, 1 min at 60 C for ET-1 and 50 C for ET-3, and finally 1 min at 72 C) using previously described ET-1 and ET-3 primers (2, 5). Amplified products were electrophoresed and stained with ethidium bromide. Both 5' primers covered splice junctions, thus excluding amplification of genomic DNA.

RESULTS

In normal anterior pituitaries immunoreactive ET-1 could not be detected, whereas ET-3 was found in 4/13 cases (31%). Nearly 50% of pituitary adenomas (28/58, 48%) contain immunoreactive ET-1, whereas only 18/58 (31%) of the tumor tissue displays ET-3 immunoreactivity. In all normal and pathological pituitaries showing positivity for ET-3 and ET-1 staining, a co-expression of ETs with all anterior pituitary hormones tested could be observed. In all five corticotrophic adenomas, a consistently expressed positive double staining for ACTH and ET-1 was found. By RT-PCR we examined ET-1 expression in 2 normal pituitaries (negative at immunohistochemistry) and 21 pituitary adenomas (16 positive for ET-1 at immunohistochemistry and 5 negative). ET-1 mRNA expression was observed in 2 normal pituitaries, in all 16 pituitary adenomas positive at immunohistochemistry and in 2 adenomas negative at immunostaining (Fig. 3A). 3 tumors negative after staining were also negative after RT-PCR examination. A similar comparison was made for ET-3 in 2 normal pituitaries and in 7 pituitary adenomas positive at immunohistochemistry. ET-3 mRNA expression was detected in all tissues studied (Fig. 3B).

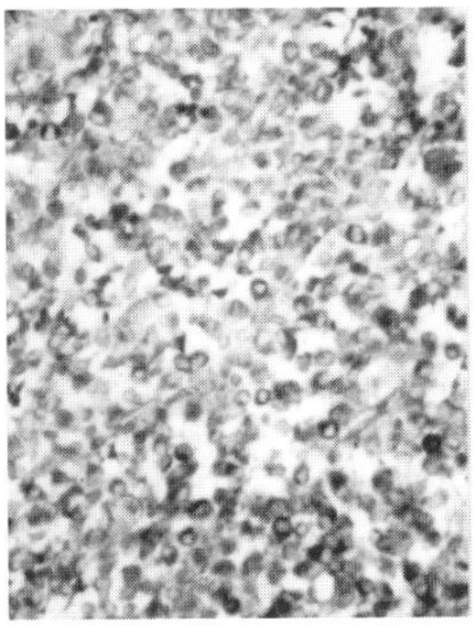

FIG. 1.

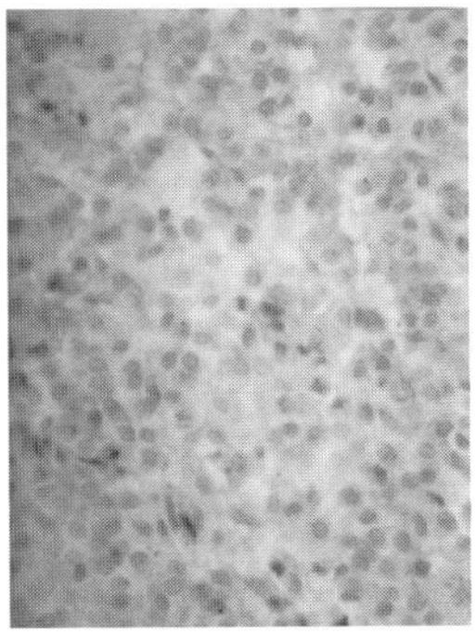

FIG. 2.

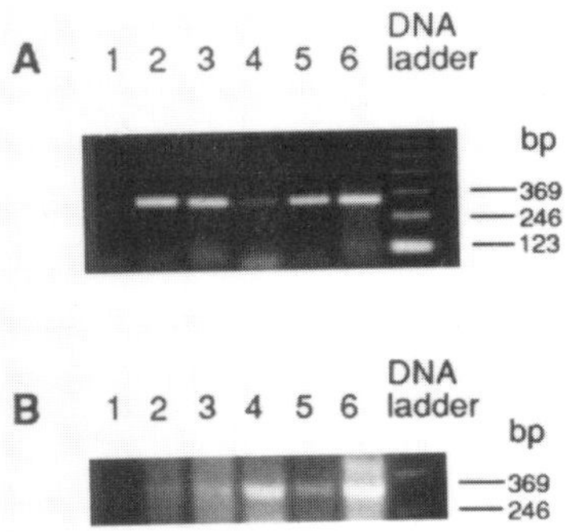

FIG. 3.

FIG.1. Section from corticotrophic adenoma. ET-1 staining (1:1600). Multiple dark stained ET-1 positive cells could be found.
FIG. 2. Same specimen as in Fig. 1. Before application of the ET-1 antibody to the section, immunoneutralization with synthetic ET-1 was performed. No ir-ET-1 staining cells are visible.
FIG. 3. ET-1 mRNA (A) and ET-3 mRNA (B) detected by RT-PCR in normal pituitaries and pituitary adenomas. PCR-cDNA gels show PCR products of 304 bp (ET-1) and 340 bp (ET-3), Lane 1: negative control (absence of specific primers), lane 2: somatotrophic adenoma, lane 3: corticotrophic adenoma, lane 4: non-functioning adenoma, lane 5: normal pituitary, lane 6: human lung (positive control)

DISCUSSION AND CONCLUSIONS

We demonstrate, for the first time, the presence of cytoplasmic immunoreactive ET-1 and ET-3 in hormone-producing cells of human pituitary adenomas, whereas, in normal human anterior pituitary, we were only able to detect immunoreactivity for ET-3. When tested, also the mRNA expression for the peptides was found. The finding of gene expression rules out the possibility that the peptides are derived from the circulation and trapped in tumor tissue. The biological significance of the peculiar ET-1 immunoreactivity in pituitary adenomas remains unclear. ET-1 is the isoform, among the family of endothelins, with the most pronounced mitogenic effects (1). The lack of immunoreactivity for ET-1 in the normal pituitary in comparison to adenoma might indicate that this endothelin plays a role in the pathogenesis of these tumors. Interestingly, we observed a high incidence of ET-1 expression in the corticotrophic cells from Cushing adenomas, this may point to a functional interaction between corticotrophic hormone and ET-1. Takahashi et al. (9) showed that ectopic ACTH secreting bronchial carcinoid tumors secrete ET-1, although the mechanisms of this interaction remains to be elucidated, it may be of relevance in agreement with our findings. As mentioned above, in normal human pituitaries only immunoreactivity for ET-3 was found; on the contrary, in the same normal tissues, using RT-PCR we could show the presence of both and ET-3 mRNA. The greater sensitivity of the PCR method in comparison to the immunohistochemical technique could explain this discrepancy. Our findings support the concept, already demonstrated by other groups (4, 8), that, among the endothelins, ET-3 is the predominant form in normal pituitary, and ET-1 is expressed at too low a level to be detected by immunological techniques.

In conclusion, our data demonstrate that, in contrast to normal human pituitaries that lack ET-1 immunoreactivity, pituitary adenomas display immunoreactivity for this peptide. In addition we have documented the intratumoral presence of mRNA for ET-1, indicating that this peptide is synthesized within the tumor and it is not acting like a circulating hormone. These data suggest that ET-1 is a unique marker of pituitary adenomas, but its potential autocrine/paracrine influence on secretion and on growth still remains unclear and requires further investigations.

REFERENCES

1. Battistini B., Chaille, P., D'Orleans-Juste P., Briere N. and Siroi, P. (1993): Peptides 14: 385-399.
2. Ehrenreich H., Rieckmann P., Sinowatz F., Weih K.A., Arthur L.O., Goebel F.D., Burd P.R., Coligan J.E. and Clouse K.A. (1993): J. Immunol. 150: 4601-4609.
3. Kanyicska B. and Freeman M.E. (1993): Am. J. Physiol. 265: E601-E608.
4. Matsumoto H., Suzuki N., Onda H. and Fujino M. (1989): Biochem. Biophys. Res. Commun. 164: 74-80.
5. McMahon L.P., Redman C.W.G. and Firth J.D. (1993): Clin. Sci. 85: 417-424.
6. Naruse M., Naruse K., Nishikawa T., Yoshihara I., Ohsumi K., Suzuki N., Demura R. and Demura H. (1992): J. Clin. Endocrinol. Metab. 74: 968-972.
7. Shichiri M., Hirata Y., Nakajima T., Ando K., Imai T., Yanagisawa M., Masaki T. and Marumo F. (1991): J. Clin. Invest. 87: 1867-1871.
8. Takahashi K., Ghatei M.A., Jones P.M., Murph, J.K., Lam H.-C., O'Halloran D.J. and Bloom S.R. (1991): J. Clin. Endocrinol. Metab. 72: 693-699.
9. Takahashi K., Satoh F., Murakami O., Totsune K., Sone M., Itoi K., Ohneda M. and Mouri T. (1993): J. Cardiovasc. Pharmac. 22 (Suppl. 8): S288-S290.

Frontiers in Endocrinology
Volume 9 - 1994

Serum Levels of Beta Subunit of Chorionic Gonadotropin as Tumoral Marker in Pituitary Tumors

P. Gil-del-Alamo, K. Saccomanno and A. Spada

Institute of Endocrine Sciences, University of Milan, Ospedale Maggiore IRCCS, Via Francesco Sforza 35, 20122 Milan, Italy

INTRODUCTION

Chorionic Gonadotropin (CG) is a glycoprotein hormone produced in high concentrations by the placenta, trophoblastic and nontrophoblastic tumors (2, 8, 9)

Previous studies have demonstrated that human pituitary gland produces not only the classical glycoproteins, i.e., TSH, LH and FSH, but also CG (4, 11, 14). More recently, it has been demonstrated that small amounts of CG are present in blood and urine of nonpregnant eugonadal women, and men. The pituitary origin of the CG present in the blood of these subjects is strongly suggested by the observation that CG is secreted in a pulsatile manner during the follicular and luteal phase of the human menstrual cycle, stimulated by GnRH and suppressed by GnRH-agonist treatment (3, 5, 6, 10, 11, 13). Several studies carried out using *in situ* hybridization in different types of human pituitary tumors, in particular GH- and PRL-secreting adenomas, have demonstrated that they frequently express the β-subunit of CG (CGβ) (1, 7, 15). Moreover, we have recently demonstrated by immunohistochemical analysis that the majority of nonfunctioning pituitary adenomas (NFPA) possess a significant number of cells positive for CGβ (12).

The aim of the present study was to evaluate circulating serum basal levels of CGβ in a large series of patients with different types of pituitary tumors with a new immunometric assay using two highly specific monoclonal antibodies against CGβ. Moreover, the possible presence of abnormal CGβ responses to TRH has been evaluated.

MATERIAL AND METHODS

Subjects The study includes 77 patients (43 women and 34 men, age 27 - 75 years) with nonfunctioning pituitary adenoma (NFPA), 22 patients with PRL-secreting macroadenoma (17 women and 5 men, age 21 - 55 years), 20 with GH-secreting adenoma (12 women and 8 men, age 27 - 65 years) and 24 healthy subjects (17 women and 7 men, age 24 - 66 years).

For the evaluation of CGß, CG, LH, FSH and α-SU levels in basal conditions samples were collected after an overnight fast. Normally menstruating women were studied during the early follicular phase. Levels of CGß after the injection of TRH were evaluated in 16 patients with NFPA (5 women and 11 men) and 3 with PRL-oma (2 women and 1 man) blood was sampled 30 minutes and immediately before TRH injection (200 μg) and 20, 30 and 60 minutes after.

Assays CGß was measured with a new one-step immunometric assay. Microtitration strip wells were coated with monoclonal antibodies specific for the CGβ. Samarium (Sm) chelates were used as reporter molecules for another set of specific monoclonals for CGβ with a Delfia® type dissociative enhancement of the fluorescence. Combining two highly specific monoclonal antibodies against CGß enabled the design of a one-step assay procedure whose cross-reactivity with complete CG is very low (<0.01%). Both monoclonal antibodies for CGß were direct against epitopes present only on the free subunit and not on the intact CG dimer. The detection limit for CGß was 0.04 U/L. Within-assay reproducibility over the whole standard ranges were less than or equal to 5%. Twenty five microliters of serum were incubated for 90 minutes at room temperature under continuous mixing with 100 ng of Sm-labelled monoclonal antibodies in 100 μL Delfia Assay Buffer.

CG was measured by a two-site fluoroimmunometric assay, with minor modifications, in which two monoclonal antibodies are directed against two separate antigenic determinants on the CG molecule (Delfia). The detection limit was less than 0.1 U/L defined as the value which is 2 standard deviations above the mean of the "0" Standard measurement values.

Statistical analysis The results are expressed as the means ± SD. Unpaired two-tailed Student t-test was used to detect the significance of the differences between two means. $p<0.05$ was accepted as statistically significant.

RESULTS AND DISCUSSION

The CGβ was undetectable in all patients except 7 NFPA (mean ± SD 0.3 ± 0.3 U/L) and 4 PRL-omas (0.09 ± 0.06 U/L). These data indicate that although the majority of nonfunctioning pituitary adenomas are immunopositive for CGβ this subunit is present in the circulation in a low number of patients, in particular in 10% of NFPA and in 17% of PRL-omas. The discrepancy between the presence of glycoprotein molecules frequently detected in nonfunctioning pituitary adenomas by morphological immunotechnique and the low circulating levels of these hormones is probably the rule in NFPA. In fact, positivity for FSH and/or LH β subunits is frequently observed in NFPA despite the fact that levels of these glycoproteins in the circulation are generally in the normal/low range. In none of the subjects with CGβ hypersecretion was an abnormal response to TRH observed. Conversely, in 2 (1 woman and 1 man) out of 11 patients with NFPA showing undetectable levels of CGβ in basal conditions, TRH caused an abnormal response (% net increase >100%). Therefore, the abnormal CGβ response to TRH was found to be a marker of the disease in a very limited number of patients. However, since in these patients neither elevated levels of subunits nor abnormal responses of FSH and/or LH to TRH were present, this test may represent an additional marker of NFPA.

Serum CG, measured in patients with detectable CGβ levels, was found to be in the normal range. Similarly, no abnormal CG response to TRH was observed in patients responsive and unresponsive to TRH with CGβ. These data suggest an unbalanced secretion of CG subunits from NFPA, as already demonstrated for other glycoproteins. The possible discrepancy between α-SU and CGβ secretion was evaluated after TRH stimulation in patients with NFPA. In fact, after stimuli, neither the simultaneous increase of the two subunits, not accompanied by the rise of the intact CG molecule, nor the dissociated response of the β or α subunits, were observed. Therefore, it is tempting to speculate that posttranslational abnormalities, such as alterations in the glycosylation process and/or in the amounts of available α-subunit molecules, may prevent the assembly of the two subunits to form the complete hormone in NFPA.

REFERENCES

1. Baz E., Saeger W., Uhlig H., Fehr S. and Ludecke D.K. (1991): Virchows Archiv. A. Pathol. Anat. 418: 405-410.
2. Beck J.S., Porteous B.G. and Ullyot J.L. (1970): J. Pathol. 101: 59-62.
3. Borkowski A. and Muquardt C. (1982): New Engl. J. Med. 30: 298-302.
4. Braunstein G.D., Kamdar V., Rasor J., Swaminathan N. and Wade M.E. (1979): J. Clin. Endocrinol. Metab. 49: 917-925.
5. Griffin J. and Odell W.D. (1987): J. Immunol. Method. 103: 275-278.
6. Hammond E., Griffin J. and Odell W.D. (1991): J. Clin. Endocrinol. Metab. 72: 747-754.
7. Jameson J.L., Lindell C.M., Husu D.W., Habener J.F. and Ridgway E.C. (1986): J. Clin. Endocrinol. Metab. 62: 1271-1278.
8. Mc Manus L.M., Naughton M.A. and Martinez-Hernandez A. (1976): Cancer. Res. 36: 3476-3481.
9. Odell W.D, Hertz R., Lipsett M.B., Ross G.T. and Hammond C.B. (1967): Clin. Obstet. Gynecol. 10: 290-302.

10. Odell W.D. and Griffin J. (1987): New. Engl. J. Med. 31: 1688-1691.
11. Odell W.D. and Griffin J. (1989): J. Clin. Endocrinol. Metab. 69: 528-532.
12. Saccomanno K., Spada A., Bassetti M., Gil-del-Alamo P. and Faglia G. (1994): J. Clin. Endocrinol. Metab. 78: 1103-1107.
13. Stenman U-H., Alfthan H., Ranta T., Vartiainen E., Jalkanen J. and Seppala M. (1987): J. Clin. Endocrinol. Metab. 64: 730-736.
14. Suginami H. and Kawaoi A. (1982): J. Clin. Endocrinol. Metab. 55: 1161-1166.
15. Uhlig H., Saege, W., Fehr S. and Ludecke D.K. (1991): Virchows Archiv. A Pathol. Anat. 418: 539-546.

Frontiers in Endocrinology
Volume 9 - 1994

24-Hour Melatonin Secretion in Acromegaly

A.A. Sinisi, A. D'Apuzzo, D. Pasquali, C. Scurini, I. Ventre, T. Venditto and A. Bellastella

Chair of Endocrinology, Facoltà di Medicina, II University of Naples, Via Pansini 5, 80131 Naples, Italy

INTRODUCTION

Findings in animals and in humans suggest a possible involvement of melatonin (MT) in GH secretion neuroregulation; but the physiological importance of the pineal gland remains controversial. In healthy young individuals no relationship has been found between endogenous nocturnal MT and GH levels (7, 14). In elderly men, MT and GH serum levels decrease, even if 24-hour profiles decline differently, MT decreasing during the nighttime only and GH both in day and nighttime (16). Data on MT levels in states of altered GH secretion are inconsistent in the literature. Idiopathic GH deficiency has been associated with the absence of MT circadian rhythm (2). There are two reports of a persistence of MT rhythm in acromegalic patients (15, 18). Another study on 8 patients with acromegaly indicates a significant increase of MT secretion during the daytime period with blunted day-night oscillations (6).

To further clarify the circadian secretion of MT in acromegaly, we investigated the MT 24-hour concentrations before and after acute somatostatin (octreotide, OCT) administration in acromegalic patients.

MATERIAL AND METHODS

Studies were carried out on seven subjects (4 M, 3 F; 24-52 years old) with active acromegaly due to pituitary adenoma, diagnosed by clinical and hormonal findings and magnetic resonance imaging. Blood samples were drawn every 2 hours over a 48-h span. After 24-h basal blood collection, OCT (Sandostatin, Sandoz) 100 μg s.c./8 was administered. As controls, 5 healthy subjects (3 M, 2 F; 26-47 years old) were studied in basal conditions over a 24-h span. Plasma MT levels were measured after ethyl-ether extraction by RIA (Nichols Institute, Wijchen, The Netherlands).

RESULTS

Plasma MT 24-h mean and absolute nocturnal MT peaks were reduced in acromegalics ($p<0.006$ and 0.001, respectively, vs controls, by ANOVA) (Table 1). Acute OCT administration restored 24-hour mean concentration but slightly increased nocturnal peak, which was still lower than in controls ($p<0.001$). Moreover, nocturnal peaks appeared earlier in acromegalics both before and after OCT (20.00-02.00 h vs 24.00-04.00 in controls).

Table 1. *MT 24-hour concentration and nighttime peak*

	24-hour mean M±SE pmol/l	nighttime peak M±SE pmol/l
Acromegalics	117.8±6.9*a,b	207.7±19.4**a
OCT treated	153.5±6.4	254.1±16.7**a
Controls	146.2±8.2	341.8±20.2

p: *<0.006, **<0.001; a vs controls; b vs OCT treated by ANOVA.

DISCUSSION

These data indicate a reduction of basal MT circadian secretion in GH-secreting adenoma, suggesting a possible inverse relationship between pituitary GH and pineal MT secretions. The increase of plasma MT concentrations after OCT could be mediated by inhibition of GH release or due to the direct stimulating effect of OCT on pineal secretion. Data on the possible influence of somatostatin on MT secretion are lacking. Several findings *in vitro* and *in vivo* suggest a possible relationship between somatostatinergic tone, GH and MT secretions. MT *in vitro* induces a release of somatostatin by rat hypothalamic fragments (9) whereas MT does not have any effect on GH release inhibition by somatostatin in rat pituitary cells (5). MT administration at high doses in man seems to play a stimulatory role on basal GH levels and on GH response to GH-RH (10, 12, 13), whereas it seems to inhibit the GH response to hypoglycemia and L-tryptophan (11, 3). Instead, exogenous MT administration at low doses seems to decrease GH levels (11) or has no effect (17). Pretreatment of MT plus pyridostigmine increases GH response to GH-

RH as well as MT or pyridostigmine alone, suggesting an action of both drugs on somatostatinergic pathway at the same level (13). Impaired MT secretion in our acromegalics after acute somatostatin administration seems to further support a possible involvement of somatostatinergic tone on pineal function.

REFERENCES

1. Dieguez C., Page M.D. and Scanlon M.F. (1988): Clin Endocrin. 28: 109-143.
2. Grugni D., Maestroni G.J.M., Lissoni P., Barbaglia M., Moreni G., Mazzilli G. and Morabito F. (1990): J. Endocrinol. Invest. 13 (suppl.3): 34.
3. Koulu M. and Lammintausta R. (1977): J. Clin. Endocrinol. Metab. 45 (4): 768-74.
4. Lissoni P., Resentini M., Mauri R., De Medici C., Morabito F., Esposti D., Di Bella L., Esposti G., Rossi D., Parravicini L., Legname G. and Fraschini F. (1986): Acta Endocrinol. 113: 12-16.
5. Martin J.E. and Sattler C. (1982): Neuroendocrinol. 34 (2): 112-116.
6. Piovesan A., Terzolo M., Borretta G., Torta M., Buniva T., Osella G., Paccotti P. and Angeli A. (1990): Chronobiol. Int. 7 (3): 259-261.
7. Rao M.L. and Mager T. (1987): Psychoneuroendocrinol. 12: 141-147.
8. Reiter R.J. (1989): In: Endocrinology, edited by Leslie J. De Groot, pp. 240-253, W.B. Saunders Company. Philadelphia.
9. Richardson S.B., Hollander C.S., D'Eletto R., Geerleaf P.W. and Thaw C. (1980): Endocrinology 107: 122-129.
10. Smythe G. and Lazarus L. (1974a): Nature 184: 230-231.
11. Smythe G. and Lazarus L. (1974b): J. Clin. Invest. 54: 116-121.
12. Valcavi R., Dieguez C., Azzarito C., Edwards C.A., Dotti C., Page M.D., Portioli I. and Scanlon M.F. (1987): Clin. Endocrinol. 26: 453-458.
13. Valcavi R., Zini M., Maestroni G.J., Conti A. and Portioli I. (1993): Clin Endocrinol. 39: 193-199.
14. Vaughan G.M., Allen J.P., Tullis W., Siler-Khodr T.M., de La Pena A. and Sackman J.W. (1978): J. Clin. Endocrinol. 47: 566-571.
15. Vaughan M.K. (1981): Int. Rev. Physiol. 24: 41-95.
16. Van-Coevorden A., Mockel J., Laurent E., Kerkhofs M., L'Hermite-Baleriaux M., Decoster C., Nev, P and Van Cauter E. (1991): Am. J. Physiol. 260: 651-661.
17. Wright J., Aldhous M., Franey G., English J. and Arendt J. (1986): Clin. Endocrinol. 24: 375-382.
18. Young I.M. (1981): In: Pineal Function, edited by Matthews C.D. and Seamark R.F., pp. 7-12, Elsevier/North Holland. Amsterdam.

Frontiers in Endocrinology
Volume 9 - 1994

Effects of Hexarelin (EP 23905-MF 6003) on Circulating GH Levels in Acromegalic Patients

M. Arosio, O. Biella, G. Casati, L. Guglielmino, E. Palmieri and G. Faglia

Institute of Endocrine Sciences, University of Milan, Ospedale Maggiore IRCCS, pad. Granelli, via F. Sforza, 35, 20123 Milan, Italy

INTRODUCTION

Growth hormone (GH) secretion is physiologically regulated by two hypothalamic hormones, one stimulatory, GH-releasing hormone (GHRH), and one inhibitory, somatostatin (SRIF). In addition a new family of peptides that specifically release GH *in vivo* and *in vitro* in multiple animal species, has been recently synthetized (4). These peptides are structurally related to enkephalin and consist of 6-7 amino acids (5). They are known as GH releasing peptides (GHRPs). Their exact mechanism of action is unknown, but probably GHRPs act at both pituitary and hypothalamic levels through mechanisms distinct from those of GHRH and SRIF (5). It is worth noting that specific receptors for GHRPs have been found in the hypophysis and the hypothalamus (6), thus suggesting the existence of endogenous peptides similar to GHRPs with a physiological role in the regulation of GH secretion. Hexarelin (His-D-2- Methyl-Trp-Ala-Trp-D-Phe-Lys-NH2) is an analogue to GHRP-6, in which D-tryptophan has been replaced by its 2-methyl derivative (10). Compared to GHRP-6, hexarelin is more stable under a number of conditions of degradation (13). In normal subjects hexarelin has been found to release GH more efficaciously than GHRH (7). A slight dose-related increase in prolactin levels in comparison to placebo has also been described (7, 10).

Aim of the present study was to compare the effects of hexarelin and GHRH on GH and PRL secretion in acromegaly. In addition, since serum GH levels in acromegalic patients are also responsive to a variety of neuropeptides, GH responses to TRH and GnRH were also evaluated.

MATERIAL AND METHODS

Ten patients (3 men and 7 women, aged 29-66 years) with active acromegaly participated in the study after giving informed consent. All patients had elevated serum GH (range: 4.0-29.3; mean±SD=12.6±10 μg/L), and IGF-I levels (range: 80 -180; mean±SD=129±32 nmol/L), while PRL concentrations were in the normal range (2.5-20; mean±SD=9.2±5 μg/L). Four patients showed an abnormal GH increase after TRH administration, and 5 an abnormal GH response to GnRH according to previously reported criteria (3). Four patients had been unsuccessfully treated by surgery. Any medical treatment with somatostatin analogs or bromocriptine was discontinued 4 weeks before the study. All patients received, in random order, on different days, a single iv bolus injection of 1 μg/Kg hexarelin (Europeptides, Argenteuil, France), or 1 μg/Kg GHRH-1-29 (Geref, Serono, Italy), or saline. Blood samples were obtained 15 min before and 15, 30, 45, 60, 90 and 120 min after the injections. Both serum GH and PRL were measured by immunofluorimetric (IFMA) method (Delfia Prolactin and Delfia hGH, Kabi-Pharmacia). Statistical comparisons were performed with non parametric tests (Wilcoxon signed rank test and Mann-Whitney test). The significance level was $p<0.05$. Unless otherwise stated, results are expressed as the mean±SD.

RESULTS

Hexarelin significantly increased GH levels in all patients from a mean of 14.6±14 μg/L to 88.7±66 μg/L. Peak levels were observed at 15 min in 9 patients and at 30 min in one. Maximal % increase of GH from basal values ranged from 80 to 3000%. GH levels gradually returned to the basal levels in 90-120 min. GHRH injection increased GH levels from 17.6±18 to 76.2±98 μg/L, with peaks between 15 and 60 min. One patient was completely unresponsive to GHRH, while in the remaining cases maximal % increase ranged from 53 to 1056%. A comparison between hexarelin and GHRH response is given in Table 1. No correlation was seen between GH response to hexarelin and GHRH. Although in patients showing an abnormal GH response to TRH the response of GH to hexarelin was greater than in TRH unresponsive patients, the difference was not statistically significant (1383±1176% vs 499±366% p: n.s.). GnRH responsive patients showed a greater response to GHRH (831±400 vs 235±310, $p<0.01$), but not to hexarelin (589±359% vs 1116±1171%; p: n.s.) than GnRH unresponsive patients.

Table 1. *GH and PRL responses to hexarelin and GHRH*

	GH		PRL	
	net increase (µg/L)	% increase	net increase (µg/L)	% increase
Hexarelin	74.1±56	853±862	5.5±3.0	79.5±62
GHRH	58.6±87	533±461	2.3±2.9	28.2±35
p	n.s.	n.s.	<0.01	<0.01

Hexarelin induced a slight, but significant PRL increase from 9.7±5.4 to 15.2±5.9 µg/L. No significant PRL modifications were seen after GHRH administration. The response of PRL to hexarelin was significantly correlated to GH response ($r=0.73$ $p<0.05$)

DISCUSSION

This study demonstrates that intravenous administration of hexarelin is able to induce a significant increase in serum GH levels in acromegalic patients. These results are similar to those obtained by other authors with GHRP-6 (2, 9). The time course of hexarelin-induced GH release is different from that observed after GHRH. Furthermore, a lack of correlation between GH response to GHRH and hexarelin is found. These observations are in keeping with the concept that hexarelin, like the other GHRPs, acts through pituitary receptors distinct from those of GHRH and through cAMP-independent intracellular mechanisms (8). This is also supported by our finding of a clear GH response to hexarelin in a GHRH unresponsive patient, probably bearing a GH secreting adenoma with a mutation in Gs and constitutively active adenylyl cyclase (12). Other authors (2) have previously demonstrated an agreement between the GH response to GHRP and TRH, suggesting that the two peptides may share a similar Ca^{2+}-mediated cellular mechanism. However, our data are not conclusive in this respect.

The discrepancy between the large GH increase elicited *in vivo* by GHRPs and their modest *in vitro* effect (5) has been attributed to the presence of an additional site of action at hypothalamic level. A disrupted hypothalamic control in acromegaly could explain why the magnitude of GH response after hexarelin is similar and not greater than that observed after GHRH, at variance with normal subjects. Lastly, a slight increase of serum PRL levels was observed after hexarelin, as reported in normal subjects (7, 10), but not after GHRH. Since all our acromegalic patients were normoprolactinemic, it is possible to hypothesize that hexarelin might also act on normal PRL-secreting cells, unlike

GHRH, that could stimulate PRL in acromegaly only from tumoral mammosomatotroph cells (11).

ACKNOWLEDGEMENTS

The Authors thank Mediolanum Farmaceutici and Europeptides for the supply of hexarelin. This work was partially supported by MURST (Rome) and Ospedale Maggiore di Milano IRCCS.

REFERENCES

1. Akman M.S., Girard M., O'Brien L.F., Ho A.K. and Chik C. (1993): Endocrinology 132: 1286-1291.
2. Alster D.K., Bowers C.Y., Jaffe C.A., Ho P.J. and Barkan A.L. (1993): J. Clin. Endocrinol. Metab. 77: 842-845.
3. Arosio M., Giovanelli M., Riva E., Nava C., Ambrosi B. and Faglia G. (1983): J. Neurosurg. 59: 402-408.
4. Bowers C.Y. (1993): J. Pediat. Endocrinol. 6: 21-31.
5. Bowers C.Y., Momany F.A., Reynolds G.A. and Hong A. (1984): Endocrinology 114: 1537-1545.
6. Codd E.E., Shu A.Y.L. and Walker R.F. (1989): Neuropharmacology 28: 1139-1144.
7. Ghigo E., Arvat A., Gianotti L., Imbimbo B.P., Lenaerts V., Deghenghi R. and Camanni F. (1994): J. Clin. Endocrinol. Metab. 78: 693-698.
8. Goth M.I, Lyons C.E., Canny B.J. and Thorner M.O. (1992): Endocrinology 130: 939-944.
9. Hanew K., Utsumi A., Sugawara A., Shimizu Y. and Abe K. (1994): J. Clin. Endocrinol. Metab. 78: 509-512.
10. Imbimbo B.P., Mant T., Edwards M., Amin D., Dalton N., Boutignon F., Lenaerts V., Wüthrich P. and Deghenghi R. (1994): Europ. J. Clin. Pharmacol. in press
11. Losa M., Schopohl S., Muller O.A. and Von Werder K. (1985): Acta Endocrinol. (Copenh) 109: 467-473.
12. Spada A., Arosio M., Bochicchio D., Bazzoni N., Vallar L., Bassetti M. and Faglia G. (1990): J. Clin. Endocrinol. Metab. 71: 1421-1426.
13. Wehrenberg W.B., Giustina A., Imbimbo B., Stagg L., Conle, L. and Deghenghi R. (1992): J. Endocrinol. Invest. 15 (Suppl 4): 45 (A37).

Frontiers in Endocrinology
Volume 9 - 1994

Responsiveness of Gonadotropins to TRH in Patients with Nonfunctioning Pituitary Adenomas: Correlation with Immunohistochemical Results

M. Losa, M.R. Terreni[1], P. Mortini, S. Acerno and M. Giovanelli

Chair of Neurosurgery and [1]Chair of Pathology, IRCCS San Raffaele, University of Milan, Via Olgettina 60, 20132 Milan, Italy

INTRODUCTION

Almost 20-30% of surgically removed pituitary adenomas are classified on the basis of the clinical picture as nonfunctioning. However, it has been reported that a substantial number of these tumors may synthesize and secrete intact glycoprotein hormones or their subunits, as demonstrated by cell culture experiments (6), analysis of specific mRNA species (3), and immunocytochemistry (1). Unlike normal subjects, patients with nonfunctioning adenomas may show an abnormal rise of gonadotropins or their subunits after the administration of thyrotropin-releasing hormone (TRH). This response has been considered to indicate specifically the presence of a gonadotropin-secreting adenoma both in men and women (2, 5).

In the present study, we correlated the responsiveness of intact gonadotropins to TRH with the immunohistochemical characteristics of the adenomatous tissue obtained at surgery in patients with nonfunctioning pituitary adenomas.

MATERIAL AND METHODS

We studied 25 consecutive patients who were treated by transsphenoidal surgery at our Department in the last 18 months on account of a clinically nonfunctioning pituitary adenoma, as confirmed by histological examination of the removed tissue. Patients with a history of pituitary apoplexy were not included. The study group comprised 13 men and 12 women (8 were postmenopausal), with a mean age of 54.4 ± 3.3 years (ranging from 16 to 73 years). Nineteen patients had never been treated before, 4 patients had already been operated, and the remaining 2 patients had received a short course of dopaminergic drugs, that was withdrawn at least one week before hormonal testing.

Before operation all patients were given 200 μg TRH iv, and blood samples for the determination of gonadotropin levels were taken at baseline and 15, 30, and 60 minutes after injection. Both gonadotropins have been measured by monoclonal antibody fluoroimmunometric assays (Delfia hFSH and Delfia hLH Spec, Pharmacia, Italy). The detection limit of both assays is 0.05 U/l and cross reactivity with TSH, ß-hCG, and with the other gonadotropin is less than 1%. In keeping with other authors (5, 7), a positive gonadotropin response to TRH has been considered as an increase of LH and/or FSH of 50% or more over baseline. Immunohistochemical analysis of the surgically removed adenoma was performed using specific antisera against LH and FSH. The exact percentage of cells showing a positive immunostaining was calculated for each adenoma.

All the results are expressed as the mean ± SE. Statistical analysis of the data was performed by unpaired Student t test, regression analysis, and chi square tables as appropriate.

RESULTS

Basal LH levels were normal in all patients, except two, one man and one postmenopausal woman, whereas basal FSH levels were elevated in 5 patients (one man and 4 postmenopausal women). Eleven patients (44%) had a significant increase of LH after TRH administration, ranging from 50% to 775% over baseline, while only 3 patients (12%) showed a significant elevation of FSH values (59%, 70%, and 300%, respectively). All had also the paradoxical response of LH to TRH. The increase in LH and FSH after TRH was significantly correlated in the whole group of patients ($r = 0.951$; $p < 0.001$). However, the correlation was strongly influenced by the presence of a single outlier that had the most marked gonadotropin response to TRH (775% for LH and 300 for FSH). After excluding this patient, the correlation still remained significant but at a much lower level ($r = 0.474$; $p < 0.02$). The gonadotropin response to TRH was not correlated to basal gonadotropin level, age, sex, presence of hyperprolactinemia, and tumor volume. Immunocytochemistry of the removed adenomas revealed the complete absence of LH and/or FSH immunostaining in 10 tumors and a varying degree of positivity in the remaining 15 adenomas. The percentage of positive cells was ≤ 5% in 5 adenomas, comprised between 5% and 20% in 3 other tumors, and > 20% in the remaining 7 adenomas. The percentages of cells positive for LH and

FSH were significantly correlated ($r = 0.689$; $p < 0.001$). With two exceptions, the patients with the strongest immunoreactivity for LH and/or FSH also showed the greatest paradoxical responsiveness of LH and/or FSH to TRH. The group of patients showing a paradoxical LH responsiveness to TRH showed a non significant trend towards a higher percentage of positive LH cells in the respective adenomas as compared with non responder patients (26.1 ± 6.3% vs. 8.4 ± 4.5%; $p < 0.10$). A similar result was obtained for FSH (33.3 ± 14.5% of positive cells in the patients with a paradoxical FSH response to TRH, vs 9.2 ± 4.1% in non responder patients; $p < 0.10$).

CONCLUSIONS

Our preliminary study shows that more than 40% and 12% of patients with clinically nonfunctioning pituitary adenomas show a paradoxical LH or FSH response to TRH, respectively, and that more than 50% of the tumors had positive immunostaining for LH and FSH. The two characteristics were not closely correlated, even though the greatest paradoxical responses tended to occur in those patients with intense immunostaining for LH and/or FSH.

Paradoxical responsiveness of gonadotropins or their subunits to TRH has long been recognized as a specific marker for the presence of a gonadotroph adenoma in both men and women (2, 4, 7). However, White et al. (8), recently reported that only 3 out of 6 patients whose tumor secreted LH *in vitro* showed an increased LH concentration following TRH administration. The interpretation of these findings is somewhat complicated since few reports describe the immunocytochemical characteristics of the tumors in detail and do not usually attempt to correlate these characteristics. Our results confirm that the presence of a preoperative paradoxical response of one or both gonadotropins to TRH is more likely to occur in patients with a positive LH and FSH immunostaining of the pituitary tumor.

The possibility to recognize the presence of a gonadotroph adenoma *in vivo* is important in several aspects. First, if the specificity of the paradoxical response is demonstrated in future studies to be near 100%, the TRH test could become an invaluable tool in the preoperative differential diagnosis of tumors of the sellar region. In some instances, in fact, it is not possible to discriminate a nonfunctioning adenoma from other lesions, for example a suprasellar meningioma, requiring different surgical approaches even with the most sophisticated neuroimaging techniques. Second, the paradoxical responsiveness of gonadotropins to TRH could represent a marker by which to ascertain the completeness of surgical removal. Finally, it would be possible to analyze whether the gonadotropin responsiveness to TRH is linked to particular characteristics of the adenoma, or more important, to the long-term outcome of the patients.

REFERENCES

1. Black P.M., Hsu D.W., Klibanski A., Kliman B., Jameson L., Ridgway E.C., Hedley-Whyte E.T. and Zervas N.T. (1987): J. Neurosurg. 66: 244-250.
2. Daneshdoost L., Gennarelli T.A., Bashey H.M., Savino P.J., Sergott R.C., Bosley T.M. and Snyder P.J. (1991): N. Engl. J. Med. 324: 589-594.
3. Jameson J.L., Klibanski A., Black P.M. et al. (1987): J. Clin. Invest. 80: 1472-1478.
4. Kwekkeboom D.J., de Jong F.H. and Lamberts S.W.J. (1989): J. Clin. Endocrinol. Metab. 68: 1128-1135.
5. Lamberts S.W.J., Verleun T., Oosterom R., Hofland L., van Ginkel L.A., Loeber J.G., van Vroonhoven C.C.J., Stepanko S.Z. and de Jong F.H. (1987): J. Clin. Endocrinol. Metab. 64: 524-530.
6. Mashiter K., Adams E. and Van Noorden S. (1981): Clin. Endocrinol. (Oxf.) 15: 103-112.
7. Snyder P.G., Muzyka R., Johnson J. and Utiger R.D. (1980): J. Clin. Endocrinol. Metab. 51: 744-748.
8. White M.C., Daniels M., Newland P., Thompson C.J., Cook D. Dewa, J., Perry R., Jewitt R., Mathias D., Murdoch A.P. and Kendall-Taylor P. (1990): Clin. Endocrinol. (Oxf.) 32: 681-688.

Frontiers in Endocrinology
Volume 9 - 1994

INTRODUCTORY REMARKS

Pituitary Adenomas: Recent Progress in Basic and Clinical Research

G. Faglia

Institute of Endocrine Sciences, Ospedale Maggiore IRCCS, University of Milan, Via F. Sforza 35, 20122 Milan, Italy

Basic and clinical studies on pituitary adenomas have literally exploded in more recent years.

The discovery that, in a subset of somatotroph adenomas, point mutations in the GTP-ase domain of the α-chain of Gs protein lead to the constitutive activation of adenylyl cyclase activity resulting in the expansion of the mutated clone (*gsp* oncogene) has given rise to extensive molecular biology investigations aimed to screen pituitary adenomas for structural genetic abnormalities. *gsp* mutations have been documented in about 40% of somatotropinomas, 10% of clinically non-functioning and 5% of corticotroph adenomas, while a *ras* mutation has been found in one malignant prolactinoma. Allele loss of chromosome 11, and mutated α-proteinkinase isoforms have also been reported.

These findings along with that obtained with the X-chromosome inactivation analysis technique, demonstrating that pituitary tumours are monoclonal in origin, have profoundly modified the current concepts concerning the pathogenesis of pituitary tumors.

Also the observation that pituitary tumours are able to produce a variety of growth factors and even neurohormones has given new insight into the mechanisms of clone expansion.

The introduction of new high resolution imaging techniques, such as dynamic TC and MRI, has allowed the diagnosis of microadenomas of 2-5 mm in diameter, while pituitary SPECT scintigraphy with labelled analogues of neurohormones and PET with appropriate labelled precursors have allowed the *in vivo* recognition of specific receptors and the study of tumour metabolism, respectively. The catheterization of inferior petrosal sinuses

(IPS), allowing the study of secretory dynamics on blood directly drained from the pituitary, has provided us with a new diagnostic tool that has been found to be extremely useful in adenomas undetectable with other procedures.

Therapeutic approaches have been further improved not only by the introduction of more refined surgical and radiotherapeutic techniques, but also by the development of novel dopamine agonists such as quinagolide and cabergoline for the medical treatment of prolactinomas, and of long-acting somatostatin analogues for acromegaly and thyrotropinomas.

From: JEI Vol. 17, Suppl. 2 to n. 3, 1994, p. 11.
Abstracts of the XXV National Congress of the Italian Endocrine Society.

Frontiers in Endocrinology
Volume 9 - 1994

Radiological Study of Intracranial Neuroendocrine Tumors

R. Floris, A. Apruzzese, T.Y. Aref, E. Fanucci, S. Masala, M. Crecco[1], A. Vidiri[1] and G. Simonetti

Department of Radiology, University of Rome Tor Vergata, Ospedale S. Eugenio, P.le dell'Umanesimo 10, 00144 Rome;
[1] Department of Radiology, Ospedale Regina Elena, Rome, Italy

INTRODUCTION

Pituitary adenomas are the most common sellar tumors arising from cells of the anterior pituitary gland. They are benign slowly-growing tumors representing 10 to 15% of all intracranial neoplasms. Pituitary adenomas are usually well delimited by a pseudocapsule of compressed glandular tissue, but not a true fibrous capsule.

CLASSIFICATION OF PITUITARY ADENOMAS

Radiological classification:

Microadenoma	Macroadenoma
less than 10 mm in diameter	more than 10 mm in diameter

Histological classification (conventional classification):

Acidophilic — Basophilic — Chromophobe

Functional classification:

Hormonally-Active Adenomas	Inactive Adenomas
75%	25%

Prolactinoma (40-50%)
Somatotrophic adenoma (20%)
Corticotrophic adenoma (20%)
Thyrotrophic adenoma (rare)
Gonadotrophic adenoma (rare)
Plurihormonal adenoma (10%): the most common form is prolactin-growth hormone producing adenoma.

IMAGING IN PITUITARY MACROADENOMAS

Computed Tomography (CT) of pituitary macroadenomas demonstrates a ballooned sella turcica, the adenoma itself being isodense with the surrounding normal gland and cavernous sinus. Hypodense areas of necrosis or cystic degeneration could be detected in 10-30% of cases. Calcifications, either curvilinear or central globular, are rarely seen. Macroadenomas cause mass distortion of the normal anatomy. They are homogenously enhanced after bolus iv injection of contrast agent.

Magnetic Resonance Imaging (MRI) of pituitary macroadenomas demonstrates a mass arising from the pituitary fossa, hypointense on T1 weighted images (T1 WI) (80-95%) compressing the normal gland, which has higher signal intensity, they may even fill the sella turcica completely compressing the gland. Less predictable is the signal intensity pattern on T2 weighted images (T2 WI): in 30-50% of cases it appears as a focal hyperintense lesion, and isointense in the remainder.

MRI of macroadenoma shows sellar ballooning on sagittal scans and extrasellar extension. MRI with its excellent tissue details, gives a better definition of tumor margins and adjacent non-osseous structures than CT. CT is superior in detecting bony details, such as sellar floor destruction, because MRI is unable to distinguish osseous invasion from remodeling or expansion of the sella.

MRI has many advantages over CT and it is actually considered the imaging method of choice in most cases. These advantages include good tissue details, excellent blood vessel depiction, direct orthogonal acquisition planes, absence of dental and petrous artifacts and lack of radiation exposure.

Direct visualization of the cavernous portion of the Internal Carotid Artery (ICA), Middle Carotid Artery (MCA) and Anterior Cerebral Artery (ACA) by MRI could replace routine preoperative angiography for patients with pituitary adenomas. Superior extension to suprasellar cistern is well delineated due to the hypointensity of CSF against the adenomatous tissue. The optic nerve, chiasma and tracts are well depicted. The medial wall of cavernous sinus is relatively thin and, in most cases, is not directly visualized and it is almost impossible to determine whether or not it is invaded or compressed by adenoma, unless ICA is encased. The lateral wall of the cavernous sinus is relatively thick and directly seen with MRI. Asymmetry of cavernous sinus may indicate their invasion and a very high blood prolactin level (> 1000 ng/ml) always indicates cavernous sinus invasion. However, constriction or obstruction of the cavernous portion of ICA by extension of pituitary adenoma is very rare. This is an important issue in differentiating meningiomas from adenomas. Extension of pituitary adenoma inferiorly is depicted as a mass of soft tissue signal intensity within air space of sphenoid sinus. Extension into the clivus is clearly revealed by MRI due to the replacement of the normal high signal of fatty bone marrow on T1 WI by a low signal intensity tissue. Moreover, MRI is far more effective than CT in detecting hemorrhages within macroadenomas as a focal area of hyper-intense signal in both T1 and T2 WI, these hemorrhages are rarely likely to produce pituitary apoplexy.

Cystic degeneration appears as a low signal intensity area on T1 WI and as a high signal intensity area on T2 WI.

IMAGING IN PITUITARY MICROADENOMAS

A careful correlation between imaging methods, endocrinological and clinical data is always needed for the detection of pituitary microadenomas due to the absence of gland distortion and the minimal difference in density and signal intensity between tumor and normal gland tissue.

A superior bulging of the pituitary gland, less than 10 mm in young women and less than 7 mm in adolescent males, is considered normal.

Pituitary microadenoma is usually in a lateral position. Contrast Enhanced (CE) CT scan demonstrates, in some patients, a focal hypodense lesion with no significant mass effect.

Indirect signs of pituitary microadenomas are focal convexity of the superior surface of the pituitary gland. Bowing of the infundibulum may be seen in 1/3 of cases, while local thinning or sloping of the sellar floor is not a reliable sign of microadenoma because of the wide variation of thickness and contour of the sellar floor.

Some patients with surgically-proven microadenoma may have normal CT findings.

MRI shows pituitary microadenomas as focal hypointense areas on T1 WI, often with asymmetrical superior bulging of the gland and stalk displacement (Fig. 1). The pituitary stalk may be tilted toward the tumor (paradoxical displacement).

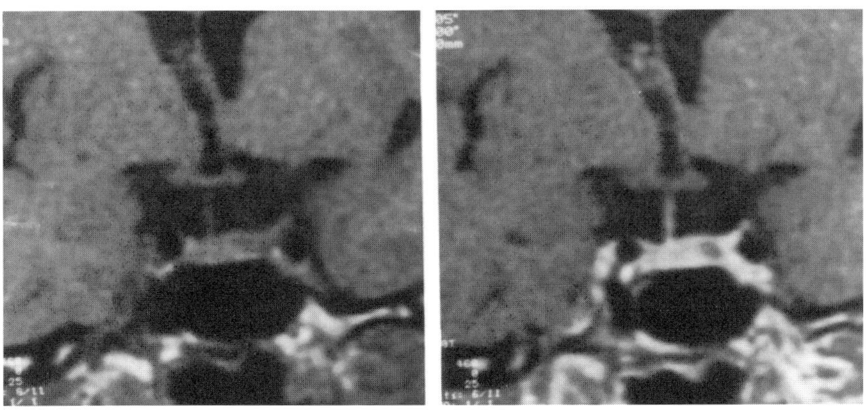

FIG. 1. Microprolactinoma. Non contrast MR T1 WI shows a focal hypointense area within pituitary parenchyma in left lateral location. The hypointense area is more evident after GD-DTPA iv administration. Pituitary stalk is tilted toward right.

Asymmetry of the sellar floor is not a reliable sign, since it may be related to the position of the sphenoid sinus septum. The normal pituitary stalk measures 4.5 mm, if it is larger than the basilar artery at the level of the dorsum sella in young patients it is a pathological finding. Up to 15% of asymptomatic patients show low signal foci on MRI of the pituitary gland, which may represent an asymptomatic microadenoma, pars intermedia cyst or colloid cyst.

High field MRI provides an accuracy rate ranging from 80% to 90% in detecting pituitary microadenomas as it results from a correlation with the surgical findings.

Gd-DTPA is indicated when plain MRI is negative or equivocal in a patient with clinically evident presentation. Immediate post-enhanced coronal MRI scan shows a well-defined hypointense lesion within normal gland, if negative or equivocal, delayed CE scans show reversed images due to an accumulation of the contrast in the tumoral cells, while washed out from the normal gland. There are no characteristic features of the different functional types of pituitary adenomas on MRI, but prolactinomas and somatotrophic adenomas are preferentially located in the lateral portion, while ACTH, TSH, LH and FSH secreting adenomas are more frequently located in the central portion.

Pituitary hyperplasia may be seen in young normally menstruating females, during puberty, pregnancy and with prolonged use of oral contraceptive pills. An enlarged pituitary gland in a child is almost always hyperplasia rather than adenoma.

Prolactinoma is the most common form of hormonally-active pituitary adenomas (40-50%). The capability to infiltrate meningeal tissue, bone and surrounding tissues is higher than other types (33% of microprolactinomas and 67% of macroprolactinomas) of adenomas, for this reason recurrences of hyperprolactinemia are seen in 50% of patients after surgery on prolactinomas. They are not enhanced after contrast injection for either CT or MR scans (Fig. 1).

Adrenocorticotrophic adenoma represents about 20% of hormonally-active pituitary adenomas. It is usually a microadenoma (2-3 mm in diameter). CT enhancement pattern is similar to surrounding gland tissue, 50-70% of surgically confirmed ACTH adenomas have normal CE-CT. MRI is more sensitive (40-80%) as ACTH microadenomas usually appear less intense than the gland on T1 WI and hyperintense on T2 WI. Gd-DTPA provides enhancement of the lesion only in delayed MR scan (1 hour), early CE scans show a non-enhanced lesion, but this pattern is not always detected.

Somatotrophic adenomas represent about 20% of hormonally-active pituitary adenomas, most of them are microadenomas.

70% of these adenomas produce excessive growth hormone, while 30% produce excess growth hormone and prolactin hormone (plurihormonal adenomas).

The other types of functional adenomas are rare and have no specific radiologic patterns.

Non-functional pituitary adenomas are usually macroadenomas with extrasellar extension, superiorly to the suprasellar cistern, optic nerve and chiasma, 3rd ventricle and foramina of Monro, laterally to the cavernous sinuses or inferiorly to the sphenoid sinuses.

POSTOPERATIVE EVALUATION OF THE PITUITARY GLAND

CT or MR examination during the first two months after pituitary surgery is helpful to detect extrasellar complications such as subarachnoid hemorrhage, hydrocephalus and infarction, but does not provide accurate information on the sellar region, on account of the progressive changes involving soft-tissues and both maxillary and sphenoid sinuses during this period.

A baseline postoperative scanning could be done three months after pituitary surgery.

MRI presents several advantages with respect to CT, to be considered the imaging method of choice for pituitary adenomas, especially microadenomas, however, CT is still more accurate in detecting bony changes associated with macroadenomas.

MRI is very sensitive for pituitary microadenomas, but not specific in differentiating the various types, since there is no evident correlation between radiological and both functional and histological types.

MRI, during the first two months after pituitary surgery, provides information only on extrasellar complications, but not on the sellar region as there are progressive postoperative sellar changes, easily leading to misinterpretation of the radiological findings during this period.

Pituitary hyperplasia may normally be seen in the young menstruating female, during puberty and pregnancy and prolonged use of oral contraceptive pills. An enlarged pituitary gland in children is almost always hyperplasia rather than pituitary adenoma.

A superior bulge in the pituitary gland of less than 10 mm in young women or less than 7 mm in adolescent males is considered normal.

MRI shows the posterior pituitary gland as a bright spot on T1 WI in 50-90% of individuals, absence of this bright spot could be normal, however, it is absent also with diabetes insipidus. Up to 15% of asymptomatic individuals show a low signal foci on MRI of the pituitary gland which may represent asymptomatic microadenomas, pars intermedia cyst or colloid cyst. All these important findings should be taken into account in interpreting MRI of the pituitary gland, considering the clinical conditions of the patients.

Hypothalamic hamartomas are rare congenital malformations composed of normal neuronal tissue and located in the region of mammillary bodies or Tuber Cinereum of the hypothalamus. The most common presenting symptom is isosexual precocious puberty, usually before the age of two years. Other symptoms consist of seizures, neurodevelopmental delay and hyperactivity. Hypothalamic hamartomas, well-defined round to oval masses, are usually attached to the mammillary bodies or Tuber Cinereum by means of a thin stalk.

They generally project into the suprasellar or the interpeduncular cistern. Histologically they consist of a heterotopic collection of small and large neuron astrocytes and oligodendroglial cells closely resembling the histological pattern of the Tuber Cinereum.

On CT, hypothalamic hamartomas appear as rounded masses isodense with brain tissue, within the suprasellar and interpeduncular cisterns. They are homogeneous and sharply delimited by the surrounding CSF. MRI features are that of a well-defined, rounded, pedunculated mass suspended from the tuber cinereum or mammillary bodies. Hypothalamic hamartomas are isointense with brain on T1 WI and isointense, to slightly hyperintense, on T2 WI.

Craniopharyngiomas are epithelially derived neoplasms that arise from remnants of the craniopharyngeal duct. They account for 3% of all intracranial tumors, 15% of supratentorial tumors and 50% of suprasellar tumors in children. Males are more commonly affected than females. Symptoms may vary with the age of the patient, they consist in visual field defects, secondary to compression of the optic chiasm and tracts, anterior pituitary dysfunction (growth failure) due to anterior pituitary and hypothalamic-pituitary portal system compression and hypothalamic dysfunction (diabetes insipidus). Craniopharyngiomas may be either largely cystic, partly solid and partly cystic, or entirely solid.

They vary greatly in size; they may extend into the third ventricle or posteriorly and inferiorly to the level of the pons or into the pituitary fossa,

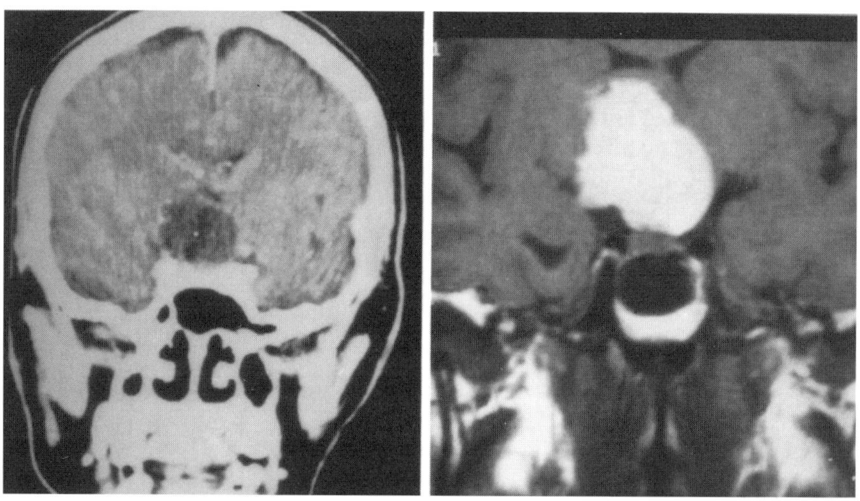

FIG. 2. A cystic craniopharyngioma in suprasellar location, spreading upward towards the diencephali, is evident, appearing as a hypodense area on CT scan (A) and hyperintense on MR T1 WI (B).

eroding both dorsum and tuberculum sellae. They may invade the surrounding brain and are frequently surrounded by considerable gliosis. Foci of calcification or even frank bone formation may be present.

CT features are peculiar. They are mostly suprasellar in location. 90% will have a cystic component, 90% will present foci of calcification, moreover, 90% will be enhanced after iv administration of contrast agent.

Craniopharyngiomas are also characteristic on MRI studies, appearing as multilobular masses extending upward from the region of diaphragma sellae.

Very rarely onset of craniopharyngiomas occurs primarily in the third ventricle or in the optic chiasm. The cystic areas may present high or low signal intensity on T1 WI while both cystic and solid components tend to be of high signal intensity on T2 WI.

REFERENCES

1. Andrews C.M. (1991): In: Handbook of Neuroradiology. edited by AG. Osborn, Mosby Year-Book. Chicago. 331.
2. Davis P.C., Hoffman J.C. and Spencer T. et al. (1987): AJNR 8: 107.
3. Grossman C.B. (1990): In: Magnetic Resonance Imaging and Computed Tomography of the Head and Spine, edited by Grayson TH, Williams & Wilkins, Baltimore. 254.
4. Kucharczyk W. and Montanera W.J. (1991): In: Magnetic Resonance Imaging of the Brain and Spine, edited by S.W. Atlas. Raven Press. New York. 625.
5. Kulkarni M.V., Lee K.F. and Ardle M.C. et al. (1988): AJNR 9: 5.
6. Peck W.W., Dillon W.P. and Norman D. et al. (1989): AJNR 9: 1085.

Frontiers in Endocrinology
Volume 9 - 1994

Hormone Receptors in Pituitary Tumors

A. Spada, P. Gil-del-Alamo and A. Lania

Institute of Endocrine Sciences, Ospedale Maggiore IRCCS, University of Milan, Via F. Sforza 35, 20122 Milan, Italy

INTRODUCTION

In the last few years particular attention has been paid to hypothalamic neurohormones as possible modulators of pituitary cell growth (14, 5, 10). In fact, these agents, originally identified on the basis of their ability to influence hormone release from the target cells, have been demonstrated to be involved in the control of several biological processes, that include coordinated cell proliferation and differentiation as well as hyperplasia and neoplastic transformation (3, 4). In this line, it has been hypothesized that abnormalities of hypothalamic hormone signalling occurring at either receptor or postreceptor level may cause uncontrolled cell growth (Table 1).

Table 1. *Abnormalities of hormonal signalling*

1.	ABNORMALITIES AT RECEPTOR LEVEL
	Alterations of number and/or affinity of receptors *(Reduction of dopaminergic receptors in resistant prolactinomas)*
	Abnormal expression of receptors for aspecific agents *(TRH receptors expressed by GH-omas, ACTH-omas and gonadotropinomas)*
	Altered regulation of receptor function *(Lack of desensitization of GHRH receptors in GH-omas)*
2.	ABNORMALITIES AT POST-RECEPTOR LEVEL
	Mutations of G-protein *(gsp oncogene in GH-omas)*
	Mutations of intracellular effector *(Mutation of protein kinase C in invasive tumors)*
	Defective second messenger generation *(Dopamine receptors uncoupled with adenylate cyclase inhibition in GH-omas)*
	Alteration of G-proteins available for receptor activation *(Stimulation of [Ca2+]i by somatostatin in nonfunctioning adenomas)*

Examples of alterations are in parentheses.

ABNORMALITIES OF HORMONE SIGNALLING AT RECEPTOR LEVEL

Hypothalamic neurohormones convey information by binding to specific receptors that belong to the superfamily of G-protein-coupled receptors since they require the recognition and activation of a single class of proteins, called G-proteins, to transduce the hormonal message (19). Specific receptors for hypothalamic hormones have, in the past, been identified and characterized in pituitary tumors by binding studies with labeled analogs. In recent years, almost all receptors for hypothalamic hormones have been identified by cloning and expression studies and it is predictable that receptor types expressed by pituitary tumors will be characterized in the near future.

Receptors for hypothalamic inhibitory hormones A reduced action of inhibitory hormones, such as dopamine (DA) and somatostatin (SRIH), has been suggested to play a role in the formation of pituitary tumors (10, 2, 13). A decreased number of DA and SRIH receptors has been observed with variable frequency in tumor tissues removed from patients resistant to the exogenous administration of neuroactive analogues while modification of receptor density seems to be unusual in the great majority of tumors. Although the reduced number of receptors is likely to be the major abnormality responsible for the resistance to specific treatment, it has been proposed that alterations, such as genetic mutations or differential mRNA splicing, may result in the expression of receptor isoforms less efficiently coupled to intracellular effectors.

To test this hypothesis, receptors expressed by pituitary tumors have recently been screened for genetic abnormalities. It has been reported that in a large series of PRL-secreting adenomas no mutations in the coding exons of the dopamine D2 receptor gene were present, all abnormalities detected being due to polymorphisms within the gene (6).

As far as SRIH receptors are concerned, the expression of two receptor subtypes, SSTR1 and SSTR2, has recently been investigated in secreting and nonsecreting adenomas (23, 7). The results demonstrate that the two SRIH receptor subtypes are heterogeneously expressed in different pituitary tumors, SSTR2 being the major form present in GH-secreting adenomas. The biological consequences of the presence of different receptor subtypes in pituitary tumors remain to be elucidated.

Receptors for hypothalamic stimulatory hormones Little attention has so far been paid to the possibility that an increased number of receptors for hypothalamic stimulatory hormones might promote pituitary tumor formation. Although it is at present unknown whether receptors for the specific releasing hormones are expressed in large amounts by pituitary tumors, pituitary tumors are frequently sensitive to hypothalamic agents that are ineffective in normal cell counterpart, as suggested by *in vivo* and *in vitro* studies. By this mechanism, pituitary adenomas acquire abnormal sensitivity to agents that have both secretory and trophic effects. In particular, since pituitary cells are programmed to replicate in response to cAMP, it is worth mentioning that the great majority of functioning and nonfunctioning adenomas show a high sensitivity to neuropeptides of the secretin superfamily, such as vasoactive intestinal peptide (VIP) and pituitary adenylate cyclase activating peptide (PACAP) which act via cAMP formation (11, 8, 15).

The amplification of stimulatory signals is also achieved by the expression of receptors generally lacking the mechanism(s) of desensitization. Although the molecular basis of these alterations is still undefined, by this mechanism tumoral cells may continue to respond to stimulatory agents, such as GHRH, GnRH and CRH, despite the continuous presence of the specific hormones (17).

Finally, following the recent demonstration that hyperfunctioning thyroid adenomas are frequently secondary to somatic mutations in the TSH receptor gene (12), it is reasonable to predict that a subset of pituitary tumors might be caused by activating mutations in receptors transducing proliferative signals. Due to the proliferative action of GHRH and CRH in target cells, the receptors for these two agents are good candidates for carrying activating mutations.

ABNORMALITIES AT POST-RECEPTOR LEVEL

Abnormality of hormonal signalling may result from postreceptor alterations. Since receptors for hypothalamic agents require coupling with one or more G-proteins to transduce the hormonal message, particular attention has been paid to these proteins as the possible site of abnormalities in hormonal signalling. Novel mutations of G-proteins have first been identified in pituitary adenomas (21, 9, 16). In fact, about a third of GH-secreting adenomas express activating mutations in the gene encoding the alpha subunit of Gs, the stimulatory regulatory protein of adenylate cyclase, leading to the constitutive activation of adenylate cyclase with consequent high rate of cAMP production, GH secretion and somatotroph replication.

By these genomic alterations, somatotroph growth bypasses the requirement for the specific growth factor, that is GHRH. Subsequently, the same mutations were found in a minority of nonfunctioning pituitary adenomas (20). Very recently, alterations have been identified in the calcium dependent pathway: mutations of protein kinase C have been reported in highly invasive pituitary tumors, further strengthening the crucial role of hormonal signalling in pituitary tumorogenesis (1).

In addition to the molecular alterations that have been recently identified, receptors expressed by pituitary tumors frequently show defective coupling with the specific G-protein. While the D2 receptor expressed by normal and tumoral lactotrophs is coupled with the inhibition of both adenylate cyclase and calcium levels (22), in GH-secreting adenomas the activation of the dopamine receptor causes the reduction of intracellular calcium levels without affecting cAMP production (18). The same abnormality seems to occur in ACTH-secreting adenomas and nonfunctioning adenomas. Since the proliferation of pituitary cells is cAMP dependent, the lack of effect of dopamine may be regarded as a defective inhibitory action of this agent.

Other abnormalities of hormonal signalling occur in pituitary tumors, although the underlying molecular defects responsible for these alterations still remain largely unknown. Example of these alterations are the paradoxical effects of both dopamine and somatostatin in a subset of nonfunctioning adenomas. In these adenomas both DA and SRIH cause an increase in cytosolic calcium levels due to calcium mobilization from the intracellular stores (17). Since these alterations involve the transduction of different hormones, it is reasonable to hypothesize that, in these tumors, quantitative/qualitative alterations of G-proteins available for receptor activation may confer stimulatory properties to inhibitory inputs.

CONCLUSIONS

Although in the last few years molecular biological investigations have revealed that the majority of pituitary tumors are monoclonal in origin, indicating the existence of genomic mutations in the progenitor cell, it is likely that promoting agents are required to cause the selective expansion of the transformed cell. Among the possible promoting agents, a crucial role might be exerted by hypothalamic neurohormones. In fact, these agents, originally identified on the basis of their ability to influence hormone release, have been demonstrated to have either proliferative or antiproliferative activity. It is, therefore, reasonable to hypothesize that either an increased or decreased action of stimulatory and inhibitory signals, respectively, might promote the clonal expansion of the transformed cell, resulting in tumor formation. It is worth noting that the abnormalities occurring at both receptor and postreceptor levels might contribute to pituitary tumorogenesis by either amplifying intracellular signals triggered by regulatory peptides with growth promoting properties or attenuating inhibitory inputs.

REFERENCES

1. Alvaro V., Levy L., Dubray C., Roche A., Peillon F., Querat B. and Joubert D. (1993): J. Clin. Endocrinol. Metab. 77: 1125-1129.
2. Bertherat J., Chanson P., Dewailly D., Enjalbert A., Jaquet P., Kordon C., Peillon F., Timsit J. and Epelbaum J. (1992): Horm. Res. 38: 94-99.
3. Billestrup N., Swanson L.W. and Vale W. (1986): Proc. Natl. Acad. Sci. USA 83: 6854-6857.
4. Billestrup N., Mitchell R.L., Vale W. and Verma I.M. (1987): Mol. Endocrinol. 1: 300-305.
5. Faglia G. (1993): Acta Endocrinol. 129, Suppl 1: 1.
6. Friedman E., Adams E.F., Hoog A., Gejman P.V., Carson E., Larsson C., Demarco L., Werner S., Fahlbusch R. and Nordenskjold M. (1994): J. Clin. Endocrinol. Metab. 78: 568-574.

7. Greenman Y. and Melmed S. (1994): J. Clin. Endocrinol. Metab. 78: 398-403.
8. Gressens P., Hill J.M., Gozes I. and Fridkin M. (1993): Nature 362: 155-158.
9. Landis C., Masters S.B., Spada A., Pace A.M., Bourne H.R. and Vallar L. (1989): Nature 340: 692-696.
10. Levy A. and Lightman S.L. (1993): Clin. Endocrinol. 38: 559-568.
11. Nicosia S., Spada A., Borghi C., Cortelazzi L. and Giannattasio G. (1980): FEBS Lett. 112: 159-164.
12. Parma J., Duprez L., Van Sande J., Cochaux P., Gervy C., Mockel J., Dumont J. and Vassart G. (1993): Nature 365: 649-651.
13. Pellegrini I., Rasolonjanahary R., Gunz G., Bertrand P., Delivet S., Jedynak C.P., Kordon C., Peillon F. and Enjalbert A. (1989): J. Clin. Endocrinol. Metab. 69: 500-509.
14. Reichlin S. (1991): Excerpta Medica International Congress Series. 961: 113-121.
15. Robberecht P., Vertongen P., Velkeniers B., de Neef P., Vergani P., Raftopoulos C., Brotchi J., Hooghe-Peters E.L. and Christophe J. (1993): J. Clin. Endocrinol. Metab. 77: 1235-1239.
16. Spada A., Vallar L. and Faglia G. (1992): Trends Endocrinol. Metab. 3: 355-360.
17. Spada A., Vallar L. and Faglia G. (1994): Eur J. Endocrinol. 130: 43-52.
18. Spada A., Bassetti M., Reza-Elahi F., Arosi M., Gil-del-Alamo P. and Vallar L. (1994): J. Clin. Endocrinol. Metab. 78: 411-417.
19. Spiegel A.M., Shenker A. and Weinstein L.S. (1992): Endocr. Rev. 13: 536-565.
20. Tordjman K., Stern N., Ouaknine G., Yossiphov Y., Razon N., Nordenskjold M. and Friedman E. (1993): J. Clin. Endocrinol. Metab. 77: 765-769.
21. Vallar L., Spada A. and Giannattasio G. (1987): Nature 330: 566-567.
22. Vallar L. and Meldolesi J. (1989): Trends Pharmacol. Sci. 10: 74-77.
23. Yamada Y., Post S.R., Wang K., Tager H.S., Bell G.I. and Seino S. (1992): Proc. Natl. Acad. Sci. USA 89: 251-255.

Frontiers in Endocrinology
Volume 9 - 1994

Octreotide Scintigraphy in the Diagnosis of Neuroendocrine Tumours

D.J. Kwekkeboom, S.W.J. Lamberts and E.P. Krenning

Departments of Nuclear Medicine and Medicine,
University Hospital Dijkzigt,
Rotterdam, The Netherlands

INTRODUCTION

Two disadvantages of conventional, radiological, imaging for tumour localization and tumour staging are that small tumours may not be identified, and that the presence or absence of enlarged lymph nodes does not ultimately prove whether nodal spread has taken place. Therefore, much effort has been given to differentiate tumorous from non-tumorous tissue by means of *in vivo* radioimmunoimaging with radiolabelled monoclonal antibodies. Although a promising and rapidly improving technique, the limitations of this type of tumour imaging are its often low sensitivity, and the low tumour to background ratio of radioactivity.

We recently developed a technique for the *in vivo* visualization of tumours that bear somatostatin receptors, which offers a powerful alternative to tumour imaging with labeled monoclonal antibodies (1, 6, 8, 9 and for reviews see 2, 3).

Instead of injecting radiolabelled antibodies against the somatostatin receptor, we labelled a somatostatin analogue which is known to bind specifically to the somatostatin receptor, and injected this labelled hormone analogue in order to visualize somatostatin receptor positive tumours.

TUMOUR LOCALIZATION USING OCTREOTIDE SCINTIGRAPHY

The somatostatin analogue octreotide has been shown to bind to somatostatin receptors on both tumorous and non-tumorous tissues. Over the past few years, it has become known that various tumours of neuroendocrine origin contain somatostatin receptors (12). [^{111}In-DTPA-D-Phe^{1}]-octreotide is a radionuclide-coupled somatostatin analogue which can be used to visualize somatostatin receptor bearing tumours efficiently after 24 h, when interfering background radioactivity is minimized by renal clearance.

Octreotide scintigraphy was performed in over 1500 patients in our hospital, without any side-effects being noticed.

In the majority of patients with neuroendocrine tumours or APUDomas, but also in patients with lymphomas or granulomas, *in vivo* somatostatin receptor imaging was successful in demonstrating tumour localizations. The results of imaging *in vivo* correlated with the somatostatin receptor status on the tumours *in vitro*.

Somatostatin receptor imaging may provide valuable information concerning the localization of the primary tumour, the secondary spread, or both, in patients with APUD-cell tumours. This is of special interest in patients with endocrine pancreatic tumours, in whom it may be very difficult, if not impossible, to localize the tumour with conventional techniques (13). Likewise, small bowel carcinoids are often hard to localize with CT scanning (14). In a large proportion of patients with carcinoids, tumour sites that were not suspected or recognized previously, were demonstrated, and in part of these patients the additional sites were thereafter confirmed with other imaging techniques or were histologically proven to be tumour deposits (5). In patients with paragangliomas, octreotide scintigraphy also frequently demonstrated more tumour localizations than did conventional imaging techniques (7). Multicentricity of paragangliomas is frequent. Because of its easy application and because of the information it provides on potential tumour localizations in the whole body, somatostatin receptor imaging, in our opinion, is the method of first choice to establish the number and localizations of tumours in patients with paragangliomas.

In APUD-cell derived tumours, the absence or presence of *in vivo* visualization of these tumours after the injection of radiolabelled octreotide is closely correlated to the presence of somatostatin receptors, as demonstrated by *in vitro* autoradiography (9). Also, the visualization of these tumours during *in vivo* somatostatin receptor imaging seems to predict the ability of octreotide therapy to control symptoms caused by hormonal secretion from these tumours (8). Apart from the medical treatment of acromegaly, octreotide is also used to control the clinical symptoms caused by overproduction of hormones from endocrine pancreatic tumours, carcinoids, and medullary thyroid carcinoma. The administration of octreotide results in a remarkable improvement in the clinical condition of most patients (10, 11). In our opinion, octreotide scintigraphy, by means of its ability to visualize somatostatin receptor positive tumours *in vivo*, could be used to predict whether octreotide therapy in the individual patient could be beneficial.

Apart from APUD-cell derived tumours, octreotide scintigraphy was also successfully applied to visualize breast cancer, lymphomas and granulomas. As octreotide scintigraphy revealed additional tumour or granuloma sites in nearly half of the patients with lymphomas and granulomas, we expect that octreotide scintigraphy may contribute to the staging of the disease in these patients. This is presently being studied in a larger group of patients.

Octreotide scintigraphy revealed the primary tumour and its metastases in all of 26 patients with Small Cell Lung Cancer (SCLC), whereas only the primary tumour could be visualized in all of 40 patients with non-SCLC. As somatostatin-receptors are absent on most non-SCLC investigated thus far, their *in vivo* visualization is probably due to uptake of radioactivity by the tissue surrounding the tumour. It was found that including octreotide scintigraphy in the staging procedure of SCLC may allow early detection of metastases, especially to the brain (4).

CONCLUSIONS

In conclusion, octreotide scintigraphy is a simple and sensitive technique to demonstrate tumour localizations in the majority of patients with APUD-cell tumours, and also in patients with lymphomas or granulomas. Apart from its merit in tumour localization, *in vivo* somatostatin receptor imaging, on account of its ability to demonstrate somatostatin receptor positive tumours, could be used to select those patients with APUD-cell tumours who are likely to respond favourably to octreotide treatment.

REFERENCES

1. Krenning E.P., Bakker W.H., Breeman W.A.P., Koper J.W., Kooij P.P.M., Ausema L., Lameris J.S. and Lamberts S.W.J. (1989): Lancet I: 242-245.
2. Krenning E.P., Bakker W.H., Kooij P.P.M., Breeman W.A.P., Oei H.Y., de Jong M, Reubi J.-C., Visser T.J., Bruns C., Kwekkeboom D.J., Reijs A.E.M., Hagen P.M., van Koper J.W. and Lamberts S.W.J. (1992): J. Nucl. Med. 33: 652-658.
3. Krenning E.P., Kwekkeboom D.J., Bakker W.H., Breeman W.A.P., Kooij P.P.M., Oei H.Y., van Hagen M., Postema P.T.E., de Jong M., Reubi J.C., Visser T.J., Reijs A.E.M., Hofland L.J., Koper J.W. and Lamberts S.W.J. (1993): Eur. J. Nucl. Med. 20: 716-731.
4. Kwekkeboom D.J., Kho G.S., Lamberts S.W.J., Reubi J.C., Laissue J.A. and Krenning E.P. (1994): Eur. J. Nucl. Med. (in press).
5. Kwekkeboom D.J., Krenning E.P., Bakker W.H., Oei H.Y., Kooij P.P.M. and Lamberts S.W.J. (1993): Eur. J. Nucl. Med. 20: 283-292.
6. Kwekkeboom D.J., Krenning E.P., Bakker W.H., Oei H.Y., Splinter T.A.W., Kho G.S. and Lamberts S.W.J. (1991): J. Nucl. Med. 32: 1845-1848.
7. Kwekkeboom D.J., Pauw B.K.H., Pauw K.H., Lamberts S.W.J., Kooij P.P.M., Hoogma R. and Krenning E.P. (1993): J. Nucl. Med. 34: 873-878.
8. Lamberts S.W.J., Bakker W.H., Reubi J.C. and Krenning E.P. (1990): N. Eng. J. Med. 323: 1246-1249.
9. Lamberts S.W.J., Hofland L.J., Koetsveld P.M., van Reubi J.C., Bruining H.A., Bakker W.H. and Krenning E.P. (1990): J. Clin. Endocrinol. Metab. 71: 566-574.

10. Mahler C., Verhelst J., De Longueville M. and Harris A. (1990): Clin. Endocrinol. 33: 261-269.
11. O'Dorisio T.M. (1986): Am. J. Med. 81: Suppl. 6B: 1-101.
12. Reubi J.C., Kvols L.K., Waser B., Nagorney D.M., Heitz P.U., Charboneau J.W., Reading C.C. and Moertel C. (1990): Cancer. Res. 50: 5969-5977.
13. Stefanini P., Carboni M., Patrassi N. and Basoli A. (1974): Surgery 75: 597-609.
14. Vinik A.I., McLeod M.K., Fig L.M., Shapiro B., Lloyd R.V. and Cho K. (1989): Gastroenterol. Clin. N. Am. 18: 865-896.

Frontiers in Endocrinology
Volume 9 - 1994

INTRODUCTION

Therapeutic Approach to Pituitary Tumors

R. Vigneri, P. Tita and C. D'Arrigo[1]

Institute of Internal Medicine, Endocrinology and Metabolism, University of Catania;
[1]Department of Neurosurgery, USL 34; Ospedale Garibaldi, 95125 Catania, Italy

Pituitary adenomas are the most frequent adult intracranial neoplasms. Any of the several types of hormone-secreting cells of the anterior pituitary can give rise to tumors which, although almost invariably benign, cause important clinical problems both because of abnormal/excessive hormonal secretion and also because of the intracranial space occupying mass. Furthermore, also pituitary adenomas, originating from non-secreting cells, may cause similar problems: the mechanical effect of tumor compression on the rest of the pituitary may, indeed, induce abnormal/defective secretion of other pituitary hormones.

RATIONALE FOR TREATMENT AND GOALS OF THERAPY

Pituitary adenomas may cause chronic debilitating conditions (such as acromegaly or Cushing's disease), may adversely affect fertility, growth, metabolic homeostasis and normal systemic functions. In addition, even when the endocrinological signs directly related to the adenoma are minor (non-secreting tumors), the tumor mass in the pituitary may cause endocrinological symptoms due to local compression and damage to the remaining pituitary function. Pituitary adenomas, therefore, lead to an increased morbidity and mortality.

It is thus important, in the patient with a pituitary adenoma, to provide an optimally effective treatment strategy to comprehensively:

a) reduce or remove the pituitary mass;

b) suppress hormone hypersecretion and/or substitute hormone deficiency;

c) prevent or correct the systemic consequences of the altered hormonal function;

d) avoid local and general disease recurrence.

TREATMENT OPTIONS

Various therapeutic options are currently available for the management of pituitary adenomas. Although each of these modes of treatment may provide unique beneficial effects, they do not necessarily fulfill all the therapeutic goals indicated above. In addition, all treatments have contraindications and may cause severe side effects. Therefore, choice of an appropriate therapeutic strategy requires balancing the possible side effects and complications of each therapeutic approach with its potential benefits.

Surgery Transsphenoidal surgical adenomectomy, after accurate NMR localization, has proved to be an effective procedure in most (more than 50%) cases. Surgery, however, seldom cures large pituitary tumors. Also in smaller tumors, recurrences and/or impaired pituitary function develop in a certain percentage of cases, reflecting incomplete removal, operative damage of the remaining normal pituitary tissue or growth tumor invasiveness. Other side effects or complications include diabetes insipidus, cerebrospinal fluid leaks, hemorrhage and meningitis. Some of these complications are transient, while others require life-long treatment. The incidence of local post-operative complications is dependent upon the size of the adenoma, its localization, the extent of local invasiveness and, last but not least, the skill of the neurosurgeon (2).

Radiation Aim of this treatment is to administer maximal radiation to the tumor with minimal damage to the adjacent normal tissue. High energy radiation can be delivered to the pituitary tumor by megavoltage sources including external deep X-ray therapy and heavy-particle (proton beam) irradiation (4). Recently, stereotactic ablation of pituitary tumors by the gamma knife has proven particularly beneficial (7).

Radiation may be used both as primary therapy as well as a second choice or adjuvant therapy for treating recurrences after surgery or also for treating patients who fail to benefit from medical treatment (on account of either unresponsiveness or intolerance). Although the tumor mass is reduced by radiation in the long-term, the effect is too slow when local (visual failure) or general conditions are severely affected.

Side effects include extended local tissue damage. One out of two patients treated with radiation will develop pituitary hormone failure within the first 10 years after treatment and will, therefore, need life-long treatment and follow-up. Other side effects may include cranial nerve palsies and tumor necrosis with hemorrhage. The serious complication of loss of vision because of optic nerve damage is very rare. The incidence of local complications has decreased with modern techniques and more precise NMR imaging in adenoma localization.

Medical treatment Anterior pituitary cell growth and function is under dual control (positive and negative) of peptide factors and neurohormones produced in the hypothalamus. This mechanism provides the rationale for the medical management of pituitary adenomas: drugs, peptides and hormones that negatively affect the function and mitogenesis of pituitary cells will reverse the abnormal/excessive secretion of pituitary tumor cells and will also induce a shrinking of the adenoma by reduction of cell size and, sometimes, cell number.

Medical treatment of pituitary adenomas (primarily prolactinomas, the most common pituitary adenoma, but also GH-secreting adenomas) has now been available for more than 20 years. More recently, effective medical treatment has been reported also in some patients with the rare TSH-secreting adenoma and in some non secretory or gonadotropin-secreting adenomas.

The two most important medical tools used for the treatment of pituitary adenomas are dopamine agonists and somatostatin and its analogs.

Dopamine and dopamine agonists The reason why these medications are effective is that dopamine and dopamine agonist ergot drugs (bromocriptine, cabergoline, pergolide and lisuride, which has also a serotonin-like activity) interact with the dopamine receptors of pituitary cells (especially PRL- but sometimes also TSH-secreting cells and non secreting cells) and inhibit their function and growth (1). In the case of GH-secreting cells, a paradoxical effect is observed: although dopamine stimulates GH secretion in normal subjects, it inhibits GH secretion in GH-secreting adenomas. Dopamine agonist medications are more effective than levo-dopa because of their longer duration of action.

Dopamine agonists are efficacious in significantly decreasing hormone hypersecretion in over 80% of prolactinomas and 20-40% of GH-secreting adenomas. A significant (over 25%) tumor mass reduction is observed in a similar proportion of patients. Therefore, dopamine agonists are often chosen as the primary mode of therapy. If they fail it is always possible to turn to other forms of medical treatment (somatostatin) or to surgery (5, 6).

The disadvantages of this form of therapy include the side effects (postural hypotension, headache, nausea, gastro-intestinal upset) which are common but usually transient and the indefinite (often life-long) duration of treatment and follow-up. Adenoma cell function and growth, in fact, is often resumed upon withdrawal of treatment.

Somatostatin and octreotide Most pituitary hormones are under the negative control of somatostatin, an inhibitory hormone that operates via specific receptors on the cell membrane. Therefore, somatostatin administration lowers pituitary hormone secretion and inhibits cell proliferation.

Octreotide is an eight amino-acid somatostatin analog that differs from the native hormone because it is more potent and has a longer duration of action. For these reasons octreotide has completely replaced somatostatin in medical treatment.

Tumor responsiveness to octreotide is determined by several factors: the most important is the number of somatostatin receptors in tumor cells. Tumor size, frequency of administration and total daily dose are also relevant factors (3).

Some pituitary tumors show a complementary responsiveness to a combination of octreotide and dopamine agonists. In these patients, combined therapy with these two medications also suppresses excessive hormone secretion and may, in addition, also cause a reduction in tumor size.

The most relevant side effects of the drug are observed at gallbladder level since it reduces contractility and delays gallbladder emptying. This may lead to particle deposits and possibly to gallstones in up to 20-25% of patients under chronic (over 1 year) treatment. Other less relevant side effects are the gastro-intestinal disorders related to the octreotide-induced reduction in pancreatic secretion and gastro-intestinal motility.

RESISTANCE TO MEDICAL TREATMENT

Hypersecretion A certain number of patients will show primary resistance to medical treatment; a certain number will develop resistance during therapy. Of the latter some, but not all, will subsequently respond to another substance of the same family (i.e. ergoline instead of ergopeptine) or to a different compound (i.e. octreotide).

Tumor volume reduction Volume reduction usually, but not necessarily, parallels hormone secretion suppression. A proportion of tumors will not regress during medical treatment. Although the percentage of these resistant tumors is probably less than 20% in terms of biology, it may be larger in terms of clinical significance. In fact, a biologically significant tumor shrinkage (> 25% of initial volume) may be insufficient to produce clinical improvement because of the initial size or the localization of the adenoma.

MEDICAL TREATMENT WITHDRAWAL

Medical treatment, with few exceptions, does not provide a definite cure for pituitary adenomas. Hormone hypersecretion will generally resume and tumor reexpansion will occur shortly after treatment withdrawal, in most cases. Early volume reexpansion is less common after long-term treatment because of late adenoma fibrosis (induced especially by dopamine agonists): tumor enlargement, however, is likely to occur in the long-term. An alternative therapeutic approach is, therefore, to continue treatment attempting to reduce the dose of the medication after control of the initial hormone hypersecretion and tumor volume has been achieved.

CONCLUSIONS

Great advancements have been made over the last decade in the treatment of pituitary tumors: a) better image localization of the tumor, more sophisticated procedures and modern technology have improved the results both of surgery and radiation and have also reduced the unfavorable consequences; b) more potent and more specific dopamine agonists and somatostatin analogs have increased the percentage of responsive patients to medical treatment and have provided effective alternative or adjuvant therapeutic approaches to pituitary tumors.

Due to the variety of therapeutic options, a comprehensive therapeutic plan is needed today for each patient with a pituitary tumor. This plan should consider first and second choice treatment and the possibility of combining various treatments. The choice and the order of the treatment protocol will be determined by the characteristics of the tumor, the characteristics of the patient, the particular experience of the physician and the availability and access to specialized and qualified facilities for both diagnostic and therapeutic procedures.

There are, however, several clinical problems that still require further therapeutic improvement based on a better understanding of the pituitary adenoma biology. These include:

a) selection of patients that may be usefully treated with life-long medical treatment;

b) selection of tumors that will not show a reduction in volume with medical treatment;

c) medical treatment of the so-called non functioning adenomas;

d) treatment of asymptomatic non-functioning intrasellar adenomas diagnosed incidentally;

e) therapeutic approach to minimal residual disease after surgical removal of a pituitary adenoma.

These and other therapeutic problems will be discussed in this Clinical Symposium. It must be pointed out, however, that this is a field in continuous and rapid progress. New drugs, new formulations of already available drugs (including longer active forms and nasal sprays) will provide further improvement for the medical treatment of pituitary adenomas. At the same time a better understanding of the biology of the different adenomas will provide a rational basis for a more extensive and effective application of medical treatment in the management of this disease.

REFERENCES

1. Bevan J.S., Webster J., Burke C.W. and Scanlon M.F. (1992): Endocr. Rev. 13: 220.
2. Fahlbusch R. (1981): In: Beardwell C. and Robertson G.L. (eds). The Pituitary. Butterworth. London. 76.
3. Gorden P., Comi R.J. and Maton P.N. et al. (1989): Ann. Inter. Med. 110: 35-50.
4. Johnston D.G., Hall K., Kendall-Taylor P., Ross W.M., Crombie A.L., Cook D.B. and Watson M.J. (1986): Clin. Endocr. (Oxf) 24: 675.
5. Liuzzi A., Dallabonzana D., Opizzi G., Verde G.G., Cozzi R., Chiodini P. and Lucarelli G. (1985): N. Engl. J. Med. 313: 656.
6. Martinez de la Escalera G. and Weiner R. (1992): Endocr. Rev. 13: 241.
7. Stephanian E., Lunsford L.D., Coffey R.J., Bissonette D.J. and Flickinger J.C. (1992): Neurosurg. Clin. N. Am. 3 (1): 207-218.

Frontiers in Endocrinology
Volume 9 - 1994

Etiopathogenesis of Pituitary Adenomas

A.A. Sinisi, A. D'Apuzzo, D. Pasquali and A. Bellastella

Chair of Endocrinology, Facoltà di Medicina e Chirurgia,
II University of Naples, Via Pansini 5, 80131 Naples, Italy

Pituitary adenomas occur in the general population with an estimated prevalence of 0.020-0.025%, but they have been found in 10-22% of unselected adult autopsies and represent 15% of intracranial tumours (4, 31, 41). These tumours are most prevalent in middle and old age (29), without significant sex-differences except for microprolactinomas and ACTH-secreting adenomas, for which the female/male ratio is 20/1 and 4/1, respectively (4, 20, 31).

Pituitary adenomas are benign neoplasms, arising from adenohypophysial cells, characterized by unrestrained cell proliferation and excessive secretion of intact pituitary hormones or/and their subunits. Adenomas determine variable clinical manifestations, depending on peptide type(s) secreted and/or mass growth. At pathology, PRL-secreting adenomas are the most commonly occurring tumour type (27%), followed by null-cell adenoma (25%), somatotroph adenomas and corticotroph adenoma (14%) (31).

PATHOGENESIS

Pathogenesis of pituitary tumours still remains elusive. Whether the basic alteration responsible for neoplastic development and growth is a primary pituitary or hypothalamic abnormality has been the object of debate for a long time and detailed discussions on this topic are reported in the literature (20, 36, 40, 50).

Recent advances on biochemical and molecular studies of pituitary tumours have clarified that a single abnormality underlying the neoplastic process is unlikely and that tumorigenesis is a multistep process in which an initial genetic transforming event on adenohypophysial cells is followed by cell proliferation and tumour progression, determined by several promoting or suppressing factors (20, 36).

CLONAL ORIGIN

Mono or plurihormonal secretion of pituitary adenomas suggests that the originating cell is an indifferentiated pluripotent stem cell, undergoing unidirectional or multidirectional differentiation (15, 27). Pituitary adenomatous cells are pluripotential, transforming their phenotype to another one (transdifferentiation) (34, 42). Moreover, a single pituitary cell may express multiple genes, as suggested by the evidence of a pituitary specific transcription factor, the Pit-1 (or GHF-1), a protein with the binding domain on promoter sequence of structurally related GH, PRL and TSH genes (34, 42). This protein is expressed also in adenomatous tissue and may have a possible role not only in the determination of cell phenotype and hormonal activity of neoplasms, but also in the regulation of tumour growth (7).

Clonality studies revealed conclusively that most, if not all, pituitary adenomas are clonal, originating in one single cell (2, 23, 24, 46). The monoclonal nature of pituitary tumours implies that a genomically altered pituitary cell undergoes clonal expansion. Instead, if hypothalamic or hormonal alteration is the cause of the initial cell transformation, cell proliferation would be expected to be polyclonal.

SOMATIC MUTATIONS AND RECEPTOR ABNORMALITIES

A mutation in a single adenohypophysial cell could be the initial step of tumorigenesis. Mutations in genes controlling cell growth and function have been disclosed in a minority of pituitary tumours In GH-secreting adenomas, a mutation in the G stimulating (Gs) gene has been firstly described which encodes protein subunits associated with the GHRH receptor (33, 54). Mutated Gs α-chain has single-point substitution (arginine 201, substituted by cysteine or histidine, and glutamine 227 by arginine or leucine, respectively) (39), inactivating GPTase and resulting in elevated adenyl cyclase activity, cAMP formation, GH production and increased cell growth (10, 11). Transgenic mice for this mutation show pituitary hyperplasia, suggesting that the G-protein mutation results in oncogenic protein, termed the gsp oncogene, that cause some pituitary tumours (13). Constitutively activated Gs mimicks GHRH rendering cells unresponsive to further GHRH stimulation (33). Tumours with gsp oncogene are smaller, with higher basal GH level unresponsive to GHRH stimulation, whereas they show TRH, dopamine, and somatostatin responsiveness, indicating that specific inhibiting G protein (Gi) is normal (49, 54). Gs mutation has been identified in about 40% of GH secreting adenomas, but also in non functioning adenoma and in ACTH-secreting adenoma (21, 53). Gs mutation has been found in McCune-Albright syndrome, which includes pituitary adenoma (58).

Other activating gene mutations have been reported in pituitary tumours.

Mutation in codon 12 of H-ras gene has been revealed in an invasive dopamine-resistant prolactinoma (30). Mutation in protein-kinase has also been described in pituitary tumours leading to inappropriate activity of this protein involved in the cAMP-dependent intracellular signalling (3). Thus the unrestrained hormone secretion and the dysregulation of cell replication in pituitary tumour may be caused by transcriptional activation, triggered by abnormal signal transduction (50).

Mutations of tumour suppressor genes have been described in other human tumours and could also be involved in the pathogenesis of pituitary adenomas. Loss of heterozigosity of the MEN-1 tumour suppression gene, mapping to chromosome locus 11q13, has been found in 3 prolactinomas (14, 25). No alteration of other known tumour suppression gene (p53, RB gene) has been reported (17, 50). Interestingly, it has been mapped to the long arm of chromosome 11, distal to the 11q13 locus, the H-ras locus and, to the pericentromeric region near to the 11q13 locus, the hst-1 gene, which express a member of fibroblastic growth factor family (FGF) (25), involved in the paracrine control of pituitary cell growth (see below).

HYPOTHALAMIC ROLE

Whilst it seems likely that the primary defect in pituitary tumour formation lies within the pituitary itself, the role of hypothalamic factors in facilitating tumour growth is supported by several observations, but remains to be further explored.

Somatomammotropic hyperplasia and GH-secreting tumours develop in GH-RH transgenic mice (6, 52) and in men with GH-RH hypersecretion (5, 60). However, no evidence of cellular hyperplasia in the tissue surrounding pituitary tumours implies an effect on sensitive cells only. Dysregulation of hormone secretion, like absent down-regulation to releasing hormones, elevated pulsatile release, normalization of paradoxical responses after ectopic GH-RH secreting tumour removal are findings supporting a role of prolonged GH-RH hypersecretion in the pathogenesis of these tumours (24, 26, 44, 48). Lack of hypothalamic inhibiting hormones could have a role in the development and progression of some pituitary tumours. However, deficiency of somatostatin is difficult to prove, and several pituitary adenomas respond to octreotide administration. Lack of dopaminergic inhibition appears to be responsible for progression of prolactinoma, but not for initial growth. Alterations in vascular supply may reduce dopaminergic inhibition at pituitary level and promote tumour progression in prolactinomas, rather than their initial growth (36).

In dopamine-resistant rat pituitary tumours, very low levels of Go protein are present, associated to D2 receptor (16), suggesting that a possible mutation of D2 receptor may be involved. In human tumours, a defective transduction mechanism has been demonstrated at D2 receptor level (51).

Nelson's syndrome development after adrenal removal in Cushing's disease, and, in rare instances, pituitary tumour growth in long-standing hypogonadism or thyroid hormone resistance syndrome suggest a possible promoting or, less likely, a transforming role of absent target hormone negative feedback (56).

PARACRINE AND GROWTH FACTORS

Evidence of the production of intrapituitary hypothalamic releasing or inhibiting hormones suggests a paracrine role of these hormones as tumour promotors: CRH, GH-RH, GH-IH, TRH and VIP expressed in tumoral tissues can stimulate or inhibit hormone secretion, increase DNA synthesis, induce c-fos expression and cell replication (9, 12, 19, 28, 36, 37, 43, 48, 55). Other paracrine factors, such as IGF-1, FGF, bFGF, TG, EGF, IL-6, produced by normal and adenomatous pituitary gland, may be involved in pituitary tumorigenesis, as transforming, promoting, or hormone secretion modulating agents (1, 8, 18, 20, 22, 32, 36, 38, 47, 50, 57, 59).

CONCLUSIONS

Recent advances in molecular biology have clarified some aspects of pituitary adenoma development, which is actually considered a multistep process. The initial step may be a somatic mutation in the primordial or differentiated adenohypophysial cell, inducing changes in genes usually regulating cell growth and function. These mutations transform the normal cell into an adenomatous cell, capable of unrestrained multiplication leading to monoclonal tumour development. Genetic mutations so far detected in a minority of pituitary tumours involve both activating oncogenes (gsp, H-ras) and anti-oncogenes (MEN-1 locus). It is possible that hypothalamic dysregulation alone may initiate pituitary tumorigenesis, but, more likely, its role may be to promote transformed cell to clonal expansion. Alternatively, hypothalamic releasing or inhibiting hormone altered secretion may lead to proliferation of normal primitive or differentiated pituitary cells, in one of which a somatic mutation may subsequently occur. Clonal proliferation follows this step.

Growth factors, receptor and post-receptor defects in adenomatous cells may have a role enhancing the effects of hypothalamic hormones.

REFERENCES

1. Alberti V.N., Takita L.C., de-Mesquita M.I., Precario S. and Macil R.M. (1991): Pathol. Res. Pract. 187: 541-542.

2. Alexander J.M., Biller B.M., Bikkal H., Zervas N.T., Arnold A. and Klibanski A. (1990): J. Clin. Invest. 86: 336-340.
3. Alvaro V., Levy L., Dubray C., Roche A., Peillon F., Querat B. and Jubert D. (1993): J. Clin. Endocrinol. Metab. 77: 1125-1129.
4. Ambrosi B. and Faglia G. (1991): Excerpta Medica Int. Congr. Ser., 961: 159-168.
5. Asa S.L., Scheithauer B.W., Bilbao J.M., Horvath E., Ryan N., Kovacs K. Randall R.B., Laws E.R. Jr., Singer W., Linfoot J.A., Thorner P.M. and Vale W. (1984): J. Clin. Endocrinol. Metab., 58: 796-804.
6. Asa S.L., Kovacs K., Stefaneanu L., Horvath E., Billestrup N., Gonzalez-Manchon C. and Vale W. (1990): Proc. Soc. Exp. Biol. Med., 193: 232-235.
7. Asa S.L., Puy L.A., Lew A.M., Sundmark V.C. and Elsholtz H.P. (1993): J. Clin. Endocrinol. Metab. 77: 1275-1280.
8. Atkin S.L. Landolt A.M. Jeffreys R.V., Diver M., Radcliffe J. and White M.C. (1993): J. Clin. Endocrinol. Metab. 77: 831-837.
9. Benlot C., Pagesy P., Peillon F. and Joubert-Bression D. (1991): Peptides 12: 945-950.
10. Billestrup N., Swanso L.W. and Vale W. (1986): Proc. Natl. Acad. Sci. 83: 6854-6857.
11. Billestrup N., Mitchel R.L., Vale W. and Verma I.M. (1987): Mol. Endocrinol. 1: 300-305.
12. Boutiller A.L., Sassone-Corsi P. and Loeffler J.P. (1991): Mol. Endocrinol. 5: 1301-1310.
13. Burton F.H., Hasel K.W., Bloom F.E. and Sutcliffe J.C. (1991): Nature 350: 74-77.
14. Bystrom C., Larsson C., Blomberg C., Sanderlin K., Falkmer E., Skogseid B., Oberg K., Werner S. and Nordenskjold M. (1990): Proc. Nat. Acad. Sci. USA 87: 1968-1972.
15. Childs G.V. (1991): Trends Endocrinol. Metab. 2: 112-117.
16. Collu R., Gravel R.A., Forget H., Painson J.C., Lagace G., Serri O., Hardy J. and Drews R.T. (1993): Progr. Endocrinol. 46: 198-204.
17. Cryns V.L. Alexander J.M. Kibanski A. and Arnold A. (1993): J. Clin. Endocrinol. Metab. 77: 644-646.
18. Denef C., Tilemans D. and Andries N. (1990): J. Endocrinol. Invest., (Suppl) 14, 205.
19. Ezzat S. and Melmed S. (1990): J. Endocrinol. Invest. 13: 691-698.
20. Faglia G. (1993): Acta. Endocrinol. 129: 1-5.
21. Friend K.E. Chiou Y.K., Laws E.R. Jr., Lopes M.B.S. and Shupnik A.M. (1993): J. Clin. Endocrinol. Metab. 77: 1281-1286.
22. Gonsky R., Herman, V., Melmed S. and Fagin J. (1991): Mol. Endocrinol. 5: 1687-95.
23. Herman V., Fagin J., Gonsky R. Kovacs K. and Melmed S. (1990): J. Clin. Endocrinol. Metab. 71: 1427-1433.
24. Herman V. and Melmed S. (1991): Endocrinol. Pathol. 2: 61-63.
25. Herman V., Drazin N.Z., Gonsky R. and Melmed S. (1993): J. Clin. Endocrinol. Metab. 77: 50-55.
26. Ho J.P., DeMott Friberg R. and Barkam, A. (1992): J. Clin. Endocrinol. Metab. 75: 812-819.
27. Horvath E., Lloyd R.V. and Kovacs K. (1990): Lab. Invest. 63: 511-520.
28. Hsu D.W., Riskind P.N. and Hedley-Whyte E.T. (1989): Am. J. Pathol. 135: 329-338.
29. Joubert D., Benlot C., Lagoguey A., Garnier P., Brandi A.M., Gautron J.P., Legrand J.C. and Peillon F. (1989): J. Clin. Endocrinol. Metab. 68: 572-577.
30. Karga H.J., Alexander J.M., Hedley-Whyte E.T., Klibanski A. and Jameson J.L. (1992): J. Clin. Endocrinol. Metab. 74: 914-919.
31. Kovacs K. and Horvath E. (1987): Endocrinol. Metab. Clin. North Am. 16: 529-551.
32. Kudlo, J.E. and Bjorge J.D. (1990): Sem. Cancer Biol. 1: 293-302.
33. Landis C.A., Masters S.B., Spada A., Pace A.M., Bourne H.R. and Vallar L. (1989): Nature 340: 692-696.
34. Lefevre C., Imagawa M., Dana S., Grindlay J., Bodner M. and Karin M. (1987): EMBO J. 6: 971-981.
35. Levy A. and Lightman S.L. (1992): J. Clin. Endocrinol. Metab. 74: 1474-1476.
36. Levy A. and Lightman S.L. (1993): Clin. Endocrinol. 38: 559-570.
37. Levy L., Bourdais J., Mouhieddine B., Benlot C., Villares S., Cohen P., Peillon F. and Joubert D. (1993): J. Clin. Endocrinol. Metab. 76: 85-90.
38. Li Y., Koga M., Kasayama S., Matusmoto K., Arita N., Hayakawa T. and Sato B. (1992): J. Clin. Endocrinol. Metab. 75: 1436-1441.
39. Lyons J., Landis C.A., Harsh G., Vallar L., Grunewald K., Feichtinger H., Kuan-Yang D., Clark O.H., Kawasaki E., Bourne H.R. and Mc Cormick F. (1990): Science 249: 655-659.
40. Melmed S. (1992): Endocrinol. Metab. Clin. North Am. 21: 539-551.
41. Molitch M.E. and Russel E.J. (1990): Ann. Intern. Med. 112: 925-931.

42. Nelson C., Albert V.R., Elsholtz H.P., Lu Li W. and Rosenfeld, M.G. (1988): Science 239: 1400-1405.
43. Pagesy P., Li J.Y., Rentier-Delrue F., Delalande O., Le Bouc Y., Kujas M., Joubert D., Martial J. and Peillon F. (1990): Acta Endocrinol. 122: 745-752.
44. Santo T., Asa S.L. and Kovacs K. (1988): Endocr. Rev. 9: 357-373.
45. Scholar E.M. and Paul S. (1991): Cancer 67: 1561-1564.
46. Schulte H.M., Oldfield E.H., Allolio B., Katz D.A., Berkman R.A. and Ali I.U. (1991): J. Clin. Endocrinol. Metab. 73: 1302-1308.
47. Silverlight J.J., Prysor-Jones R.A. and Jenkins J.S. (1990): Clin. Endocrinol. 32: 669-676.
48. Spada A., Elhai F.R., Arosio M., Sartorio A., Guglielmino L., Vallar L., and Faglia G. (1987): J. Clin. Endocrinol. Metab. 64: 585-591.
49. Spada A., Arosio M., Bochicchio D., Bazzoni N., Villar L., Bassetti M. (1990): J. Clin. Endocrinol. Metab. 71: 1421-1426.
50. Spada A., Vallar L. and Faglia G. (1994): Eur. J. Endocrinol. 130: 43-52.
51. Spada A., Bassetti M., Elhai R.F., Arosio M., Gil-del-Alamo P. and Vallar L. (1994): J. Clin. Endocrinol. Metab., 78: 411-417.
52. Stefaneanu L., Kovacs K. and Horvath E. (1989): Endocrinology 125: 2710.
53. Tordjman K., Stern N., Ouaknine G., Yossiphov Y., Razon N., Nordenskjold M. and Friedman E. (1993): J. Clin. Endocrinol. Metab. 77: 765-69.
54. Vallar L., Spada A. and Giannattasio G. (1987): Nautre 330: 566-568.
55. Wakabayashi I., Inokuchi K., Hasegawa O., Sugihara H. and Minami S. (1992): J. Clin. Endocrinol. Metab. 74: 357-361.
56. Watanabe K., Kameya T. Yamauchi A., Yamamoto N., Kuwayama A., Takei I., Maruyama H. and Saruta T. (1993): J. Clin. Endocrinol. Metab. 76: 1025-1030.
57. Webster J., ten Horn C.D., Bevan J.S., Ham J. and Scanlon M.F. (1991): J. Clin. Endocrinol. Metab. 72: 687-692.
58. Weinstein L.S., Shenker A., Gejman P.V., Merino M.J., Friedman E. and Spiegel A.M. (1991): N. Engl. J. Med. 325: 1688-1695.
59. Yamashi R.S. Weiss M. and Melmed S. (1986): J. Clin. Endocrinol. Metab. 63: 730-735.
60. Zimmermann D., Young W.F., Ebersold M.J., Scheithauer B.W., Kovacs K., Horvath E., Whitaker M.D., Eberhardt N.L., Downs T.R. and Frohman L.A. (1993): J. Clin. Endocrinol Metab. 76: 216-222.

Frontiers in Endocrinology
Volume 9 - 1994

Medical Treatment of Pituitary Adenomas

R. Cozzi, P. Orlandi, D. Dallabonzana, S. Strada, R. Attanasio and G. Oppizzi

Division of Endocrinology, Ospedale Niguarda, 20162 Milan, Italy

INTRODUCTION

The first reports in the 70s of tumor regression and improvement in visual damage induced by bromocriptine (Br) (8, 34) in macroprolactinoma (MP) heralded a new era in the approach to the treatment of prolactinomas and, later on, of the other pituitary tumors. At present, the inhibition of hormonal secretion by the adenoma has a well established role only in the treatment of hypersecreting tumors. In these cases, neuroactive drugs may exert their effects at different levels in the biosynthesis and/or secretion of pituitary hormones, i.e. increasing inhibitory inputs, by exerting agonist effect on inhibitory neurohormones, and/or counteracting stimulatory neurohormones.

MACROPROLACTINOMAS

Bromocriptine, and similarly the other dopamine agonists (DA), induce normalization of PRL in more than 80% of the patients, a significant shrinkage of the tumor in about 60% of patients, and an occasional improvement in pituitary function.

The reduction in size of the tumor occurs only in those patients in whom DA inhibit PRL secretion by stimulating D2 dopamine receptors, that are retained on tumoral lactotrophs; it is due to a lactotroph cell size reduction. Dopamine receptors are negatively coupled with adenylate cyclase with reduction in intracellular cAMP levels, that is an important mechanism whereby dopamine and DA inhibit hormone release. Although in prolactinomas the PRL secreting cells usually remain sensitive to DA, these drugs do not provide a definite cure for MP. It is still debated whether the DA treatment can be stopped after its therapeutic effects have been consolidated (17). Immediate tumor reexpansion after drug withdrawal may occur after short or medium term therapy; on the contrary, early tumor reexpansion is less common after long-term treatment. In our series of long-term treated MP patients, a stable return to normal of PRL was obtained in 28 cases (empty sella demonstrated in 20). After a very gradual Br dose reduction, PRL reincreased in 10 cases; in the remaining 18 who could completely withdraw Br PRL levels remained normal only in 2 but reincreased in the other 16 patients. Therefore it seems that MP are not completely cured even by a very prolonged treatment and DA have to be administered lifelong to the majority of these patients. Improvement in vision is a very common concomitant occurrence of tumor size reduction in patients with chiasmal compression and may precede the radiological changes.

Thus it is mandatory to use DA therapy as primary treatment in MP, whereas surgery should be reserved only to DA-resistant or -intolerant patients.

After bromocriptine many other DA have been introduced in clinical practice, such as lisuride, lergotrile, terguride, quinagolide (CV 205-502), and cabergoline. The main differences between Br and these other more recent DA compounds concern quinagolide, that has been shown to be able to suppress PRL levels in 50% of DA-resistant patients (22) and cabergoline, that possesses a very long-lasting inhibitory effect on PRL secretion, so that it can be given in weekly doses (19). Somatostatin (SS) receptor autoradiography has shown the presence of SS receptors in only one PRL secreting tumor out of 5 cases (37); on a clinical ground, neither SS nor octreotide (OC) showed an acute inhibitory effect on PRL levels in prolactinomas (30). It is unlikely that OC therapy is effective in the control of hyperprolactinemia in patients with prolactinoma, as compared to the successful effect of DA. Pituitary scintigraphy by ^{111}In-OC (pentetreotide) has shown a slight visualization of the adenoma in 3 out of 4 patients and in two of them PRL levels decreased by 20-50% after the acute OC administration. At present no clinical studies have shown any effectiveness of OC in the treatment of patients with MP.

ACROMEGALY

The clinical availability of the long-acting SS analogue OC has greatly increased the efficacy of medical treatment of patients with acromegaly, particularly when compared to Br that has been the first effective drug for this disease.

Most GH secreting pituitary adenomas maintain, at least qualitatively, a normal sensitivity to the hypothalamic regulatory hormones SS and GHRH.

The chronic administration of OC results in stable GH and IGF-I decrease in the majority of the patients. The effect of the drug is soon evident at the beginning of the treatment and persists until OC is given. Escape phenomena are not generally observed and in patients whose GH levels are suppressed OC may induce tumor shrinkage.

In the past, serum GH levels of less than 10 ng/ml were used as the cut-off point in defining "cure" for acromegaly. IGF-I is a very sensitive indicator of

GH hypersecretion and it is highly reliable to assess the success of therapy, since a good correlation has been found with the mean 24 h GH levels. Nowadays, the criterion of cure in acromegaly has become stricter: the term of biochemical cure means (near) normal IGF-I levels. Normal IGF-I levels are reached in acromegalic patients when the mean 24-h GH levels range near to 3.3 ng/ml.

During treatment, therefore, it appears sufficient to follow only IGF-I levels and to adjust the OC dose and/or the number of injections on this basis, together with the improvement in clinical symptomatology.

Today, firm conclusions regarding the use of OC in acromegaly have been reached thanks to several reports showing its high clinical and biochemical efficacy in this disease. The problems on which there is nowadays a general consensus will be considered here.

Forecasting the effectiveness of OC therapy The pathophysiological basis for treating acromegaly with OC is that most GH secreting human pituitary tumors retain a normal sensitivity to the hypothalamic regulatory hormone SS due to the presence of specific receptors on tumor cell membranes. In fact, high affinity SS binding sites were found on virtually all acromegalic tumors investigated, but their number and distribution vary considerably. The number of receptors closely predicts the success of SS analogue therapy (37).

Two predictive tools are clinically available to assess the effect of OC therapy on GH secretion. First of all, the effects of chronic OC treatment can soon be predicted since there is a close relation between GH decrease after the first acute sc administration of 50-100 γ OC and the values of mean plasma GH and of IGF I levels that will be reached during long-term treatment (7) . Secondly, SS receptors can now be visualized *in vivo* by scintigraphy. The close relation reported between the *in vivo* sensitivity of GH secretion to OC and the *in vitro* presence of SS receptors on GH-secreting adenomas (38) has been found even *in vivo* by ^{111}In-pentetreotide pituitary scintigraphy (12). In conclusion, it is clear that the acute inhibitory effect of OC on GH levels reflects the number and affinity of the SS analogue receptors on a tumor.

Dose and administration schedule A daily dose of 100 γ tid sc is the optimal effective dose of OC in more than 50% of patients. This view was confirmed in large European retrospective studies (20, 39), and more recently also by Ezzat et al. (16) in a double blind randomized trial in 115 acromegalic patients. Some investigators have studied prospectively whether a further increase in OC dose (up to 1500 γ/day) might induce a greater control of GH hypersecretion, but no additional effectiveness was reported by increasing the daily dose to more than 300 γ/day. Each sc administration is followed, after a rapid decline in plasma GH levels, by a gradual reincrease after 5-7 h. OC therapeutic effect is improved by continuous sc infusion by portable pump (9, 10): this schedule, in fact, obtains a greater reduction of plasma GH values when compared to intermittent administration, a stable suppression of GH levels, and the normalization of IGF I levels in most patients (at 200-300 γ/day). A good control of GH hypersecretion has been reported to occur also during long-term therapy with OC at the same dose (11, 27): the reincrease of GH values a few hours after each injection is attenuated and the continuous slow but greater decrease of mean GH and of IGF I levels is obtained. In addition to lowering IGF-I levels, OC also stimulates IGF-binding protein 1 (IGFBP-1), which competes with the IGF-I receptor and attenuates IGF-I action (15).

To avoid daily multiple sc OC injections, new formulations of OC and other SS analogues have recently been developed: OC nasal powder leads to the control of GH hypersecretion close to that obtained with sc OC administration, but its poor nasal tolerability does not allow chronic use at present. Preliminary results of LAR OC (long-acting repeatable) or of lanreotide (BIM 23014) show that after im injection a long-lasting inhibition of GH and IGF I levels up to 14-28 days may be achieved.

In only a few patients may a true refractoriness to the drug activity be demonstrated, even if high doses such as 1500 γ/day are used (11). Reubi and Landolt (38) have shown, in these conditions, a low capacity and/or affinity of SS receptors in tumoral cells.

Tumor shrinkage OC therapy reduces the size of adenoma in 37-70% of patients according to different series (2, 7, 29). The degree of tumor shrinkage of GH-secreting pituitary adenomas is less than that observed in macroprolactinomas during Br treatment; nevertheless, the degree of shrinkage is variable, ranging from 20% of the basal tumor area to the disappearance of the adenoma. In addition, the withdrawal of OC therapy is followed by a slow return to pretreatment GH levels and tumor size in most patients.

The mechanism of the effects of OC on tumor size is not clear: electron microscopy and *in vitro* studies show a decrease in tumor cell size, in intracellular GH content, as well as an increased lysosomal development . These findings are consistent with an increased intracellular breakdown of hormones and chronic suppression of GH synthesis, rather than a cytotoxic or vascular effect of the drug. However, in some cases, electron microscopy also reveals some necrotic cells and fibrotic changes (41).

The explanation for the rather variable degree of shrinkage of GH-secreting tumors during OC treatment has recently been suggested by Hofland et al. (21) by the reverse hemolytic plaque assay; a marked heterogeneity of pituitary adenoma cells has been observed, whereby it seems that in GH adenoms only the small portion of high secretory tumor cells, that are responsible for most of hormone secretion, are highly sensitive to OC. This finding may explain the dissociation between GH suppression and variable tumor size reduction.

OC and the outcome of surgery The improvement of clinical conditions by OC before surgery may make anesthesia management easier and lower mortality and/or morbidity due to surgical risks. As for tumor removal, Landolt's group (31) first reported that in five acromegalic patients, previously treated for 1-4 weeks with OC, the tumor appeared extraordinarily soft on operation and that the removal of pathological tissue was easier without damaging the remaining normal pituitary tissue. These data have been confirmed by Barkan et al. (3) who found a higher remission rate following presurgical OC treatment in ten patients with invasive macroadenoma as compared to untreated patients. On the contrary, Stevanaert et al. (42) reported that the complete removal of the adenoma was observed only in patients with "enclosed" adenomas, whereas in the invasive tumors the removal was incomplete, although more extensive. Therefore, whether presurgical OC treatment could become a major indication as routine treatment in patients with GH secreting adenomas has still to be confirmed in a larger series.

Comparison with bromocriptine Before OC was available, DA were the only effective medical treatment of acromegaly. Br still remains the most widely and extensively used ergot derivative. Its GH lowering effect was first described by Liuzzi et al. in 1974 (32) and confirmed by several studies (1, 13): Barkan (1), reviewing the biochemical efficacy of Br in 514 acromegalics from several series, reported that plasma GH was reduced to less than 5 ng/ml in 21%, and IGF I normalized in only 8% of assessed patients. DA rarely induce major shrinkage of GH secreting adenomas, that usually occurs only in a minority of patients, who present a marked response of plasma GH to DA and high basal PRL levels, suggesting that DA exert, similarly to observations in MP, their effects by reducing the cellular volume of PRL-secreting cells largely represented in mixed GH-PRL adenomas. In this type of patient DA might still be considered as the primary medical treatment.

By comparing the effects of Br with those of OC, it is clearly evident that the results obtained with the latter agent are far better: the percentage of patients with normal of GH and IGF-I levels, of improvement of clinical and metabolic conditions, and of tumor shrinkage are indeed higher when OC is used (Table 1).

Table 1. *Comparison of effectiveness of octreotide and bromocriptine treatment in acromegaly (% of patients)*

	Octreotide %	Bromocriptine %
GH reduction > 50%	87	56
GH < 10 ng/ml	75	40
GH < 5 ng/ml	46-53	21
IGF-I normal	36-68	8
Tumor shrinkage	37-70	18
Metabolic improvement	87	59

A few patients are, however, more sensitive to the GH lowering effect of Br (7). Lamberts (25) has reported that the combination of both drugs might be of value in the few acromegalic patients who do not respond to either drug alone.

In conclusion, we suggest the following indication for therapy with OC in acromegaly: A) treatment of patients with active disease in whom surgery and radiotherapy have been unsuccessful or during the period in which the clinical effects of radiotherapy are not yet manifest; B) preoperative therapy to improve the outcome of surgery; C) as primary treatment in elderly patients.

TSH-SECRETING ADENOMAS

TSH-secreting adenomas lead to inappropriately elevated TSH levels and may cause hyperthyroidism but the diagnosis of pituitary tumor is frequently delayed until visual disturbances or neurological defects appear. Moreover, the surgical removal of these tumors is usually incomplete. OC has been used for the treatment of these tumors since a high number of SS receptors are expressed *in vitro* in most of them and SS inhibits TSH secretion in these patients (36). Chronic OC treatment of TSH-secreting tumors has been reported to be successful (5): 50-100 γ OC bid or tid normalized TSH levels in more than 70% of the patients, whereas thyroid hormone levels decreased in all and were normalized in 78%. Comparable results have recently been obtained by lanreotide. Since, in some cases, during OC TSH levels remain high in spite of the normalization of thyroid hormones, it has been suggested that OC has also an effect on TSH bioactivity. In addition, OC treatment has been reported to reduce tumor volume in more than 30% of patients treated; on the contrary, only very few patients remained partially resistant and remained thyrotoxic during OC treatment or showed a tachyphylaxis to OC (25).

Pentetreotide scintigraphy shows a clear visualization of TSH secreting adenomas, suggesting the presence of SS receptors and forecasting the control of tumoral TSH hypersecretion with OC treatment. In conclusion, OC represents the medical treatment of choice in patients with TSH-secreting adenoma not cured by surgery or radiotherapy; the medical shrinkage of these tumors might be useful to improve the result of surgery.

"NON SECRETING" PITUITARY ADENOMAS

Non secreting pituitary tumors, now better called "clinically non functioning" adenomas (NFPA), represent, in the field of pituitary tumors, the most frequent neurosurgical failure, with a high number of recurrences, and with the frequent need for postoperative radiotherapy. A consistent proportion of them is able to produce glycoproteic hormones or their subunits, as revealed by modern techniques of immunohistochemistry and in situ hybridization. The extensive studies recently performed on the pathophysiology of these tumors have not yet improved the therapeutic approach, and the medical treatment of these is still a open problem. These neoplasms contain a heterogeneous population of anterior pituitary cells, with different receptorial characteristics; in fact, in up to 40% of patients TRH administration may cause an increase of FSH, or LH, or their subunits. In the majority of patients, there is not a distinct hormone marker useful in monitoring the results of a specific medical treatment, and the pharmacological trials so far performed have been based only on the theoretical pathophysiological knowledge. The β-subunit release after TRH may be a future marker for the gonadotropin secreting tumors, but, at present, it is only speculative.

Dopamine agonists, and Gonadotropin Releasing Hormone (GnRH) agonists are the drugs that have been employed until now.

Dopamine agonists Br was the first agent employed and the rationale for its use was based on the frequent evidence of a mild hyperprolactinaemia, the finding of dopaminergic membrane receptors on adenoma cells of NFPA, and the supporting evidence reported by Johnston and Wollesen in 1981 (23, 44), which demonstrated tumor shrinkage during chronic Br administration. Later, Br was shown to be able to reduce the levels of FSH and α-subunits, that are often synthesized in patients bearing these adenomas (43). Since then, several studies have been published on the Br effects on these tumors, and from an extensive review of the literature comprising 179 patients a 20% figure of tumor shrinkage during DA treatment is evident (33). Bevan et al. (4) reviewed seven series for a total of 84 patients, with documented size reduction in 7, and claimed that it is more useful to treat these patients longer rather than to increase Br dosage above 20 mg/day. However, the degree of tumoral reduction that Br may induce is never so impressive as in MP, but sometimes it may be enough to change the degree of optic nerve compression by the tumor: indeed a clear-cut improvement of visual fields has been reported even in the absence of neuroradiological evidence of tumor size reduction (43). The relatively low occurrence of tumor shrinkage in the spite of presence of dopaminergic receptors on cell membranes, may be explained by the presence of a low number of cells with secretory activity. Accordingly, the density of dopamine receptors in NFPA is lower than in prolactinomas, and abnormalities in transduction signals are present in the dopaminergic receptors of these tumoral cells.

Octreotide The rationale for the use of OC in the medical treatment of NFPA was based on the *in vitro* evidence of SS receptors in a high proportion of these tumors (35, 37). Recently this finding has been confirmed also by the *in vivo* detection of SS receptors with 123-I labelled OC and with ^{111}In pentetreotide (18, 24) by pituitary scintigraphy. In addition, *in vitro* studies have shown the inhibitory effect of SS on glycoproteic hormone secretion and/or their subunits by cultured NFPA.

However, preliminary data on the clinical use of OC in NFPA are not very promising at present: indeed from a review of the literature OC, at doses from 300 to 1500 γ/day, only occasionally induces a tumor size reduction (33, 40); in addition, it has been shown that even patients with pituitary scintigraphy positivity may be unresponsive to the treatment (12, 18).

On the contrary, a marked improvement of visual field defects rapidly occurs in a consistent proportion of patients treated with OC, even if it is not followed by the neuroradiological demonstration of tumor reduction. In the French Multicentre Sandostatin Study Group, 65% of patients showed a rapid improvement in chiasmal compression, within a few hours or days (40), that was long-lasting in 30% of cases. The different behaviour of visual defects and tumoral size under OC treatment might be explained by suggesting that OC possesses a direct effect on the retina, optic nerve, and cerebral cortex. Indeed, Ducati et al. (14) reported an improvement in visual-evoked potentials in 60% of their series in parallel with a subjective improvement in vision. To support this hypothesis, even patients with negative pituitary scan have been reported to improve visual damage during OC treatment. However, tumor size has also been reported to increase: a paradoxical stimulatory effect of OC (similar to that observed in meningioma *in vitro*) cannot be excluded, since *in vitro* data have shown a defect in the SS receptor coupling-transduction process (18).

GnRH analogues NFPA are frequently constituted by gonadotrope cells; most patients with NFPA have detectable levels of gonadotropins and/or their subunits responsive to GnRH test. On the basis of this rationale GnRH analogues have been used in NFPA. However, on considering the effects of these peptides on tumor size, only in 3 out of 23 cases reviewed by Liuzzi et al. (33) was an appreciable result obtained. In our experience in 11 patients there was heterogeneous pattern of gonadotropin and α-subunit behaviour, in one patient elevated basal LH, FSH, and α-subunit levels progressively increased during treatment; in 3 other patients no changes or a slight reduction in hormonal levels were seen, whereas tumor reduction was observed in two patients.

As far as concerns the data collected with GnRH antagonists, these are preliminary and it is not possible to draw any definite conclusions concerning their long-term effects.

In conclusion, medical treatment of NFPA is, at present, a discouraging affair for the clinician, who does not possess any effective way to treat this entity. Therefore, surgery is still the treatment of choice, with postsurgical radiotherapy when indicated. When medical treatment has to be planned (i.e. in cases of recurrence with minor or stable disturbances or surgical failure or after a cycle of radiotherapy to arrest the tumor growth) DA have to be employed as the drugs of choice. In addition, pituitary imaging by SPET with 123 I-iodobenzamide, by visualizing pituitary dopamine D2 receptors, might identify patients most amenable to the effects of DA treatment. OC, in our opinion, does not respond to the rational criteria of an effective ratio between costs (i.e. the discomfort for 3 subcutaneous injections, the side effects sometimes present, and the actual daily cost) and benefits; however this drug should be given to patients with very large NFPA, impairing the vision, when the decision to reoperate is still under discussion, since OC treatment represents a temporary alternative with the improvement of visual disturbances in nearly 30% of cases. Better results might be obtained with the use of SS analogues with stronger affinity for SS receptors. At present, the administration of GnRH agonists or antagonists is not proposable.

However, apart from the need for larger series of patients, it would be of great importance to characterize the receptorial status of the adenoma in order to select patients who would potentially benefit from treatment; the lack of these studies could explain, at least in part, the low success rate of these therapies observed so far in these tumors.

REFERENCES

1. Barkan A.L. (1989): Endocrinol. Metab. Clin. North Am. 18: 292-310.
2. Barkan A.L., Kelch R.P., Hopwood N.J. and Beitins I.Z. (1988): J. Clin. Endocrinol. Metab. 66: 16-23.
3. Barkan A.L., Lloyd R.V. and Chandler W.F. (1988): J. Clin. Endocrinol. Metab. 67: 1040-8.
4. Bevan J.S., Webster J., Burke C.W. and Scanlon M.F. (1992): Endocrine Rev. 13: 220-40.
5. Chanson P. and Warnet A. (1992): Metabolism 41(suppl. 2): 62-65.
6. Chiodini P.G., Cozzi R., Dallabonzana D., Oppizzi G. and Liuzzi A. (1989): In: Advances in Growth Hormone and Growth Factor Research, edited by E.E. Muller, D. Cocchi and V. Locatelli. pp 423-36. Pithagora Press. Berlin.
7. Chiodini P.G., Cozzi R., Dallabonzana D., Oppizzi G. and Liuzzi A. (1987): J. Clin. Endocrinol. Metab. 64: 447-53.
8. Chiodini P.G., Liuzzi A., Cozzi R., Verde G. and Oppizzi G. (1981): J. Clin. Endocrinol. Metab. 53: 737- 42.
9. Christensen S.E., Weeke J., Orskov H. and Moller (1987): N. Clin. Endocrinol. 27: 297-306.
10. Cozzi. R., Chiodini P.G., Dallabonzana D., Petroncini M., Verde G, Oppizzi G. and Liuzzi A. (1986): International Conference on Somatostatin, Abst p. 64.
11. Cozzi R., Liuzzi A. and Dallabonzana D. (1989): J. Endocrinol. Invest. 11: 737-40.
12. Cozzi R., Oppizzi G., Orlandi P., Dallabonzana D., Strada S., Benini Z., Chiodin, I., Possa M. and Spinelli F. (1994): 76th Ann. Meet. Endocr. Soc. (in press).
13. Craig A., Jaffe M.D. and Barkan A.L. (1992): Endocr. Metab. Clin. N. Am. 21: 713-27.
14. Ducati A., Losa M., Fava E., Cenzato M. and Giovannelli M. (1991): J. Endocrinol. Invest. 14 (suppl. 1): 120.
15. Ezzat S., Ren S.G., Braunstein G.D. and Melmed S. (1992): J. Clin. Endocrinol. Metab. 75: 1459-1463.
16. Ezzat S., Snyder P.J. and Young W.F. (1992): Ann. Int. Med. 117: 711-718.
17. Faglia G. (1991): Clin. Endocrinol. 34: 173-174.
18. Faglia G., Bazzoni N., Spada A., Arosio M., Ambrosi B., Spinelli F. and Sara R. (1991): J. Clin. Endocrinol. Metab. 73: 850-856.
19. Ferrari C., Barbieri C. and Caldara R. (1986): J. Clin. Endocrinol. Metab. 63: 941-5.
20. Harris A.G., Prestele H., Herold K. and Boerlin V. (1988): In: Sandostatin in the Treatment of Acromegaly, edited by S.W.J. Lamberts, pp. 117-27. Springer-Verlag. New York.
21. Hofland L.J., van Koetsveld P.M., van Vroonhoven C.C.J., Stefanko S.Z. and Lamberts S.W.J. (1989): J. Clin. Endocrinol. Metab. 68: 613-20.
22. Jaquet P., Brue T. and Morange I. (1991): In: Pituitary Adenomas: New Trends in Basic and Clinical Research, edited by G. Faglia, P. Beck-Peccoz, B. Ambrosi et al., pp 287-92. Excerpta Medica. Amsterdam.
23. Johnston D.G., Hall K., Mc Gregor A., Ross W.M., Kendall-Taylor P. and Hall R. (1981): Am. J. Med. 71: 1059-1061.

24. Kwekkeboom D.J., Krenning E.P. and Lamberts S.W.J. (1991) In: Pituitary Adenomas: New Trends in Basic and Clinical Research, edited by G. Faglia, P. Beck-Peccoz, B. Ambrosi et al., pp. 359-364. Excerpta Medica. Amsterdam.
25. Lamberts S.W.J. (1988): Endocr. Rev. 9: 417-36.
26. Lamberts S.W.J. (1988): J. Clin. Endocrinol. Metab. 9: 417-435.
27. Lamberts S.W.J., Uitterlinden P. and del Pozo E. (1987): J. Clin. Endocrinol. Metab. 65: 703-10.
28. Lamberts S.W.J., Uitterlinden P., Schuijff P.C. and Klijn J.G.M. (1988): Clin. Endocrinol., 29: 411-29.
29. Lamberts S.W.J., Uitterlinden P., Verschoor L., van Dongen K.J. and del Pozo E. (1985): N. Engl. J. Med. 313: 1576-80.
30. Lamberts S.W.J., Hofland L.J. and De Herder W.W. (1993): Front. Neuroendocrinol. 14: 1, 27-55.
31. Landolt A.M., Osterwalder V., Jantzer R. and Stuckmann G. (1985): Neuroendocrinol. Letters 7: 94-9.
32. Liuzzi A., Chiodini P.G., Botalla L. and Silvestrini F. (1974): J. Clin. Endocrinol. Metab. 38: 910-12.
33. Liuzzi A., Dallabonzana D., Oppizzi G., Cozzi R., Strada S., Benini Z., Chiodini I. and Chiodini P.G. (1991): In: Pituitary Adenomas: New Trends in Basic and Clinical Research, edited by G. Faglia, P. Beck-Peccoz, B. Ambrosi et al., pp. 383-390. Excerpta Medica. Amsterdam.
34. McGregor A.M., Scanlon M.F., Hall K., Cook D.B. and Hall R. (1979): N. Engl. J. Med. 300: 291-95.
35. Oppizzi G., Dallabonzana D., Cozzi R., Benini Z., Liuzzi A. and Chiodini P.G. (1993): In: 3rd Int. Pituitary Congress, Marina del Rey, CA, USA, June 13-15, Abst. TA-6.
36. Reschini E., Giustina G., Cantalamessa L. and Paracchi M. (1976): J. Clin. Endocrinol. Metab. 43: 924-27.
37. Reubi J.C., Heitz P.U. and Landolt A.M. (1987): J. Clin. Endocrinol. Metab. 65: 65-72.
38. Reubi J.C. and Landolt A.M. (1989): J. Clin. Endocrinol. Metab. 68: 844-50.
39. Sassolas G., Harris A.G. and James-Dedier A. (1990): J. Clin. Endocrinol. Metab. 71: 391-7.
40. Sassolas G., Trouillas J., Treluyer C. and Perrin G. (1993): Acta Endocrinol. 129 (suppl. 1): 21-6.
41. Spinas G.A., Zapf J., Landolt A.M., Stuckmann G. and Froesch E.R. (1987): Acta Endocrinol. 114: 249-56.
42. Stevanaert A. and Beckers A. (1993): Acta Endocrinol. 129 (suppl. 1): 18.
43. Vance M.L., Chester Ridgway E. and Thorner M.O. (1985): J. Clin. Endocrinol. Metab. 61: 580-585.
44. Wollesen F., Andersen T. and Karle A. (1982): Ann. Int. Med. 96: 281-286.

Frontiers in Endocrinology
Volume 9 - 1994

Therapeutic Perspectives for Neuroendocrine Tumors

A. Liuzzi, S. De Cosmo, S. Bacci, I. Chiodini, M. Zingrillo, R. Boffi[1] and V. Soresi[1]

Division of Endocrinology, Casa Sollievo della Sofferenza IRCCS, 71013 S. Giovanni Rotondo; [1]Service of Pneumology, Ospedale Niguarda, 20162 Milan, Italy

INTRODUCTION

The concept of APUD cells, as normal or tumoral cells originating from common ancestral cells of neural origin, has gradually expanded and been replaced by that of neuroendocrine cells; these cells are characterised by neuroendocrine markers and have a far wider distribution than previously thought (5). In particular, it has been appreciated that neuroendocrine tumors are not always well differentiated such as carcinoids, medullary thyroid carcinomas, paragangliomas, but that also a consistent proportion of non well differentiated tumors, namely those of ovary, breast, colon, lung, can be considered as neuroendocrine.

The availability of the long-lasting somatostatin (SS) analog octreotide has allowed, mainly due to the work performed by the group led by Lamberts and Reubi, to reveal, both *in vitro* and *in vivo*, that the expression of SS receptors is a very specific marker of neuroendocrine tumors; furthermore, *in vitro* studies have provided evidence that SS may exert a powerful antiproliferative effect on several non classical endocrine tumor cell lines (10). These studies indicated that non endocrine tumors with neuroendocrine markers might benefit also from an approach with SS analogs (SSA).

The aim of this report is to briefly review the data on the mechanisms of the antitumor activity of SS and its analogs and to consider the preliminary clinical data on the use of octreotide and other SSA as antitumor agents.

Antiproliferative effects of somatostatin and its analog An impressive number of studies (10) have shown that SS and its analogs (SSA) inhibit the growth of a large number of tumor cell lines *in vivo* and *in vitro*. The various steps at which SSA act remain to be established but several mechanisms of action have been identified (22).

A) SSA may exert its antitumor effect by inhibiting the release of the hormones involved in the control of the tumor growth, such as growth hormone (GH) insulin, and gastrointestinal hormones e.g. gastrin, secretin, cholecystokinin (CCK). The importance of this level of action is uncertain, also considering that, in a number of studies, the inhibitory effect of octreotide on GH release seems to be lost during prolonged administration (24).

B) SSA may inhibit the activity of growth factors exerting this effect at different levels. First of all, circulating levels of IGF1 are reduced indirectly by octreotide through the inhibition of GH release; moreover, octreotide increases the circulating levels of IGF Binding Protein 1 (13) and, by this mechanism, can reduce the availability of this growth factor to the tumor cells. More directly, in gerbil fibroma, SS-14 inhibits DNA replication induced by the Epidermal Growth Factor (EGF) by blocking EGF-induced centrosomal separation (13). In the MIA $PaCa^2$ human pancreatic cell line, SS reverses the stimulatory effect of EGF on the phosphorylation of the tyrosine kinase portion of the EGF receptor and this reduction appears to correlate with the decrease in pancreatic tumor growth and volume during chronic administration (8). SS might also inhibit the local generation of Growth Factors. This step could be one of the mechanisms of action of these agents on cells lines *in vitro* devoid of SS receptors (34).

C) SS and its analogs also act directly on the tumor cells; it has been demonstrated that most of the neuroendocrine cells have SS receptors. Octreotide inhibits the growth of pancreatic tumors (AR4-2J) which are very rich in SS receptors and there was a parallelism between the inhibitory effect and the dissociation constant of these receptors. Moreover, in the same cell line, octreotide activates a phosphotyrosine phosphatase, a finding, that may partially explain its antitumor effect (33). Recent studies have provided evidence that both octreotide and IRC-160 stimulate tyrosine phosphatase activity and inhibit tumor growth in relation to their affinity for SSTR1 and SSTR2 receptor subtype (3).

D) SS receptors have been found in a number of cell types of the immune system and octreotide has been shown to stimulate the activity of the reticuloendothelial cells in rat and produce changes in the killer cell activity in man (2).

E) A very interesting mechanism of action of SSA is the inhibitory effect on angiogenesis, in chorioallantoic membranes of chick embryo a dose dependent inhibition of angiogenesis, up to 68% of the control, was observed in the membranes implanted with methylcellulose disks containing SS (4). In this respect, some interesting data have emerged (20) showing the presence of high density SS receptors in the peritumoral vessels of colonic carcinomas, carcinoids, renal carcinomas and malignant lymphomas whereas the neoplastic tissue was devoid of receptors. On the contrary, well differentiated tumors were rich in receptors, whereas the perivascular tissue was poor.

In summary, the mechanisms of the antitumor effect of SS and its analogs are complex and still to be fully elucidated: they involve both the direct effect on the tumor cells and indirect effect through inhibition of the secretion of hormones involved in tumor growth and of synthesis and action of circulating or autocrine growth factors.

CLINICAL STUDIES

SS receptors have been demonstrated in several human tumors both *in vivo* and *in vitro* (10). Clinical experience on the effects of SS analogs has been collected in only a few of them and no conclusive results have been obtained as yet.

Data on the most investigated tumor lines are discussed in the attempt to summarize present knowledge and to envisage possible developments.

Pancreatic tumors The use of SSA as antitumor agents in patients with pancreatic cancers is supported by several experimental data. SS inhibits both spontaneous and stimulated pancreatic growth and there is an inverse relationship between SS pancreatic content and the growth of the gland so that SS has been defined as an antigrowth factor of the pancreas (14). Approximately 95% of all pancreatic tumors occur within the exocrine portion of the gland; the most common form is the ductal adenocarcinoma which accounts for about 80% of all pancreatic cancers and has a survival rate at 5 years of about 1-2%. SSA inhibit the growth of experimentally induced pancreatic tumors in the rat (19); in addition, the growth of human pancreatic tumors transplanted in nude mice is inhibited by the intraperitoneal injection of octreotide (31). Although the etiology of pancreatic cancer is unknown, various factors have been implicated in its growth. GH, secretin, CCK, and other gastrointestinal peptides, inhibited by SSA stimulate the growth of ductal pancreatic adenocarcinoma (6) Pancreatic tumor cells express and produce TGF which is over expressed by the human pancreatic cell line, acts through EGF receptor, and is 10 - 100-fold more active than EGF (30).

In spite of these data supporting the potential usefulness of the treatment of human pancreatic cancer with SSA, the clinical results obtained so far are not conclusive. In 15 patients given 1.5 mg of BIM 23014 day no effect was obtained on tumor progression; however, this dose did not suppress GH levels. Six mg/day of this compound determined, in two of five patients, a clear-cut inhibition of CA 19-9 and a good symptomatic improvement. In 14 patients with metastatic cancer, an objective antitumor effect could not be observed with 100-200 mcg/day of octreotide (17). The importance of the dose is stressed by the recent finding (7) showing that 2000 mcg t.i.d. of octreotide increased the mean survival to 6 months and in 4/10 patients determined a disease stabilization; the quality of life scoring of these 4 patients was comparable to that of healthy controls.

Lung tumors Small Cell Lung Cancer (SCLC) comprises 30% of the total lung cancers and exhibits marked neuroendocrine features (10); since half of the patients at presentation have metastates and the survival rate at 2 years is only 5% in spite of initial response to chemotherapy, there is a strong need for new therapeutic approaches. There are several reasons to test SSA in such patients: EGF receptors have been demonstrated in this tumor (23) and IGF1 has been shown to be a potent mitogen for SCLC (17). *In vitro* inhibition of growth of human SCLC has been demonstrated by BIM 23014 (29). SS receptors have been detected in biopsy samples of human tumors in the majority of SCLC but not in non SCLC and similar results have been obtained by *in vivo* scintigraphy for SS receptors which allows both the primary sites and the metastases to be identified (10).

Since SCLC are characterized by several neuroendocrine tissue and circulating markers and, in particular, by high serum levels of NSE, Soresi et al. (27) have studied the effects of short-term administration of octreotide on NSE levels in ten patients with SCLC and found a significant inhibition of this marker. To test whether octreotide can enhance the effects of chemotherapy, the same group (26) treated 21 patients with limited or extensive SCLC with a seven-day trial of 1500 mcg/day of octreotide before starting the conventional chemotherapy. They noticed a very low rate of brain metastases i.e. 4.5% versus 21.3% of a historical group of 103 patients. Further studies will be carried out using higher drug doses.

Breast tumors A consistent proportion of human breast cancer seem to be of neureondocrine origin and express receptors of SS. Autoradiographic studies (20) have shown that in a large series of biopsy samples 46% of the specimens are SS-R positive and a far higher (75%) percentage of positivity has recently been reported *in vivo* (32). A large body of experimental studies *in vitro* have provided evidence of antitumor activity of SS and its analogs on breast tumor cell lines both estrogen positive and negative (18). This direct effect, which involves the phenomenon of apoptosis (16), requires the presence of SS receptors on the cells; however, SS can also bring about its antiproliferative activity by indirect mechanisms i.e. inhibition of local or systemic growth factors such as EGF and IGF1. In particular, most breast cancers are IGF1 receptor positive and monoclonal antibodies anti IGF1 block the tumor growth (18). The evidence for indirect activity has been provided by Noguchi et al. (15) studying an androgen dependent mouse mammary tumor (Shionogi carcinoma 115) devoid of SS receptors. The administration of octreotide determined a dose-dependent inhibition of tumor growth which was overcome by the treatment with GH; since this tumor line seems to be independent of EGF and IGF1, GH itself seems to be a primary regulator of the growth of this tumor.

Clinical studies with octreotide in patients with breast cancer are so far not conclusive. Low doses of octreotide (100-200 mcg/day) given alone or in combination with bromocriptine have determined disease stabilization only in a few patients (11). More interestingly (28), short-term treatment, but with higher doses (up to 1000 mcg/day) in 10 patients, resulted in partial responses i.e. reduction of metastatic lymph nodes and skin nodules over the breasts in two patients and reduction of the primary site in a third: moreover, a reduction in edema and cyanosis as well as a reduction of pain was observed in most cases. Stabilization of the disease for up to 34 weeks was observed in 2 out of 20 patients treated with up to 2000 mcg/day and in one of them a 47% reduction of the metastases (25). Other trials have attempted to investigate the effects of the combined treatment of effective doses of octreotide given with PRL inhibitors. Arrest of disease progression for up to 6 months (1) and in one patient (9), complete remission of a recurrence were observed.

Other tumors There are uncontrolled clinical trials on the effects of octreotide in patients with prostate or colon cancer with not conclusive results (17). Another major problem is that of brain tumor, such as meningiomas or glial tumors which possess a high density of receptors for SS but, at least *in vitro*, their growth seems to be stimulated by octreotide (10).

CONCLUSIONS AND PERSPECTIVES

The data reported here show that, in spite of the very convincing experimental evidence of the antiproliferative effect of SS and its analogs, attempts to prove the therapeutic value of these peptides is still at the beginning. Virtually all nonendocrine tumors with neuroendocrine markers could benefit from treatment with SSA. We feel, however, that further studies are needed to clarify the question of the heterogeneity of the receptors for SS and, in particular, if there are definite receptors that mediate this activity (34); hopefully, by this approach, a ß emitting isotope-coupled SSA will lead, in the future, to a specific radiotherapy of these tumors (10).

At present, from the clinical point of view there are two basic questions: the optimal doses that have to be employed and whether SSA are effective as primary therapy or whether they are to be used in combination with chemotherapy. Only studies in very controlled conditions will provide an answer to these questions but the data collected so far are promising.

REFERENCES

1. Anderson E., Ferguson J., Morten H., Shalet S.M., Robinson E.L. and Howell A. (1993): Eur. J. Canc. 29A: 209-217.
2. Baxter J.N., Jenkins S.A. and Shields R. (1985): J. Surg. 72: 1005-1008.
3. Buscail L., Delesque N., Esteve, J.P., Saintlaurant N., Prats H., Clerc P., Robberecht P., Bell, G.I., Liebow C., Schally A.V., Vayasse N. and Susini C. (1994): Proc. Nat. Acad. Sci. Am. 91: 2315-2319.
4. Danesi R., Benelli U., Del Bianchi S., Campagni A., Costa M., Agen C. and Del Tacca M. (1993): Proc. Am. Ass. Canc. Res. 34: p. 354 (abs 2109).
5. De Lellis R.A. and Tiscler A.S. (1990): The dispersed neuroendocrine cell system: In: Functional Endocrine Pathology edited by K. Kwac, S.A. Asa, pp 493-512. Blackwell Scientific Publications. Boston.
6. Debinski A.B. and Johnson L.R. (1980): Endocrinology 106: 323-328.
7. Ebert M., Friess H., Beger H.G. and Buchler M.W. (1994): Digestion 55 (Suppl 1): 48-51.
8. Hierowski M.T. Liebow C., Du Sapin K. and Schally A.V. (1985): Febs Lett. 179: 252-256.
9. Hotkamp W. and Nagel G.A. (1990): Europ. J. Canc. 26: p. 177 (abs 122).
10. Lamberts S.J.W., Krenning E.P. and Reubi J.C. (1991): Endocr. Rev. 12: 450-482.
11. Manni A., Boucher A.E., Demers M.L., Harvey H.A., Lipton A., Simmonds M.A. and Bartholomew M. (1989): Breast Cancer Research and Treatment, 14: 289-298.
12. Mascardo R.N. and Sherline P. (1982): Endocrinology, 3: 1394-1396.
13. Melmed S. (1992): In: Acromegaly. Edited by S. Melmed pp. 539-551. Endocr. Metab. Clin. N. A., vol. 21, n. 3. Saunders Company. Philadelphia.
14. Muller K., Runzi M., Laye, P. and Goell H. (1988): Pancreas 3: 609A.
15. Noguchi S., Nishizawa Y., Motomura K., Inaji H., Imaoka I., Koyama H. and Matsumoto K. (1993): Jpn J. Canc. Res. 84: 656-663.
16. Pagliacci M.C., Tognellini R., Grignani F. and Nicoletti A. (1991): Endocrinology 129: 2555-2562.
17. Parmar H., Phillips R.H. and Lightman S.L. (1992): In: Peptides in Oncology II-Somatostatin Analogues and Bombesin Antagonists, edited by K. Hoffken, pp. 2-24. Springer Verlag. Berlin.
18. Prevost G. and Israel L. (1992): In: Peptides in Oncology II - Somatostatin Analogues and Bomesin Antagonists, edited by K. Hoffken, pp. 31-38. Springer Verlag. Berlin.
19. Redding T.W. and Shally A.V. (1984): Proc. Natl. Acad. Sci. USA 81: 248-252.
20. Reubi J.C., Waser B., Foekens J.A., Klijn J.G.M., Lamberts S.W.J. and Laissue J. (1990): Int. J. Canc. 46: 446-420.
21. Reubi J.C., Horisberger U. and Laissue J. (1994): Exper. Biol. Med. 56 681-688.
22. Schally A.V. (1988): Cancer Res. 48: 69-77.
23. Sherwin S.A., Minna J.D., Gazdar F. and Todaro G.J. (1981): Cancer Res., 41: 3538-3542.
24. Siegel R.A., Tolcsvai L. and Rudin M. (1988): Cancer Res., 48: 4651-4662.
25. Somlo G. Vogel C., Flamm Honig F., Linnartz R., Israel R. (1993): Proc. Am. Soc. Clin. Onc. 12: p93 (abs. 172).
26. Soresi E., Invernizzi G., Boffi R., Liuzzi A., Borghini U. and Mantellini P.V. (1993): XVII World Congress on Disease of the Chest., Amsterdam, May 1993, (Abstr. 88).
27. Soresi E., Invernizzi G., Boffi R., Borghini U., Sciraldi G., Mantellini P.V., Gramegna G. and Liuzzi A. (1994): Tumori (in press).
28. Stolfi R., Parisi A.M. and Jacobelli S. (1990): Anticanc. Res., 10: 203-204.
29. Taylor J.E., Coy D.H. and Moreau J.P. (1988): Biochem. Biophys. Res. Comm., 153: 81-86.

30. Todaro G.J., Fryling, C. and De Laro J.E. (1980): Proc. Natl. Acad. Sci. USA 77: 5258-5262.
31. Upp J.R., Olson D., Poston G.J., Alexander R.W., Townsend C.M. and Thompson J.C. (1988): Am. J. Surg. 155: 29-35.
32. van Eijck C.H.J., Krennig E.P., Bootsma A., Oei H.Y. van Pei R., Lindemans J., Jeekel J., Reubi J.C. and Lamberts S.W.J. (1994): Lancet 343: 640-643.
33. Viguerie N., Tashiri-Jout N., Ayal A.M., Cambillau C., Scemana J., Bastie M.J., Khnutsen S., Estev J.P., Pradayrol L., Susini C. and Vayasse N. (1989): Endocrinology 124: 1017-1021.
34. Weckbecke, G., Raulf F., Stolz B. and Bruns C. (1993): In: Pharmacological Therapies. edited by D. Shugar, pp. 245-264, Elsevier Sciences. Great Britain.

Frontiers in Endocrinology
Volume 9 - 1994

INTRODUCTION

Diagnostic and Therapeutic Aspects of GH Deficiency in Adults

A. Bellastella and B. Boscherini[1]

Chair of Endocrinology, II University of Naples,
[1]Pediatrics Clinic II, University of Rome Tor Vergata, Rome, Italy

Treatment with growth hormone (GH) is usually limited to GH-deficient short children until puberty. However, the availability of recombinant human GH (rhGH) has promoted several therapeutic trials in GH-deficient adults (GHDA). In fact, physiological GH secretion is still present after puberty and, in adults, it plays an important role in regulating carbohydrate metabolism and promoting anabolism and lipolysis. However, GH secretion declines with increasing age during adult life (5, 11): this reduction was estimated to be about 14% per decade (6). GHDA can show several changes in body composition (2); moreover, they are at higher risk of premature mortality for cardiovascular disease (10), probably due to alterations in cardiac structure and function caused by GH deficiency (1, 7). The aim of this Workshop is to evaluate the progress in studies on GH deficiency in adults.

Problems in diagnosing GH deficiency in children and in adults will be discussed by Camanni who will illustrate, in particular, the usefulness of GHRH+pyridostigmine test. The most common alterations related to the GH deficiency in adults and the effect of rhGH treatment will be subsequently illustrated by Sartorio and Faglia (bone turnover, muscle size and strength), Lombardi (heart and lung structure and function), Delitala (metabolic problems). So far, the following alterations have been described in the literature (9):

Decrease of lean body mass and of its hydration with fat mass increase.
Changes in bone density and osteoblastic activity;
Changes in cardiac structure and function;
Alterations in carbohydrate, lipid, protein and electrolyte metabolism;
Changes in renal function;
Psychological impairment with decreased social adaptability.

The more serious and early the deficiency of GH and IGF1 secretion, the more marked the impairment. Replacement GH therapy in prepubertal age prevents these alterations improving also the final stature. However, the withdrawal of therapy after puberty causes relapse of metabolic, cardiac, renal, body and bone alterations. Thus a prolonged replacement therapy with rhGH should be reliable in these patients but some problems must be considered. In particular, treatment must be scheduled in order to reverse the impairment of the above-mentioned parameters, subsequently improving the quality of life of GHDA and the cost/benefit ratio without causing side or adverse effects.

In the first protocols, the doses of rGH used in GHDA were those commonly employed in the treatment of GH-deficient children (4), but many adverse effects were reported (arthralgias, fluid retention, carpal tunnel syndrome, etc.), which disappeared when the dose was reduced (3, 4). Recent studies have demonstrated that significantly lower doses are able to reverse the alterations due to GH deficiency without causing adverse effects (1, 8).

In particular, low doses of rGH therapy in GHDA can induce:
Return to normal of IGF1 levels and significant improvement of abnormalities in body composition, bone metabolism and cardiac structure and function, subsequently improving the psychological well-being and the quality of life without causing side or adverse effects (1, 8). Since the patients show a return to pretreatment conditions after stopping therapy, an indefinite replacement rGH administration might be suggested.

REFERENCES

1. Amato G., Carella C., Fazio S., La Montagna G., Cittadini A., Sabatini D., Marciano-Mone C., Saccà L. and Bellastella A. (1983): J. Clin. Endocrinol. Metab. 77: 1671-6.
2. Bengtsson B.A., Eden S., Lonn L., Kvist H., Stokland G., Lindstedt G., Bosaeus I., Tolli J., Syostrom L. and Isaksson (1993): J. Clin. Endocrinol. Metab. 76: 309-17.
3. Binnerts A., Swart G.R., Wilson J.H.P., Hoogerbrugge N., Pols H.A.P., Birkenheger A. and Lamberts S.W.J. (1992): Clin. Endocrinol. (Oxf.) 37: 79-87.
4. Cuneo R.C., Salomon F., Mc Gauley G.A. and Sonksen P.H. (1992): Clin. Endocrinol. (Oxf.) 37: 387-97.
5. Ho K.Y., Evans W.S. Blizzard R.M., Veldhuis J.D., Merriam G.R., Samojlik E., Furlanetto R., Rogol A.D., Kaiser D.L and Thorner M.O. (1987): J. Clin. Endocrinol. Metab. 64:51-8.
6. Iranmanesh A., Lizzaralde G. and Veldhuis J.D. (1991): J. Clin. Endocrinol. Metab. 73: 1081-8.
7. Merola B., Cittadini A., Colao A., Longobardi S., Fazio, S., Sabatini D., Saccà L. and Lombardi G. (1993): J. Clin. Endocrinol. Metab. 77: 1658-61.
8. Orme S.M., Sebastian J.P., Oldroyd B., Stewart S.P., Grant P.I., Stickland M.H., Smith M.A. and Belchetz P.E. (1982): Clin Endocrinol. (Oxf.) 37: 453-9.
9. Rosen T. (1994): Growth hormone deficiency in adults. Tryckt & Bunden. Vasastadens Bokbinderi, A.B.
10. Rosen T. and Bengtsson B.A. (1990): Lancet 336: 285-8.
11. Zadik Z., Stuart A.C., Mc Carter R.J., Meistas M. and Kowarski A.A. (1985): J. Clin. Endocr. Metab. 60: 513-16.

Frontiers in Endocrinology
Volume 9 - 1994

Diagnosis of Growth Hormone Deficiency

F. Camanni, E. Ghigo, G. Aimaretti, L. Gianotti, J. Bellone and E. Imperiale[1]

Division of Endocrinology, Department of Pathophysiology, University of Turin;
[1]Division of Internal Medicine, Chieri Hospital, Chieri, Italy

INTRODUCTION

The pathophysiology of growth hormone (GH) deficiency includes either a primary pituitary failure or hypothalamic dysfunction. A GH deficiency may also be sustained by secretion of biologically inactive GH or by different types of peripheral insensitivity to GH or somatomedins (20, 21).

In childhood the diagnosis of GH deficiency (GHD) is based on auxological and hormonal investigations. In adults, on the other hand, this diagnosis is based only on hormonal investigations, i.e. assessment of serum levels of IGF-I and its binding protein and testing GH secretion after pharmacological stimuli, or spontaneous GH secretion, or both. However, there is no consensus as to which test or combination of tests should be used to assess GH status either in children or in adults.

SERUM IGF-I AND IGF-I BINDING PROTEIN CONCENTRATIONS

The serum concentration of insulin-like growth factor I (IGF-I) provides an overall index of GH secretion, and assay of IGF-I is now widely used for screening in patients with suspected GHD. It is important, however, to recognize that the IGF-I concentration is dependent on the nutritional status of the patient (21). Furthermore, the limits of the normal range of IGF-I are age-related and not yet well defined. IGF-I concentrations increase slowly in early childhood, with a further steep increase during puberty. After puberty, a subsequent fall in serum IGF-I concentrations is apparent (14).

We studied IGF-I concentrations in 272 healthy adults (181 females and 91 males, age 20-86 years) and in 36 patients with GHD (20 females and 16 males, age 20-74 years). In normal subjects, serum IGF-I levels decreased significantly ($p < 0.00001$) during the life span, with no significant sex difference. IGF-I concentrations were lower than 2.5 percentile of the normal values in 27 out of 36 (75%) patients with GHD. However, IGF-I levels in GHD patients and normal subjects were more frequently overlapped, from 40 to 80 years, than from 20 to 40 years (61.5 vs 4.4%). In 25 children and adolescents with GHD (5 females and 20 males, age 5-16 years) low IGF-I concentrations were shown in 60% of cases.

The assessment of serum levels of IGF-I binding protein (IFGBP-3) has also been shown to be valuable in screening for GH deficiency (4). However IGFBP-3 was recently reported to be less reliable than IGF-I for differential diagnosis, in adults (13).

SPONTANEOUS GH SECRETION

The evaluation of spontaneous GH secretion should be performed over 24 hours, sampling every 10 min in order to obtain maximal reliability of this approach. Since these modalities are difficult to follow in clinical practice, it is generally agreed at present that nocturnal, 8-12 hours sampling, every 30 min, is sufficiently reliable (1).

It is generally held that the measurement of spontaneous GH secretion is the best approach to detect the existence of low GH secretion in childhood (1, 18, 22). On the other hand, some authors (15, 17) emphasized that there is a great overlap in mean 24-hour GH levels between normal and GH deficient children, if they are matched for age and puberal development. Moreover, spontaneous GH secretion alone is unable to distinguish between GH deficiency due to pituitary and hypothalamic pathogenesis.

In adults, more than in childhood, the enormous variation in the secretion rate of GH associated with physiological variables, including age, sex, body mass index, food intake, nutritional states and physical activity makes diagnosis of GHD very difficult in all but the most extreme cases, in which spontaneous GH secretion is virtually undetectable. In a recent report (13), the overlap in mean 24-hour GH levels was accounted for by the occurrence of undetectable values (<0.2 ng/ml) in 16% of control subjects, as compared with 80% of the GH-deficient group.

To evaluate spontaneous GH secretion over the day, the urinary assay is promising but its diagnostic reliability has still to be definitely proven.

GROWTH HORMONE STIMULATION TESTS

It is well known that GH secretion is increased by physiological and pharmacological stimuli using insulin-induced hypoglycemia, arginine, glucagon, levodopa, clonidine (8, 20, 21). The limits for normal responses to these stimulation tests have not been properly established; therefore, the minimum normal GH peak has been arbitrarily considered to range between 7 and 10 μg/L. The high frequency of low or absent GH responses to these stimuli in normal children (8, 19, 21, 22) greatly reduces the diagnostic reliability also of these tests and has suggested the need to take into consideration the response of at least two pharmacological tests in order to diagnose GHD on the basis of the failure to achieve a "normal" GH level. In adults, however, the insulin tolerance test seems more reliable (13). The availability of GHRH in clinical practice has led to the demonstration that some GHD children, non responders to classical pharmacological stimuli, are responders to the neurohormone (5, 12). However, it has been clearly shown that even the GHRH test does not discriminate between normal and GHD subjects. In fact, great inter- and intra individual variability and absent GH responses to the maximally effective dose of GHRH occur frequently also in normal subjects (16).

The wide variability of the GH response to GHRH is likely due to variations of the endogenous somatostatinergic tone. In fact, as with somatostatin antiserum in rat, in man drugs that may inhibit hypothalamic somatostatin release are able to enhance the GH response to GHRH even unmasking it when absent (10). Among these substances pyridostigmine, a cholinesterase inhibitor, and arginine have been more extensively studied for diagnostic purposes. In contrast to observations using all known GH secretagogues, in normal children the combination of pyridostigmine or arginine with GHRH gives no false negative responses, the GH response always being higher than 20 μg/L (3, 9, 16). Thus, when combined with substances inhibiting hypothalamic somatostatin release, GHRH is able to better explore the maximal secretory capacity of somatotrope cells, thus indicating the existence of a pituitary pool of GH, very much greater than hitherto assumed. Moreover, the enhancing effect of pyridostigmine on the GH response to GHRH does not vary in the various pubertal stages (6) and does not present significant sex differences.

In children with short stature of varying etiology testing with pyridostigmine+GHRH demonstrated a low GH response (<20 μg/L) in all subjects with organic GHD as well as in half of those with so-called idiopathic GHD, and in some children with constitutional growth delay, indicating the existence of a pituitary pathogenesis (9). In the remaining patients with idiopathic GHD and in some with constitutional growth delay, a normal GH response to pyridostigmine + GHRH test, together with low spontaneous GH and IGF-I levels, indicated the presence of a neurosecretory dysfunction, i.e. GH deficiency due to hypothalamic pathogenesis. In another study (7), GH secretion was evaluated in 214 children and adolescents with short stature by assessing mean spontaneous overnight GH concentrations and responsiveness to stimulation with GHRH combined with pyridostigmine. Forty-five subjects (21%) were shown to present GH deficiency. This prevalence was considerably higher than that reported for short children evaluated using conventional testing protocols.

In adults, both pyridostigmine and arginine enhanced the GH response to GHRH to the same extent shown in children. However, in elderly subjects only arginine is able to totally restore the reduced GH responsiveness to GHRH (Figs. 1, 2).

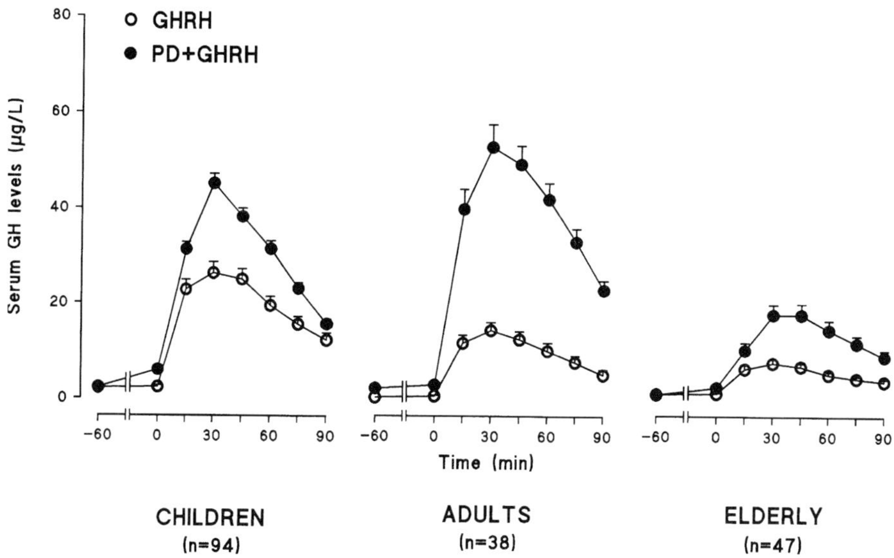

FIG. 1. Serum GH response (mean ± SEM) to GHRH alone and to pyridostigmine (PD) plus GHRH in healthy children, adults and elderly subjects.

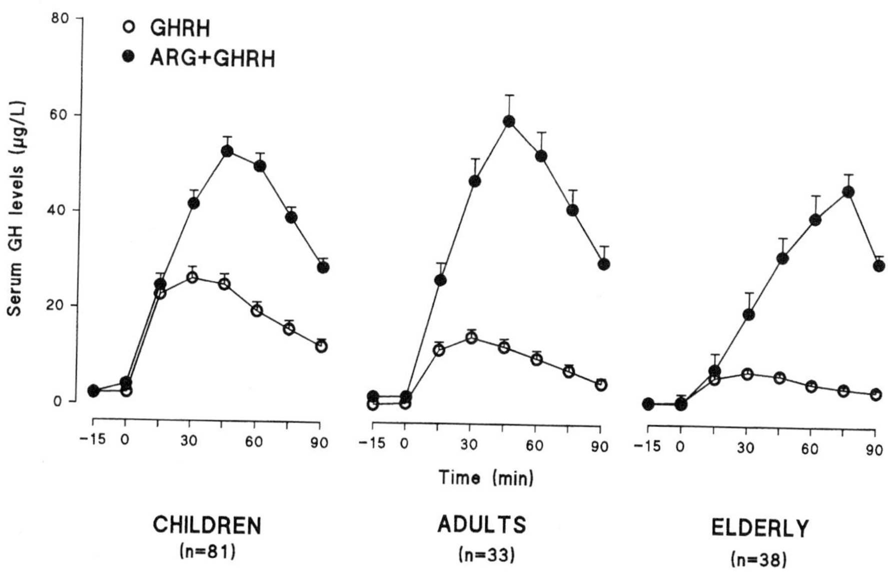

FIG. 2. Serum GH response (mean ± SEM) to GHRH alone and to arginine (ARG) plus GHRH in healthy children, adults and elderly subjects.

Peak GH responses to pyridostigmine+GHRH and arginine+GHRH tests shown in normal adult and elderly subjects are reported in Table 1. In adults the peak GH response to these tests is markedly higher than that to insulin-induced hypoglycemia reported by Hoffman et al. (13). Moreover, the minimum normal GH peak is 17.7 and 16.9 μg/L for pyridostigmine+GHRH and arginine+GHRH tests, respectively, and 5.3 μg/L for insulin tolerance test. Since GHRH combined with pyridostigmine or arginine induces markedly higher and reproducible GH increase, these new tests are also able to detect even minor defects in GH secretion, likely unrevealed by insulin. However, unlike findings in adults, in elderly subjects, the GH increase observed after combined administration of pyridostigmine and GHRH was lower ($p<0.0001$) than that elicited by arginine plus GHRH, suggesting that in aging only the arginine combined with GHRH test is reliable.

Table 1. *Peak GH responses (mean±SEM, range) to pyridostigmine (PD)+GHRH, arginine (ARG)+GHRH and insulin-induced hypoglycemia (ITT) in adult and elderly subjects*

Test	Subjects (n)	Age (yrs)	Peak GH (μg/L)
PD+GHRH	38	27.3±0.7	57.9±4.5 (17.7-114)
PD+GHRH	47	74.7±0.8	20.4±2.3 (3.4-79.4)
ARG+GHRH	33	27.7±0.7	61.0±5.3 (16.9-119)
ARG+GHRH	38	75.8±0.9	48.3±4.4 (11.1-135)
ITT*	25	46.5±3.1	16.3±1.8 (5.3-42.5)

* from Hoffman et al., Lancet, 1994 (13). In brackets = range.

We evaluated the usefulness of the pyridostigmine+GHRH test in 21 adults with suspected GHD. Most patients had major structural lesions of the pituitary requiring hormone replacement therapy. All presented, a stimulated GH peak below the lower normal range, ranging from 0 to 12 μg/L.

The possibility that new synthetic GH-releasing peptides could be useful for diagnostic purposes should also be considered. Recently, one of these peptides, hexarelin,was reported to have a very strong and reproducible GH-releasing activity both in adults (11) and in children with normal or familial short stature (2).

CONCLUSIONS

Definition of GH deficiency is clearly more challenging in adults than in children. Conventional provocative tests of GH secretion, extensively used so far, should be considered obsolete on account of their low diagnostic efficacy as shown by the frequent occurrence of false negative results. Some of the new neuro-pharmacological tests assessing pituitary somatotrope function, i.e., the combined administration of GHRH and pyridostigmine or arginine that induce suppression of hypothalamic somatostatin release must, indeed, be considered more reliable.

Auxological investigations, IGF-I, spontaneous 24-hour GH secretion and the new GH stimulation tests are reliable indicators of sufficiency or insufficiency of GH secretion in children. Moreover, it is now possible using the new GH stimulation tests, combined with evaluation of spontaneous GH secretion, to distinguish between GH deficiency due to pituitary and hypothalamic pathogenesis.

In adults, particularly over 40 years of age, there is a considerable overlap of mean 24-hour GH concentrations and serum IGF-I levels, between normal and GH-deficient subjects, thus making these measurements unreliable in the diagnosis of GHD. Pyridostigmine+GHRH and arginine+GHRH testing should be considered the most reliable biochemical means of measuring GH deficiency in adults and elderly, respectively. These new tests are also able to assess the true secretory capacity of somatotrope cells allowing us to detect even subjects with partial GH deficiency.

REFERENCES

1. Albertson Wikland K. and Rosberg S. (1988): J. Clin. Endocrinol. Metab. 67: 493-500.
2. Bellone J., Ghigo E., Aimaretti G., Benso L., Bartolotta E., Imbimbo B.P., Deghenghi R. and Camanni F. (1993): J. Endocrinol. Invest. 16 (suppl. 1): 157.
3. Bellone J., Valente F., Aimaretti G., Loche S., Cappa M., Bartolotta E., Dammacco F., Camanni F. and Ghigo E. (1993): Pediatr. Res. 5 (suppl): S25.
4. Blum W.F., Ranke M.B., Keitzmann K., Gauggel E., Zeisel H.J. and Bierich J.R. (1990): J. Clin. Endocrinol. Metab. 70: 1292-1298.
5. Borges JLC., Blizzard R.M., Gelato M.C., Furlanetto R., Rogol A.D., Evans W.S., Vance M.L., Kaiser D.L., Mac Leod R.M., Merriam G.R., Loriaux D.L., Spiess J., Rivier J., Vale W.W. and Thorner M.O. (1983): Lancet 2: 119-123.
6. Cappa M., Loche S., Salvatori R., Faedda A., Borrelli P., Cella S.G., Pintor C. and Muller E.E. (1991): J. Endocrinol. Invest. 14: 41-45.
7. Dammacco F., Boghen M.F., Camanni F., Cappa M., Ferrari C., Ghigo E., Giordano G., Loche S., Minuto F., Mucci M., Muller E.E. and the Italian Collaborative Group of Neuroendocrinology (1993): J. Clin. Endocrinol. Metab. 77: 68-72.
8. Frasier S.D. (1974): Pediatrics 53: 929-937.
9. Ghigo E., Imperiale E., Boffano G.M., Mazza E., Bellone J., Arvat E., Procopio M., Goffi S., Barreca A., Chiabotto P., Lala R., De Sanctis C., Boghen M.F., Muller E.E. and Camanni F. (1990): J. Endocrinol. Invest. 13: 307-316.
10. Ghigo E. (1992): In: Regulation of Growth Hormone and Somatic Growth, edited by E.F. De La Cruz, pp. 103-136. Elsevier Science Publishers. Amsterdam.
11. Ghigo E., Arvat E., Gianotti L., Imbimbo B.P., Lenaerts, Deghenghi R. and Camanni F. (1994): J. Clin. Endocrinol. Metab. 78: 693-698.

12. Grossman A., Savage M.O., Wass J.A.H., Lytras N., Sueiras-Diaz J., Coy D.H. and Besser G.M. (1983): Lancet 2: 137-138.
13. Hoffman D.M., O'Sullivan A.J., Baxter R.C. and Ho K. K.Y. (1994): Lancet 343, 1064-1068.
14. Juul A., Bang P., Hertel N.T., Main K., Dalgaard P., Jorgensen K., Muller J., Hall K. and Skakkebek N.E. (1994): J. Clin. Endocrinol. Metab. 78: 744-752.
15. Lanes R. (1989): Am. J. Dis. Child 143: 1284-1291.
16. Mazza E., Ghigo E., Goffi S., Procopio M., Imperiale E., Arvat E., Bellone J., Boghen M.F., Muller E. and Camanni F. (1989): J. Endocrinol. Invest. 12: 795-798.
17. Rose S.R., Ross Y.L., Uriarte M., Barnes K.M., Cassorla F.G. and Cutler G.B. (1988): N. Engl. J. Med. 319: 201-207.
18. Spiliotis B.E., August G.B., Hung W., Sonis W., Mendelson W. and Bercu B.B. (1984): JAMA 251: 2223-2230.
19. Tassoni P., Cacciari E., Can N., Colli C., Tosti M.T., Zucchini S., Cicognani A., Pirazzoli P., Salardi S., Balsamo A., Frejaville E., Cassio A. and Zappulla F. (1990): J. Clin. Endocrinol. Metab. 71: 230-234.
20. Thorner M.O., Vance M.L., Horvath E. and Kovacs K. (1992): In: Williams Textbook of Endocrinology, 8th edn., edited by J.D. Wilson and D.W. Foster, pp. 221-310. W.B. Saunders Co. Philadelphia.
21. Underwood L.E. and Van Wyk J.J. (1992): In: Williams Textbook of Endocrinology, 8th edn., edited by J.D. Wilson and D.W. Foster, pp. 1079-1138. W.B. Saunders Co. Philadelphia.
22. Zadik Z., Chalew S.A., Gilula Z. and Kowarsky A.A. (1990): J. Clin. Endocrinol. Metab. 71: 1127-1130.

Frontiers in Endocrinology
Volume 9 - 1994

Growth Hormone Treatment in Adults with GH Deficiency: Effects on Muscle Size, Strength and Bone Turnover

A. Sartorio[1,2], A. Conti[1,2], M. Monzani[1,2],
M. Narici[3], F. Morabito[2] and G. Faglia[1]

[1]*Institute of Endocrine Sciences, Via F. Sforza 35, 20122 Milan;*
[2]*Italian Auxological Center, Via L. Ariosto 13, 20145 Milan;*
[3]*Institute of Advanced Biomedical Technology, CNR,*
Via A.M. Ampere 56, 20131 Milan, Italy

INTRODUCTION

It is well established that growth hormone (GH) is necessary for normal infant and childhood growth; in children with GH deficiency (GHD), treatment with GH not only results in acceleration of linear growth, but also in increases of skeletal muscle mass and lean tissue (18). On the contrary, the physiological role of GH, once skeletal growth is complete, is still poorly understood, although it has been demonstrated that GH secretion continues in normal adults more or less lifelong (13). Furthermore, little information is available on the effects exerted by GHD in adulthood, although promising studies (1, 2) seem to confirm the notion that GH is also of critical importance during adult life. Nevertheless, before lifelong GH replacement therapy can be recommended to adults with GHD, further long-term studies are needed to establish the overall potential benefits of this treatment.

An analysis is made of our recent results, concerning the effects of GH therapy on muscle function (16) and bone turnover (14, 15) in adults with childhood onset GHD, and compared with those from the literature.

MUSCLE FUNCTION

It is well known that adults with hypopituitarism, although able to carry out normal daily activities, frequently suffer from general fatigue, low physical capacity and muscle weakness (4), which have been attributed to the chronic uncorrected GHD. In this respect, a significant reduction of the torque during isokinetic flexion and extension has been reported in adults with GHD (4). The presence of a reduced muscle mass was confirmed by Jorgensen et al. (9), who found a significant reduction in mid-thigh muscle to fat ratio, as assessed by CT scan. Recently, Cuneo et al. (2) have demonstrated a reduction of skeletal cross sectional area of thigh muscle/body weight, of quadriceps force/weight and quadriceps force/muscle area ratios in adults with the acquired form of GHD (2). The reduced skeletal muscle force has been alternatively attributed to altered muscle mass, contractile elements/muscle fibre, anaerobic energy supply, neural recruitment of fibres, or to a combination of these (2). However, despite the lack of the anabolic effects of GH, it has been reported that these patients have relatively normal mean skeletal muscle fibre areas and proportions of type I and II fibres, without obvious features of myopathy (3).

Since the majority of clinical studies have been performed on patients with the acquired form of GHD, while few data are available in adults with childhood onset GHD, we have recently evaluated the muscle function (cross-sectional area, lower limb volume, quadriceps strength, neural activation of the dominant vastus lateralis muscle) in a group of adults with childhood onset GHD (16).

These patients had significantly lower thigh cross sectional area (CSA) muscle plus bone and lower limb volume (LLV) muscle plus bone than in normals (Fig. 1). This finding is in keeping with the observation that also patients' isometric maximal voluntary contraction (MVC) of the dominant quadriceps was also significantly lower than in controls.

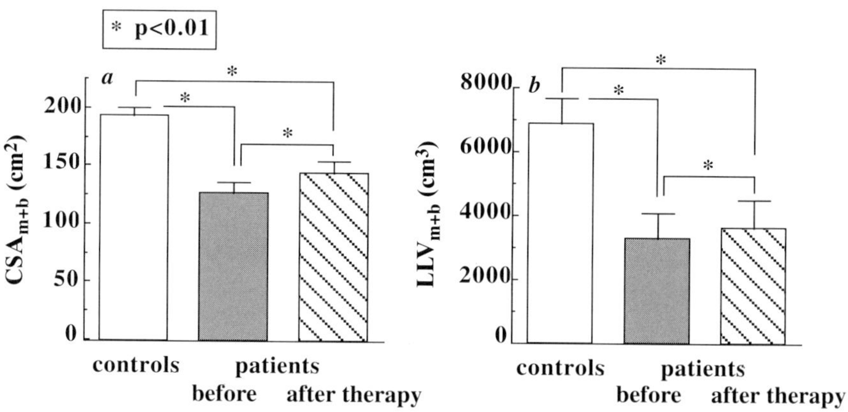

FIG. 1. Thigh cross sectional area muscle plus bone (CSA $_{m+b}$, panel a) and lower limb volume (LLV $_{m+b}$, panel b) of controls and patients.

However, it is interesting that the quadriceps force expressed per unit area (F/CSA) and per body mass (F/BM) were not different from those recorded in normals, thus suggesting that the differences observed in the muscle function between adults with GHD and controls might be due to a simple dimensional scaling. Nevertheless, it is worth noting that six months GH treatment resulted in a significant increase in muscle CSA and force, the increase in CSA being also reflected by a significant rise in LLV, as shown in Figure 1. Muscle hypertrophy alone probably accounted for the increase in muscle strength, since the maximal neural activity did not change after the treatment.

BONE TURNOVER AND BONE MASS

It is well known that GH plays a relevant role on bone turnover, its effects being mediated at least in part by IGF-I (6, 7). The negative effects of GHD on bone (that is, osteopenia, low bone remodeling) have been evaluated in children with GHD (8, 14, 17), while the importance of the metabolic effects of GH has been appreciated only recently in adults with GHD. In these patients the chronic absence of GH seems to exert less relevant effects on bone turnover, as demonstrated by a normal bone resorption activity, in the presence of a reduced bone formation (14, 15). The negative equilibrium between bone formation and resorption might contribute to explain the finding that adults with childhood onset GHD have a low bone mass, in particular at the forearm site (10), probably due to a deficient build-up of bone during childhood and adolescence (10). Recently, Rosen et al. (12) have confirmed the negative effects of GHD on bone in adults with the acquired form of GHD, although the clinical implications of this finding still remain unknown (increased incidence of fractures?). As far as concerns the effects of GH therapy on bone metabolism, recent short-term studies with GH have shown promising results. Several Authors (1, 5, 19) reported that recombinant GH treatment significantly increases the indexes of bone formation i.e., total alkaline phosphatase (T-AP), bone Gla protein (BGP). However, the positive effect exerted by GH on bone formation might be counteracted, at least in part, by the simultaneous increase of bone resorption markers, such as urinary hydroxyproline excretion (19) or carboxyterminal cross-linked telopeptide of type I collagen (ICTP) (15). In our experience (15), GH treatment caused a significant and rapid rise in serum BGP, bone alkaline phosphatase isoenzyme (B-AP), T-AP and ICTP levels in adults with childhood onset GHD (Table 1), confirming the notion that GH increased, although to a different extent (more pronounced for bone formation), the two components of bone remodeling.

Table 1. *Serum BGP, B-AP, T-AP and ICTP levels of patients with GHD before and after recombinant GH treatment*

	before GH	after 3 months GH	after 6 months GH
BGP (ng/ml)	3.8±1.3	28.4±15.0	25.1±14.1
B-AP (IU/L)	44.9±19.6	173.6±113.1	194.4±113.1
T-AP (IU/L)	119.5±41.8	229.5±134.1	247.6±121.3
ICTP (ng/ml)	4.7±2.3	17.5±7.9	15.0±5.4

Normal values (mean±SD) : BGP: 5.4±0.7 ng/ml; B-AP: 58.2±10.6 IU/L; T-AP: 122.3±21.2 IU/L; ICTP: 4.1±2.0 ng/ml.

The ultimate meaning of the GH-induced increase of bone turnover on bone mineral content remains to be elucidated, since the results are partially conflicting. In fact, Ernst and Froesch (6) were unable to detect a significant increase in bone mineral content after GH therapy, not excluding, however, that more prolonged treatment might have positive effects on bone; as pointed out by the Authors themselves, the treatment duration might have been too short and, therefore, the trial design suboptimal to detect any effects. On the contrary, Degerblad et al. (5) have shown a significant increase in the reduced BMD of adults with the acquired form of GHD after GH therapy, although it remains to be clarified whether this effect might be able to modify the risk of fractures of these patients (with a complete "normalization" of BMD). The discrepancies between the different studies might be explained by the degree and the duration of GHD, the trial design, the presence of concomitant risk factors (diet regimen, alcohol consumption, smoking, etc.) and of substitutive therapies for the associated hormonal defects. In our experience, mean lumbar spine BMD and whole proximal femor BMD did not significantly change after six months of GH treatment; on the contrary, the throcanteric subregion showed a significant 4.8% increase, while other hip subregions showed minor changes. Bone mass and bone density of the whole skeleton and of its subregions did not show any significant variation. Although six months of treatment do not seem to exert relevant effects on BMD, it can not be ruled out that the use of recombinant GH, probably at a lower dosage and/or in association with drugs able to counteract the GH-induced increase of bone resorption, might improve the bone mineral content of adults with GHD.

DISCUSSION

The physiological relevance of the metabolic effects exerted by GH in adulthood is still poorly understood, probably due to the fact that until now GH treatment has been strictly limited to children with GHD and withdrawn once skeletal growth is complete. The recent widespread availability of GH obtained by recombinant DNA technology has led us to reconsider the possibility of a substitutive GH treatment in adults with GHD.

Several recent studies have demonstrated that these patients, despite adequate replacement therapy for hormonal deficiencies but not for GHD, have persisting clinical problems which seem to be positively influenced by recombinant GH therapy (1, 2, 5, 19). Furthermore, the recent observation that these patients have a decreased life expectancy, due to an increased risk of premature death from cardiovascular disease (11), emphasizes the need for further controlled studies.

Whether long-term GH treatment of adults with GHD was able to change the prognosis of these patients and clearly improve their health status (quality of life, exercise capacity, lipid homeostasis, etc), the indication for replacement therapy with GH in this clinical condition should be reconsidered.

ACKNOWLEDGEMENTS

Supported by Progetti di Ricerca Corrente, Centro Auxologico Italiano, IRCCS, Milan, Italy. Part of the results produced in the Authors' laboratories referred to in this paper have been published elsewhere (ref. 14-16). The Authors wish to thank Dr Sergio Ortolani for the analysis of BMC.

REFERENCES

1. Bengtsson B.A., Edén S., Lönn L., Kvist H., Stokland A., Lindstedt G., Bosaeus I, Tölli J., Sjöström L. and Isaksson O.G.P. (1993): J. Clin. Endocrinol. Metab. 76: 309-317.
2. Cuneo R.C., Salomon F., McGauley G.A. and Sonksen P.H. (1992): Clin. Endocrinol. 37: 387-397.
3. Cuneo R.C., Salomon F., Wiles C.M., Round J.M., Jones D., Hesp R. and Sonksen P.H. (1992): Horm. Res. 37: 23-28.
4. Degerblad M., Almkvist O., Grunditz R., Hall K., Kaijser L., Knutsson E., Ringertz H. and Thoren M. (1990): Acta Endocrinol. 123: 185-193.
5. Degerblad M., Elgindy N., Hall K., Sjoberg H.E. and Thoren M. (1992): Acta Endocrinol. 126: 387-393.
6. Ernst M. and Froesch E.R. (1988): Biochem. Biophys. Res. Commun. 151: 142-147.
7. Hock J.M., Centrella M. and Canalis E. (1988): Endocrinology 122: 254-260.
8. Johansen J.S., Giwercman A., Hartwell D., Nielsen C.T., Price P.A., Christiansen C. and Skakkebaek N.E. (1988): J. Clin. Endocrinol. Metab. 67: 273-278.
9. Jorgensen J.O.L., Pedersen S.A., Thuesen L., Jorgensen, J., Ingemann-Hansen T., Skakkebaek N.E. and Christiansen J.S. (1989): Lancet i: 1221-1225.
10. Kaufman J.M., Taelman P., Vermeulen A. and Vandeweghe M. (1992): J. Clin. Endocrinol. Metab. 74: 118-123.

11. Rosen T., Eden S., Larson G., Wilhelmsen L. and Bengtsson B.A. (1993): Acta Endocrinol. 129: 195-200.
12. Rosen T., Hansson T., Granhed H., Szucs J. and Bengtsson, B.A. (1993): Acta Endocrinol. 129: 201-206.
13. Rudman D., Feller A.G., Nagraj H.S., Gergans G.A., Lalitha P.Y., Goldberg A.F., Schenkler R.A., Cohn L., Rudman I.W. and Mattson D.E. (1990): N. Engl. J. Med. 323: 1-6.
14. Sartorio A., Conti A. and Monzani M. (1993): Postgrad. Med. J. 69: 846-850.
15. Sartorio A., Conti A., Monzani M., Morabito F. and Faglia G. (1993): J. Endocrinol. Invest. 16: 893-898.
16. Sartorio A. and Narici M. (1994): Clin. Physiol. (in press).
17. Shore R.M., Chesney R.W., Mazess R.B., Rose P.G. and Bargman G.J. (1980): J. Pediatr. 96: 393-396.
18. Tanner J.M., Hughes P.C.R. and Whitehouse R.H. (1977): Acta Endocrinol. 84: 681-696.
19. Whitehead H.M., Boreham C., Mc Ilrath E.M., Sheridan B., Kennedy L., Atkinson A.B. and Hadden D.R. (1992): Clin. Endocrinol. 36: 45-52.

Frontiers in Endocrinology
Volume 9 - 1994

Effects of GH Treatment on Cardiac and Ventilatory Function in Adult Patients with GH Deficiency

G. Lombardi, B. Merola, A. Colao, S. Longobardi, M. Sofia[1], A. Cuocolo[2], A. Cittadini[3], S. Fazio[3] and L. Saccà[3]

Departments of Clinical and Molecular Endocrinology and Oncology; [1]Respiratory Disease; [2]Nuclear Medicine; [3]IV Division of Internal Medicine, Federico II University, School of Medicine, Via Pansini 5, 80131 Naples, Italy

INTRODUCTION

Patients with hypopituitarism generally receive life-long replacement therapy with thyroxine, corticosteroids and sex hormones. Conversely, substitutive growth hormone (GH) therapy is usually withdrawn after epiphysial fusion (19). In normal subjects after that time, however, GH still continues to be secreted acting on glucose and lipid metabolism, muscle and bone mass and adipose tissue (5, 7, 13, 16). In fact, adults with GH deficiency (GHD), submitted in the past to hypophysectomy for metastatic breast carcinoma, diabetes mellitus with retinopathy and acromegaly, presented several impairments related to renal blood flow, heart rate, blood volume and basal metabolism. These modifications remain after conventional replacement therapy (10). Recently with the introduction of recombinant GH (rGH), it is possible to evaluate the benefits of replacement treatment with GH in adults with GHD (2, 15). In fact, an improvement of muscle mass and a decrease of fat tissue, an increase of renal plasma flow and glomerular filtration rate have been described (3, 9, 12, 18). On the other hand, little information is available concerning heart and lung structure. Recently, we reported an impairment of heart structure and function in 11 patients with GHD (6, 14). The effects of low doses of GH treatment on heart structure and function were reported in adults with GHD (1).

Aim of this study was to evaluate heart and lung structure and function using echocardiography, gated blood pool cardiac scintigraphy and spirometry before and after rGH treatment.

MATERIAL AND METHODS

Five patients (2 males, 3 females, 19-32 years old) previously diagnosed as GHD children and 5 healthy subjects entered the study, after giving informed consent. All the patients had adequate recordings for analysis. Four patients requiring hormone replacement took their usual medication on the morning of the study. All the patients were submitted to GHRH with pyridostigmine (GHRH+PD) and clonidine tests. The following criteria were used for inclusion in the study: 1) GH response after GHRH+PD and clonidine tests below 5 µg/L, and 2) plasma Insulin-like-growth factor-I (IGF-I) levels below the normal range for age. The 5 patients had been treated with extractive GH over a 9-year period and had stopped therapy at least 3 years before entering the study. Clinical and hormonal data from these 5 patients are shown in Table 1.

Table 1. *Clinical and hormonal data of the 5 patients with GH deficiency*

Patient (sex/age)	Height (cm)	Weight (Kg)	GH Peak (µg/L) after GHRH+PD	after Clonidine	IGF-I (µg/L)	Diagnosis
1(M 32)	157.7	64	1.7	1.2	146.8	MD
2(M 24)	151.0	44	2.2	1.8	145.8	MD
3(F 32)	164.0	63	1.3	0.7	173.0	MD
4(F 19)	153.0	62	1.7	1.2	151.0	IGHD
5(F 27)	141.5	51	1.7	1.6	162.1	MD

MD: Multiple pituitary deficiency; IGHD: Isolated Growth Hormone Deficiency; PD: Pyridostigmine.

Echocardiography Complete M-mode and two-dimensional analyses were performed using an ultrasound mechanical system equipped with 3.5 mHz transducer (Apogee CX, Interspec, Ambler, CA). M-Mode and two-dimensional recordings were made with the subjects in a lateral recumbent position according to the standardization of the American Society of Echocardiography (17). Interventricular septal and left ventricular posterior wall thickness and left ventricular end-diastolic and end-systolic cavity dimensions were measured by mean values of four consecutive cycles. As ejection phase indices, the percentage of left ventricular fractional shortening was calculated using internal end-diastolic dimension minus internal end-systolic dimension divided by internal end-diastolic dimension multiplied by 100.

Gated blood pool cardiac scintigraphy All subjects underwent a symptom-limited supine exercise testing on a bicycle ergometer. Exercise load was increased by 25 W every two minutes until limiting dyspnea or fatigue developed. Equilibrium radionuclide angiography was performed at rest and during maximal supine bicycle exercise using red blood cells labelled *in vivo* with 15-20 mCi technetium-99m and a small field-of-view gamma camera (Starcam 300 A/M, GE) equipped with a low-energy all purpose collimator. Left ventricular ejection fraction (%), peak ejection rate (EDV/s), and peak filling rate (EDV/s) were measured as previously described (8). End-diastolic volume (ml), end-systolic volume (ml), stroke volume (ml) and cardiac output (L/min) were measured according to the attenuation corrected count-based distance method (20). Volumes and cardiac output were indexed to body size by dividing by body surface area.

Pulmonary function tests All the subjects were submitted to chest-X-ray examination to exclude respiratory disease. Pulmonary function was evaluated in each subject using the same standard approach, consisting in preliminary assessment of respiratory strength, routine spirometry with measurement of lung volumes and recordings of flow-volume curves and measurement of lung diffusing capacity. Strength of the respiratory muscles was assessed under static conditions measuring maximal inspiratory (IPmax) and Expiratory (EPmax) pressures by Mouth Pressure Meter (Chest Scientific Instruments Ltd, Markos Italia). Values were recorded in cm H_2O and were expressed as percent of predicted values taken from Black and Hyatt (4). Lung volumes and flow-volume curves were recorded using a computerized system (2200 Computerized Function Laboratory, Sensor Medics Italia). The subjects, seated first performed three acceptable forced vital capacity (FVC) manoeuvres and flow signals were electronically integrated to obtain volume measurements. The best of flow-volume loops, reflecting the largest FVC and forced expiratory volume at 1 sec from the expiration (FEV1), was selected according to the American Thoracic Society (ATS) criteria (11). The subjects were then asked to perform two slow capacity (VC) manoeuvres the best one being taken into account. VC and expiratory reserve volume (ERV) were then computed. Functional Residual Capacity (FRC) was measured by the nitrogen wash-out method, using a rapid response analyzer mounted inside the breathing valve assembly and measuring breath by breath instantaneous nitrogen concentrations. Residual volume (RV) was computed subtracting ERV from FRC; total lung capacity (TLC) was computed adding RV to VC. Lung diffusing capacity of carbon monoxide was measured in duplicate and mean values obtained using the single breath method (System 2200 Sensor Medics, Milan).

Assays Plasma FSH, LH, PRL, T3, T4, FT3, FT4 and Cortisol were assessed by RIA, while TSH and ACTH were assessed by IRMA using commercial kits. Serum GH levels were assessed by RIA using Radim kits (Pomezia, Rome). The normal range was 0-5 μg/L in males and 0-10 μg/L in females. The intra- and inter-assay coefficient of variation were 6.5 and 5% and 6.7 and 8.9%, for low and high points of the curve, respectively. Serum IGF-1 levels were assessed by IRMA, using commercial kits (DSL, Diagnostic System Laboratories, Inc., Webster, TX). The normal range was 247.2-261.6 ug/L. All samples were run in the same assay.

Statistical Analysis Data are expressed as mean ± SD. Differences between continuous variables were determined using non parametric tests (Wilcoxon and Rank sum test).

RESULTS

In comparison to sex- and age matched healthy subjects, these patients had significantly lower values of interventricular septum (IVS: 7.6±1 vs 9±1 mm, $p<0.01$), left ventricular mass index (LVMi: 53.4±11.3 vs 85±15 g/m2, $p<0.001$) and fractional shortening (FS: 35±3 vs 38±5%, $p<0.03$) using echocardiography. Cardiac parameters were normalized after 6 months therapy with rGH at a dose of 0.05 IU/kg/die (IVS: 7.6±1 vs 9.2±1 mm, $p<0.03$; LVMi: 53.4±11.3 vs 77±4.5 g/m2, $p<0.01$; FS: 35±3 vs 42±3%, $p<0.03$).

These data were confirmed using a more reliable evaluation: the Gated Blood Pool Cardiac Scintigraphy both at rest and during exercise. In fact, the ejection fraction rose from 66±6 to 76±7% during exercise in healthy subjects, whereas in GHD patients it remained unchanged or even decreased, 55±6 and 54±9%, at rest and after exercise, respectively.

After rGH treatment, the ejection fraction significantly improved at rest (61±8%) and during exercise (64±8%), with a $p<0.01$ when compared to baseline value (Fig. 1).

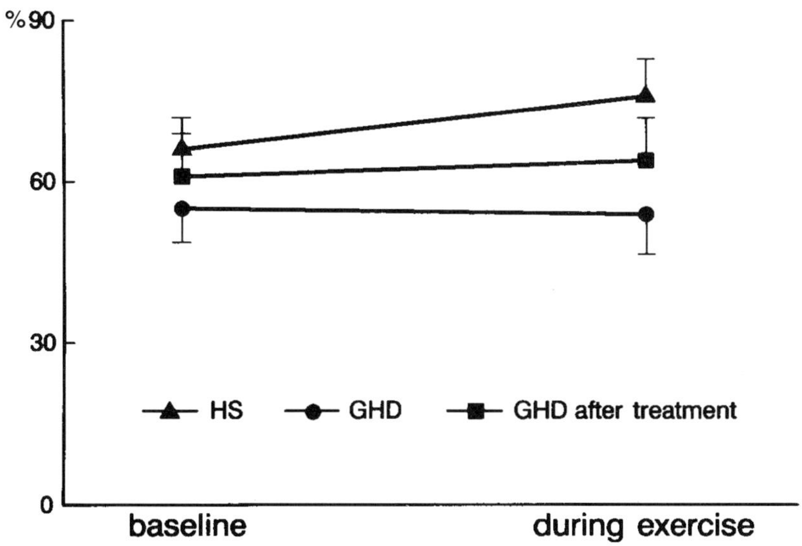

FIG. 1. Ejection fraction. HS = healthy subjects; GHD = GH-deficient patients.

As far as ventilatory function was concerned, both IPmax and EPmax were significantly ($p<0.05$) decreased in GHD when compared to healthy subjects. Lung volumes (Forced Vital Capacity; Forced Expiratory Volume at 1 sec; Total Lung Capacity) were significantly ($p<0.05$) reduced in GHD when compared to healthy subjects while Residual Volume and Diffusing Lung Capacity to CO did not show any significant change (Table 2). After short-term treatment no significant changes were observed in lung volumes and respiratory pressures of these patients (Table 2).

Table 2. *Ventilatory parameters of healthy subjects and patients with GH deficiency (GHD) before and after treatment (± SD)*

	Healthy subjects	GHD before treatment	GHD after treatment
FVC	4.4±1.0 L	3.3±0.9	3.7±1.0
FEV1	3.8±0.9 L	2.7±0.8	2.9±0.8
TLC	6.1±0.9 L	4.6±1.3	5.0±1.2
RV	1.8±0.4 L	1.6±0.7	1.6±0.8
DLCO	26.1±10.9 ml/mmHg/min	20.5±5.8	23.2±7.7
IPmax	113.3±11.9 cm H_2O	93.3±27.0	95.5±26.3
EPmax	158.0±39.0 cm H_2O	96.4±33.8	99.0±30.7

FVC: Forced Vital Capacity; FEV1: Forced Expiratory Volume at 1 sec; TLC: Total Lung Capacity; RV: Residual Volume; DLCO: Diffusing Capacity to CO; IPmax: Maximal Inspiratory Pressure; EPmax: Maximal Expiratory pressure.

DISCUSSION

GH has been shown to maintain substantial skeletal muscle integrity and body composition. In fact, GH treatment induced a rapid increase in lean body and skeletal muscle mass and strength as well as a decrease in fat tissue. Results of this study demonstrated cardiac structural and functional abnormalities in adult patients with GHD. The major findings are a decrease in the wall thickness leading to a reduced LV mass index and low values of ejection phase indices, such as fractional shortening and ejection fraction, compared to the sex-, age-, weight-, and height-matched control group using echocardiography. These data were confirmed using gated blood pool scintigraphy. Cuneo et al. (7) and Jorgensen et al. (12) reporting on cardiological data in GHD adults before and after rGH therapy, found no relevant changes in cardiac mass and function, although Cuneo et al. described a not too well explained significant reduction in fractional shortening in one GHD patient group. Our findings are not in keeping with these reports, and this discrepancy may be partly explained by the different inclusion criteria employed. Cuneo et al. studied patients with adulthood onset GHD, whereas our patients had a childhood onset GHD.

However, Amato et al. found that cardiac structure and function impairment was fully restored after GH treatment at low doses (1). These beneficial effects stopped upon withdrawal of treatment. Furthermore, taking into account that lung volumes are also conditioned by muscle function, we attempted to establish whether any change occurs in spirometric indices in these patients. Routine pulmonary function studies showed, in almost all patients, an abnormal pattern consisting of a mild ventilatory defect of restrictive pattern, characterized by the reduction of vital capacity accompanied by a proportional drop in the FEV1 and corresponding reduction of TLC in spite of relatively preserved RV. The factors responsible for this abnormality may be related inter alia to: poor cooperation of the patients, functional loss of pulmonary parenchyma, constrictive disease of the pleura and chest wall, neuromuscular disease that could decrease respiratory force. However, since, these conditions were excluded at the beginning of the study, this respiratory pattern is probably due to an impairment of respiratory muscle strength. After six months of treatment with rGH, at a dose of 0.05 IU/Kg/die, cardiac parameters improved with an increase in cardiac muscle mass and ejection phase indices, whereas ventilatory parameters showed only an insignificant improvement.

These data suggest that GH treatment in adult patients with GHD improves cardiac function. However, taking into account data reported in the literature (1) further studies are necessary to indicate the appropriate dose of GH replacement. The failure to induce ventilatory improvement may be due to the short-term treatment and further studies are in progress to evaluate the efficacy of long-term treatment to restore ventilatory function.

CONCLUSIONS

In conclusion, patients with GHD show impairment of cardiac structure and performance that were fully restored after 6 months treatment with rGH. On the other hand, impairment of ventilatory function, characterized by the reduction of FVC, accompanied by a proportional drop in the FEV1 and a corresponding reduction of TLC, in spite of relatively preserved RV, was observed. After short-term treatment this impairment is still present even if there is a slight tendency to increase.

REFERENCES

1. Amato G., Carella C., Fazio S., La Montagna G., Cittadini A., Sabatini D., Marciano-Mone C., Saccà L. and Bellastella A. (1993): J. Clin. Endocrinol. Metab. 77: 1671-1676.
2. Bengtsson B.A. (1993): Acta Endocrinol. 128 (Suppl 2): 2-5.
3. Bengtsson B.A., Eden S., Lonn L., Kvist H., Stokland A. and Lindstedt G. (1993): J. Clin. Endocrinol. Metab. 76: 309-17.
4. Black L.F. and Hyatt R.E. (1996): Am. Rev. Respir. Dis. 99: 696-702.
5. Blackett P.R., Weech P.K., Mc Conathy W.J. and Fesmire J.D. (1982): Metabolism 31: 117-120.

6. Cittadini A., Cuocolo A., Merola B., Fazio S., Sabatini D., Nicolai E., Colao A., Longobardi S., Lombardi G. and Saccà L. (1994): Am. J. Physiol. 267: E219-E225.
7. Cuneo R.C., Salomon F., McGauley G.A. and Sonksen P.H. (1992): Clin. Endocrinol. (Oxf) 37: 387-97.
8. Cuocolo A., Sax F.L., Brush J.E., Maron B.J., Bacharach S.L. and Bonow R.O. (1990): Circulation 81: 978-986.
9. Degerblad M., Elgindy N., Hall K., Sjoberg H.E. and Thoren M. (1992): Acta Endocrinol. 126: 387-93.
10. Falkheden T. and Sjogren B. (1987): Acta Endocrinol. 46: 80-88.
11. Gardner R.M., Hankinson J.L., Clausen J.L., Cropo R.O., Johnson R.L. and Eples G.R. (1987): Am. Rev. Respir. Dis. 136: 1285-1298.
12. Jorgensen J.O.L., Thuesen L., Ingemann-Hansen T., Pedersen S.A., Jorghensen J., Skakkebaek N.E. and Christiansen J.S. (1989): Lancet 2: 1221-6.
13. Lamberts S.W.J., Valt N.K. and Binnerts A. (1992): Clin. Endocrinol. (Oxf) 37: 111-15.
14. Merola B., Cittadini A., Colao A., Longobardi S., Fazio S., Sabatini D., Saccà L. and Lombardi G. (1993): J. Clin. Endocrinol. Metab. 77: 1658-1661.
15. Rosen T. and Bengtsson B.A. (1990): Lancet 336: 285-288.
16. Rosen T., Bosaeus I., Tolli J., Lindstedt G and Bengtsson B.A. (1993): Clin.Endocrinol. (Oxf) 38: 63-71.
17. Sahn D.J., De Maria A., Kissio J. and Weiman A. (1978): Circulation 58: 1072-1083.
18. Salomon F., Cuneo R.C. Hesp R. and Sonksen P.N. (1989): Engl J Med. 321: 1797-803.
19. Sonksen P.H. (1990): Horm. Res. 33 (Suppl 4): 45-51.
20. Starling M.R., Dell'Italia L.J., Walsh R.A., Little W.C., Benedetto A.R. and Nusynowitz M.L. (1984): J. Am. Coll. Cardiol. 3: 789-798.

Frontiers in Endocrinology
Volume 9 - 1994

Metabolic Effects of Growth Hormone in GH Deficient Adults

G. Delitala, G. Fanciulli, M. Giusti[1] and G. Giordano[1]

Istituto di Patologia Speciale Medica, University of Sassari;
[1]DISEM, Chair of Endocrinology, University of Genova, Italy

INTRODUCTION

The Growth Hormone Deficiency (GHD) syndrome in adults has only very recently been defined even if it had already been demonstrated that GH is secreted in adult life, and some of the physiological consequences of GH deficiency in adults have been known for many years (20).

GHD affects many physiological functions in addition to growth, all of which may have an impact on the quality of life. A number of clinical and biochemical features might suggest the GHD syndrome: thus reduced muscle volume and strength, changes in body mass, reduced basal metabolic rate, decreased physical mobility with increased abdominal adiposity, lack of energy, low sexual drive, depressed mood and impaired cognitive function, may all be consequences of GHD in adults (8).

SYSTEMIC EFFECTS OF GH ADMINISTRATION

Body composition GH has marked effects on body composition, through its anabolic, lipolytic and anti-natriuretic actions (9). Adults with GHD have significantly more body fat compared with that predicted, for age, height, weight and sex, and is distributed more in a central than peripheral pattern (18). Thus, the waist:hip ratio is increased compared with that in control subjects (2).

Adults with GHD also show a reduced lean body mass: in particular, the muscle area is smaller, and extracellular fluid is reduced in GHD compared to healthy matched controls. However, muscle histology showed normal fibre type proportions and areas, with individual muscle fibre type function qualitatively normal (6).

Adults with non childhood-onset GHD have also been shown to have a decreased bone mineral content both in the lumbar spine and in the forearm (12). The cause of osteopenia in these patients is considered to be a deficient build-up of bone mass during childhood and adolescence, and maintenance of peak bone mass. Nevertheless, a low bone mineral content, compared with matched controls, is also observed in adults with GHD (4).

GH is known to stimulate osteoblast proliferation and differentiation and local bone remodelling. However, other GH-dependent mechanisms (increase in muscle mass, strength and exercise capacity, increases in mobility and improvement in quality of life, increases in the mechanical properties in bone) may contribute to the anabolic action of GH in bone and calcium metabolism.

Physical performance Adults with GHD do not perform as well as expected in exercise capacity tests.

This poor physical performance is probably due to reduced cardiac function and to the reduction in muscle mass and strength in these patients. Exercise capacity and maximal heart rate was reported to be 70% and 90%, respectively, of expected values. Quadriceps muscle strength is also reduced in GHD adults when compared with age matched controls (7).

Although the reduction of exercise capacity is due, at least in part, to the reduction in muscle mass, some data suggest impairment in muscle function in patients with GHD. The decreased cardiac output combined with a reduced volume of the extracellular water could also explain the depressed renal function, assessed by glomerular filtration rate and renal plasma flow, observed in the GHD patients (11).

Metabolic abnormalities Untreated GHD in adults appears to increase the risk of premature death from cardiovascular disease (17).

Patients between the ages of 40 and 60 years show major differences in the mean intima thickness and in the number of atherosclerotic plaques in the common carotid and femoral arteries as reflected by the arterial ultrasound score. These findings likely reflect the known metabolic action of GH on lipid metabolism.

Adults with GHD have a mild increase in the circulating level of total and of the more atherogenic fraction LDL cholesterol (10). GH also appears to play a role in regulating the levels of ApoB and ApoE in plasma and promoting triglyceride removal through an increase in lipoprotein lipase activity.

In adults with GHD, fasting plasma glucose values are usually normal but fasting hypoglycaemia may be present. Hypoglycaemia responsiveness to iv insulin is normal, but the recovery is usually delayed. Some degree of insulin resistance may, however, still be present in obese patients with GHD (8). The role of GH in the regulation of whole body protein metabolism in adults is well established (4).

GH has protein anabolic effects: GH increases RNA, DNA and protein synthesis. Increases in amino acid incorporation have been clearly demonstrated *in vitro* on isolated cells or organs. Incorporation of leucine and glycine into proteins of diaphragmatic muscle is less in tissues of hypophysectomised animals (9).

Adult patients with GHD have reduced lean body mass with a reduced muscle mass as assessed by cross-sectioned computed tomography of the thigh (4).

GHD also affects mineral metabolism inducing a reduction in potassium, magnesium amd phosphate in the body. Total exchangeable sodium and calcium are reduced in GHD patients. Glomerular filtration rate and renal blood flow are reduced in GHD patients.

Finally, growth hormone can affect the 1-hydroxylation of 25-hydroxy-vitamin D_3 and the peripheral metabolism of T_4 (8). The metabolic abnormalities observed in adult patients with GHD usually reverse to normal following hGH replacement therapy.

Metabolic benefits of GH replacement in adult Administration of GH in patients with GHD syndrome became a feasible option after the introduction of biosynthetic GH. Several Authors, studying GH therapy in GHD adults, have revealed a series of beneficial effects on certain physical, biochemical, and physiological parameters (19). However, the dose regimes used have been assessed empirically and were often based on those established in children. This has resulted in a relatively high incidence of side effects (e.g. arthralgias, fluid retention and/or carpal tunnel symptoms), which were reduced when the dose was lowered. The differences in dose regimes also makes comparison of the published results rather difficult.

In general, various dose-schedules ranging from 2 to 2.9 IU/m^2 were used and the higher dose resulted in side-effects and often in supranormal IGF-I levels (19).

Recent studies have attempted to define a dose response to GH in GHD patients. The results would suggest that a dose of 1-2 $IU/m^2/day$ (a dose which is less than that used in previous studies on GH replacement) is probably adequate for inducing definite clinical and metabolic improvement in these patients (15). Some of the dramatic effects of rhGH treatment in GHD involve alterations in body composition with rapid changes in body water and body fat. Results obtained with CT clearly illustrate the specific effect of GH in mobilizing fat in the abdomen, by an average of 30%, while subcutaneous adipose tissue was reduced by an average of 10% (2). The decrease in adipose tissue mass is balanced by an increase in muscle volume and by a significant increase in lean body mass of about 10%, with a significant increase in total body nitrogen. These effects are observed during the first month of therapy, but tend to be maintained with long-term treatment (3).

In GHD patients, rhGH therapy can also alter serum levels of lipid and lipoproteins with potential therapeutic benefit, total cholesterol and LDL decreases, while HDL cholesterol levels increase during treatment.

Apolipoprotein A_1 and A_2 also tend to increase, while apolipoprotein B decrease, during rhGH administration (5). The data, taken together, suggest a possible beneficial effect of GH treatment by reducing the risk of cardiovascular diseases in adults with GHD.

The effect of hGH therapy on carbohydrate metabolism is less marked, particularly when low doses of GH are used.

In general, blood glucose and insulin levels remain unchanged with 1 IU/kg/day of GH (15).

However, rhGH caused a dose-dependent increase in serum insulin. The relative insulin resistance after rhGH given in high doses, together with the beneficial effects of low doses of GH, clearly add further support for the use of the lower dose of rhGH (1-1.5 IU/m^2/day) since hyperinsulinaemia is considered an additional risk for cardiovascular diseases.

GH replacement exerts anabolic actions through a direct stimulation of protein synthesis, thus providing a mechanism for the changes in body composition and increased lean body mass found during therapy (13). GH seems to produce its anabolic action without affecting proteolysis. The basal metabolic rate also increases by approximately 10-15% during rhGH treatment: these changes could be accounted for by the modifications in body composition (lipolysis and anabolism) (16).

The increase in peripheral conversion of T_4 to T_3 also appears to contribute to the increase in basal metabolic rate. According to several recent reports, GHD patients treated with rhGH show some improvement in their exercise capacity (4-10). This seems to be related to an increase both in skeletal muscle mass, and cardiac function (as suggested by echocardiographic data (11), as well as to the significant increase in stroke volume (14, 1).

These positive effects of rhGH therapy are evident during the first months of treatment, but appear to continue during the whole period of rhGH administration.

rhGH treatment normalizes total body water, apparently by an increase in extracellular water. The effect may be accounted for by an increase in sodium retention likely mediated by a stimulation of sodium-potassium ATPase in the kidney.

CONCLUSIONS

Only recently has the importance of GHD syndrome in the adult been recognized. Even though some of the signs and symptoms of the syndrome in adults were known many years ago, only since the recent introduction of recombinant human GH has it been possible to treat GH deficient adults.

Since the aim of therapy is to maximize the benefits with minimal side effects, selection of the optimal dose of GH still represents a clinical problem. This means that the initial and maintenance doses should be tailored according to the requirements and responses of individual patients.

The results of clinical experience available would suggest that a low dose (probably not higher than 0.01 IU/kg/day (which can be increased, if necessary) should be used at the beginning of treatment.

However, the clinical and metabolic responses to GH replacement are expected to be different in GHD patients, on account of the varying degrees of GH deficiency in these patients.

These aspects, the potential long-term risks of overtreatment together with the appropriate dose regimes, which will also have to be changed with increasing age, will probably represent the future direction of clinical trials in patients with GHD.

ACKNOWLEDGEMENTS

This work was supported by grants from CNR (Contract n. 9100344 P.F. 40) to G.D.

REFERENCES

1. Amato L., Carella C., Fazio S., La Montagna G., Cittadini A., Sabatini D., Marciano-Mone C., Saccà L. and Bellastella A. (1994): J. Clin. Endocrinol. Metab. 77: 1671-1676.
2. Bengtsson B.Å., Brummer R.J.M., Edén S., Rosén T. and Sjöstrom L. (1992): Acta Paediatr. 383: 62-65.
3. Bengtsson B.Å., Edén S., Lönn L., Kvist H., Stokland A., Lindstedt G., Bosacus I., Tölli J., Sjöstrom L. and Isaksson O.G.P. (1993): J. Clin. Endocrinol. Metab. 76: 309-327.
4. Bengtsson B.Å. (1993): Acta Endocrinol. 128, suppl. 2, 2-5.
5. Brosnan E., Laski J. and Devlin J.C. (1993): Acta Endocrinol. 128, suppl. 2, 68.
6. Cuneo R.C., Salomon F., Wile, C.M. and Sönsken P.H. (1990): Horm. Res. 33 suppl. 4, 55-60.
7. Cuneo R.C., Salomon F., Wiles C.M., Hesp R. and Sönksen P.H. (1991): J. Appl. Physiol. 70: 769-700.
8. Cuneo R.C., Salomon F., Mc Gauley G.A. and Sönksen P.H. (1992): Clin. Endocrinol. (Oxf) 37: 387-397.
9. Delitala G., Oliva O., Fanciulli, G., Fresu P. and Uggias B. (1992): In: Advances in Pediatric Endocrinology, edited by C. Pintor, E.E. Müller, S. Loche, M.I. New, pp. 31-44, Springer-Verlag. Berlin.
10. Edén S., Bengtsson B.Å., Oscarsson J. and Wiklund O. (1993): Acta Endocrinol. 128 suppl. 2, 67.
11. Jørgensen J.O.L., Thuesen L., Ingemann-Hansen T., Skakkebaek N.E. and Christiansen J.S. (1989): Lancet 1: 1221-1226.
12. Kaufman J.M., Taelman P., Vermeulen A. and Vandeweghe M. (1992): J. Clin. Endocrinol. Metab. 74: 118-123.
13. Lundeberg S., Belfrage M., Wernerman J., von der Decken A., Thunell S. and Vinnars E. (1991): Metabolism 40: 315-322.
14. Merola B., Cittadini A., Colao A., Longobardi S., Fazio S., Sabatini D., Saccà L. and Lombardi G. (1994): J. Clin. Endocrinol. Metab. 77: 1658-1661.
15. Møller J., Jørgensen J.O.L., Lauersen T., Frystyk J., Naeraa R.W., Orskov H. and Christiansen J.S. (1993): Clin. Endocrinol. (Oxf) 39: 403-408.
16. Møller N., Møller J., Jørgensen J.O.L., Ovesen P., Schmidtz O., Alberti K.G.M.M. and Christiansen J.S. 1993): Clin. Endocrinol. (Oxf) 39: 577-581.
17. Rosén T. and Bengtsson BÅ. (1990): Lancet 2: 285-288.
18. Rosen T., Bosaeus I., Tîlli J., Lindstedt G. and Bengtsson B.Å. (1993): Clin. Endocrinol. (Oxf) 38: 63-7.
19. Ross R.J.M. (1993): Clin. Endocrinol. (Oxf) 39: 401-402.
20. White H.L.B., Heinbecker P. and Rolf G. (1947): Am. J. Physiol. 149: 404-417.

INFERTILITY

Alterations of Gametogenesis (Workshop)

SOCIETA'
ITALIANA
DI ENDOCRINOLOGIA

Frontiers in Endocrinology
Volume 9 - 1994

INTRODUCTORY REMARKS

New Aspects in the Field of Gametogenesis and its Disorders

G. Giordano

DISEM, Chair of Endocrinology, University of Genova, Viale Benedetto XV, 6, 16132 Genova, Italy

Clinical evaluation of infertility is based on the assumption that reproductive problems affect couples and that the cause of reproductive failure may lie with the man, woman or both. Hence, the infertile couple has to be examined as a single unit.

General evaluation of infertile men includes history, physical examination, routine laboratory tests, semen analysis and hormonal studies. Sperm analysis rarely provides definitive proof of infertility, primarily because sperm parameters vary considerably in a same individual.

To prevent subjectivity and eliminate the effect of potentially confounding influences it is, therefore, recommended to carry out at least two examinations of the sperm. Even if in the clinical evaluation of the infertile couple the basic test is semen analysis, new information could emerge from computer-assisted analysis and electron microscopic analysis of the sperm. These new techniques seem to be very sensitive tools in revealing abnormalities related to spermatogenesis. Without going into detail, it should be stressed that the assessment of FSH levels is the crucial hormonal parameter. Testicular biopsy adds further important information on the evaluation of infertile man.

The work-up of the female patient should include reproductive and marital history, gynaecological examination and other studies including hormonal and immunological evaluation, imaging to visualize genital organs and related abnormalities.

Reproductive function is critically dependent on an intact and fully integrated hypothalamic-pituitary gonadal axis, which acts as the central regulator and coordinator of complex endocrine and paracrine effects and feed-back mechanisms.

In the last 10 years, pulsatile LHRH administration by portable pump has confirmed that follicular maturation is a gonadotrophin-regulated process. LHRH therapy induces ovulation in hypogonadotropic hypogonadism and improves the ovulatory rate in polycystic ovary syndrome. However, gonadotrophins are the most used drug in the clinical management of the infertile patient, both male and female. Recombinant gonadotrophins or specific hormonal isoforms with well-defined biological activity could be a future choice.

More recently, studies have been focused on the role of paracrine and autocrine factors in the regulation of the ovarian follicular cycle. GH and GHRH seem to be effective in protocols for induction of ovulation by activation of the intragonadal IGF-I. On the other hand, further research is necessary to elucidate the role of the GH/IGF-I axis in spermatogenesis.

From: JEI, Vol. 17, Suppl. 2 to n. 3, 1994, p. 10.
Abstracts of the XXV National Congress of the Italian Endocrine Society.

Frontiers in Endocrinology
Volume 9 - 1994

Clinical Evaluation of the Infertile Couple

F. Romanelli, A. Fabbri and A. Isidori

Chair of Andrology, Institute of Internal Medicine V,
University of Rome La Sapienza,
Via del Policlinico 155, 00161 Rome, Italy

Infertility is a problem concerning the couple, and both partners should be assessed at the same time. It is defined as the failure to initiate a pregnancy after at least 12 months of unprotected sexual intercourse and affects approximately 15% of married couples (14). In the past, the female was thought to be mainly responsible for infertility but during the last decade this concept has changed and it is now estimated that in 40-50% of these infertile couples the man is infertile. The approach to the infertile couple is obviously multidisciplinary, and mutual cooperation of the gynecologist and of the andrologist in this field is mandatory (4, 6).

From the operative viewpoint, the diagnostic workup of the two partners is essentially the same, since the causes leading to infertility in both sexes (i.e. genetic, anatomical, secretory or hormonal and excretory) are fundamentally the same. After a careful study of the case history and physical examination, special attention being paid to the primary and secondary sex organs, functional tests must be performed. The assessment of the sperm-cervical mucus interaction (post-coital test) is still a good and simple preliminary assessment of the peripheral situation of a given couple. The study of sperm-oocyte interaction through the evaluation of sperm-zona pellucida and sperm-oolemma binding ratios (11) represents a more sophisticated approach. Thereafter, the algorithmic diagnostic protocol is differentiated for the two members of the couple.

For the female, the integrity of the hypothalamic-pituitary-gonadal axis and the validity of the ovulatory process must be ascertained, and the anatomy of the genital tract assessed to exclude pelvic, tubal, uterine and vaginal factors (3, 6), a fascinating aspect dealt with elsewhere in this Volume.

As far as the male is concerned (Table 1), the basic test is a semen analysis properly carried out and considering not only the classic parameters (volume, sperm concentration, motility and morphology) and the biochemistry of seminal fluid (fructose, carnitine, citric acid, etc.) but in particular the immunopathology (sperm antibodies) and the functional aspects, i.e. fertilizing potential of the sperm through the evaluation of sperm membrane integrity, sperm nuclear maturity, acrosome assessment, etc. (16). Computer-assisted analysis (CASA) and electron-microscopy studies could also be very useful in this respect on account of the great variability in semen parameters. Three semen analyses should, therefore, be performed with an adequate interval between collections. Thereafter, attempts should be made to establish the causes in those cases of azoo-oligodyspermia, considering the present evidence of a decreased quality of semen during the past 50 years (2).

Table 1. *Evalutation of infertile male*

Case history	medical diseases, surgery, drugs, etc.
Physical examination	general and urogenital
Semen analysis	classic parameters (concentrations, motility, etc.) CASA (computer assisted sperm analysis) electron microscopy biochemistry (fructose, carnitine, phosphates, etc.) immunology (antisperm antibodies) microbiology (cultural analysis of semen, urine) fertilizing potential (acrosome assessment, etc.)
Hormonal assays	free T, LH, FSH, PRL, E2, SHBG, 17OHP, FT4, TSH biological assay of gonadotropins dynamic tests (GnRH, HCG, clomiphene, naloxone)
Morphological studies	echosonography doppler velocimetry thermography phlebography VDG computed tomography magnetic resonance
Histological study	testicular biopsy, fine needle aspiration
Genetic study	karyotype, chromosome mapping

Hormonal studies are a crucial, although often neglected point, spermatogenesis being a hormone-dependent process also in its functional aspects, and the assessment of the FSH secretion being a cornerstone in the diagnostic, prognostic and therapeutic management of the infertile patient, especially in the very numerous cases of idiopathic oligo-azoospermias. Hormonal evaluation is carried out through the study of the hypothalamic-pituitary-testicular axis, by means of basal evaluation and specific tests (13).

The pituitary gonadotropins FSH and LH are stimulated by the episodic release of hypothalamic GnRH and are, in turn, modulated by gonadal feedback mechanisms; yet they are not secreted as single molecular species but in multiple molecular forms. These isohormones have different molecular weights, overall charge, circulating half-lives and biological properties. This heterogeneity appears to be due to the difference in the carbohydrate content of each isohormone. In this regard, the biological and not only the radioimmunological activity of gonadotropins should be evaluated (5). The GnRH test has an important prognostic function in oligospermic patients. An exaggerated excretion of FSH following iv injection of 100 mcg GnRH indicates inhibin deficiency and Sertoli cell insufficiency. An exaggerated response of LH to GnRH administration has been found in some patients affected by varicocele, thus indicating Leydig cell insufficiency. The lack of sufficient response to GnRH indicates gonadotropin deficiency either primary, due to pituitary, or secondary, due to hypothalamic insufficiency. Other endocrine tests to evaluate the integrity of the hypothalamic-pituitary axis utilize antiestrogens (tamoxifen, clomiphene) and antiopioids (naloxone and naltrexone) (15).

The basal and dynamic evaluation of the other pituitary hormones (particularly prolactin and thyrotropin) should be performed where necessary. Nighttime melatonin levels could be useful in certain conditions.

At testicular level, the interstitial activity is assessed by the assay of the steroid compounds both in basal conditions and after stimulation. Serum total and free testosterone, estradiol, SHBG, 17 alpha-hydroxyprogesterone in basal conditions and after 5000 IU hCG at 4, 24, 48, 72 and 96 hours, which may also indicate, in some patients, estrogen- or other substance-mediated enzyme block at the 17-20-desmolase level or blunted response (7).

Special attention is focused nowadays on the activity of the intratesticular auto- and paracrine factors (activins/inhibins, CRF/endorphins, GHRH, endothelin), which can be shown by means of immunohistochemical procedures. In this regard, testicular biopsy (surgical or by needle aspiration) is now usefully employed. Chromosomal studies are useful in cases of idiopathic azoospermias with high FSH levels. Excretory and post-testicular causes of infertility can be detected with conventional laboratory tests (bacteriological and immunological) and by non-invasive and invasive procedures (e.g. echosonography, Doppler velocimetry, VDG etc) (12). Other morphological tools are computed tomography and magnetic resonance imaging particularly in the study of the hypothalamus and pituitary.

The final strategy for improving fertility of the patient *in vivo* may be attempted through three approaches:
1) new criteria of efficacy (sophisticated sperm and oocyte functional test);
2) new criteria in the use of known substances (i.e. FSH);
3) use of new substances (antiopioids, growth factors, etc.) to remove excess inhibiting factors or to increase the levels of stimulating elements (1, 9).

REFERENCES

1. Baker H.W.G. (1993): Int. J. Androl. 16: 343-8.
2. Carlsen E., Giwereman A., Keiding N. and Skakkebaek N.E. (1992): Brit. Med. J. 305: 609-13.
3. Carr, B.R. (1992): In: Williams Textbook of Endocrinology edited by Wilson J.D. and Foster D.W., pp.733-798. W.B.Saunders. Philadelphia.
4. Crosignani P.G., Collins J., Cooke I.D., Diczfaluzy E. and Rubin B. (1992): Hum. Reprod. 8: 977-980.
5. Fabbri A., Jannini E.A., Ulisse S., Gnessi L., Moretti C., Frajese G. and Isidori A. (1988): J. Clin. Endocrinol. Metab. 67: 867-75.
6. Glass R.H. (1992): In: Reproductive Endocrinology, edited by R.B.Jaffe and S.S.C.Yen, Third edn., pp. 689-709. W.B. Saunders. Philadelphia.
7. Griffin J.E. and Wilson J.D. (1992): In: Williams Textbook of Endocrinology edited by Wilson J.D. and Foster D.W., pp. 799-852. W.B. Saunders. Philadelphia.
8. Howell R. (1992): In: Clinical Endocrinology, edited by A. Grossman, pp.763-772. Blackwell Scientific Publications. Oxford.
9. Isidori A., Conte D., Nordio M., Fillo S. and Romanelli F. (1992): In: The Fourth Advanced Course on Clinical Reproductive Endocrinology and Infertility, edited by P.C. Wong, pp.1-5. Excerpta Medica. Hong Kong.
10. Jaffe S.B. and Jewelewicz R. (1991): Fertil. Steril. 56: 599-613.
11. Liu D.Y. and Baker H.W.G. (1992): Fertil. Steril. 58: 465-83.
12. Nieschlag E. (1993): Clin. Endocrinol. 38: 123-33.
13. Romanelli F., Di Luigi L. and Isidori A. (1994): In: Endocrinologia della Riproduzione Umana, edited by G. Benagiano, M. Negri, pp. 559-572. UTET. Torino.
14. Swerdloff R.S., Wang C. and Kandeel F.R. (1988): Endocrinol. Metab. Clin. N. A. 17(2): 301-337.
15. Wang C. and Swerdloff R.S. (1992): Bailliere's Clin. Endocrinol. Metab. 6 (2): 405-34.
16. WHO (1992): Laboratory Manual for the Examination of Human Semen and Semen Cervical Mucus Interaction, Third edn., Cambridge University Press. Cambridge.

Frontiers in Endocrinology
Volume 9 - 1994

Mathematical Evaluation of Ultrastructural Characters in Spermatozoa of Infertile Men

B. Baccetti, G. Bernieri[1], A.G. Burrini, S. Capitani, G. Collodel, M. Mirolli, P. Piomboni and T. Renieri

Institute of General Biology of the University, and Center for the Study of Germinal Cells, C.N.R., via T. Pendola 62, 53100 Siena;
[1]Department of Mathematics, University of Siena, Italy

INTRODUCTION

The mathematical evaluation of the entire complex of submicroscopical defects occurring in spermatozoa, each of which able to produce infertility, is a very difficult problem, as most of the sperm defects are interdependent, and the probability of a spermatozoon being healthy, i.e., completely devoid of defects, is related to the degree of the interdependece of each defect with the others. We have recently proposed a formula which allows a precise numerical appraisal of the entire spectrum of the characters studied, and a means to determine the number of spermatozoa free from defects.

The various kinds, degrees and direction of interdependence in all the sperm characters have been estimated according to our experience, and the percent of the single defects resulting from the electron microscopic examination of the sperm sections able to contain them is calculated, reported in a form, and introduced into the programmed computer.

In practice, in order to find the probability for a spermatozoon to be healthy, we have used the formula:

$$\Pi = P(\mathrm{Me}) \cdot P(\mathrm{Sp}) \cdot P(\mathrm{Fi}) \cdot P(\mathrm{Mi}_2) \cdot P(\mathrm{Mi}_1|\mathrm{Mi}_2) \cdot P(\mathrm{Ac}_2) \cdot P(\mathrm{Ac}_1|\mathrm{Ac}_2) \cdot P(\mathrm{Ac}_3|\mathrm{Ac}_2) \cdot P(\mathrm{Nu}_1|\mathrm{Ac}_2) \cdot P(\mathrm{Nu}_2|\mathrm{Nu}_1) \cdot$$

$$\cdot P(\mathrm{Ax}_2) \cdot P(\mathrm{Re}|\mathrm{Ac}_1 \wedge \mathrm{Ac}_2) \cdot P(\mathrm{Ac}_4|\mathrm{Re}) \cdot P(\mathrm{Ax}_1|\mathrm{Ax}_2 \wedge \mathrm{Re}) \cdot P(\mathrm{Ax}_3|\mathrm{Re} \wedge \mathrm{Ax}_1) \cdot P(\mathrm{Sh}|\mathrm{Re} \wedge \mathrm{Ax}_3),$$

where symbols like Me or Mi_2 refer to the various defects for each pair D_1 D_2 of defects, we have set:

$$P\left(\overline{D_1}\,|\,\overline{D_2}\right)=\int_0^1\int_0^1 \vartheta_1 \cdot f_{\Theta_1}(\vartheta_1,\vartheta_2)\,d\vartheta_1 d\vartheta_2$$

$$=\frac{\int_0^1\int_0^1 \vartheta_1\cdot\vartheta_1^{p_1}(1-\vartheta_1)^{q_1}\vartheta_2^{p_2}(1-\vartheta_2)^{q_2}\left(\vartheta_1\cdot\pi+\vartheta_2\cdot(1-\pi)\right)^h\cdot\left((1-\vartheta_1)\cdot\pi+(1-\vartheta_2)\cdot(1-\pi)\right)^{n-h}d\vartheta_1 d\vartheta_2}{\int_0^1\int_0^1 \vartheta_1^{p_1}(1-\vartheta_1)^{q_1}\vartheta_2^{p_2}(1-\vartheta_2)^{q_2}\left(\vartheta_1\cdot\pi+\vartheta_2\cdot(1-\pi)\right)^h\cdot\left((1-\vartheta_1)\cdot\pi+(1-\vartheta_2)\cdot(1-\pi)\right)^{n-h}d\vartheta_1 d\vartheta_2}.$$

and

$$P\left(\overline{D_2}\right)=\frac{h+1}{n+2},$$

In the preceding formula n is the number of sections considered, h is the number of sections in which the defect has been detected, while π, p1, p2, q1 and q2 are chosen in order to take into account the opinion of an expert.

This formula has been applied to calculate the number of healthy spermatozoa in the ejaculates of several patients affected by varicocele and of subfertile men, in view of assisted reproduction.

In the first case, a direct relationship has been found beween the degree of varicocele and the number of spermatozoa free from defects: moreover, their number signficantly increases after surgical repair of the varicocele condition.

In the second case, a good correlation between the quality of the semen resulting from the mathematical evaluation and the success of different procedures of assisted reproduction (FIVET, SUSM, ICSI) has been observed.

In conclusion, quantitative electron microscopy may be considered a valid tool by which to estimate sperm quality. With this method we can easily obtain information concerning the basal status of the semen, the degree of improvement in pathological conditions treated pharmacologically or surgically, and we can better predict the success of assisted insemination.

Frontiers in Endocrinology
Volume 9 - 1994

Clinical Effects of GRF plus pFSH in Poor-Responder Patients

A.R. Genazzani, P.G. Artini, C. Battaglia, F. Droghini, A.C. Mancini and G. D'Ambrogio

Department of Obstetrics and Gynecology, University of Modena, Via del Pozzo 71, 41100 Modena, Italy

INTRODUCTION

Recently, it has been shown that some growth factors play an important role in modulating the ovarian follicular cycle and the response of ovarian cells to gonadotropins (Gn). In fact, insulin-like growth factor-I (IGF-I) seems to exert a stimulatory action on the replication of granulosa cells (1, 13) and on the aromatase activity directly and by synergizing with Gn (9). Growth hormone (GH) stimulates the synthesis and release of IGF-I (7, 8). GH-releasing factor (GRF) greatly stimulates GH release by the human pituitary gland (12) and might be employed to increase endogenous GH release during superovulation induction, as it has been shown that GRF plus Gn administration improves the clinical response in patients resistant to Gn alone undergoing an IVF/ET-GIFT programme (18).

In view of these findings, we have evaluated, in this study, the different results of two protocols of superovulation induction with only purified follicle stimulating hormone (pFSH) or pFSH plus GRF in poor-responder patients.

MATERIAL AND METHODS

A retrospective study was performed on the files of women included in our IVF programme to select a population with a poor response to a protocol of superovulation induction with pFSH alone. This qualification was assigned to patients showing a slow rise or a low plateau in plasma oestradiol (E2) levels and a small number of follicles >1.6 cm recruited on the human chorionic gonadotropin (hCG) day of administration. 50 poor-responder patients (aged 23-40 years) were studied. Length of infertility was 2-11 years. All patients presented a normal body mass index and height ≥160 cm. None showed endocrine abnormalities or hypertension. All patients were recruited after giving written informed consent and the protocol of the study was approved by the Ethics Committee of the Medical School of the University of Modena.

In the first cycle, all patients were administered a gonadotropin-releasing hormone analogue (GnRHa) long-term protocol (Decapeptyl, Triptorelin 3,75 on the first day of a spontaneous cycle). The superovulation was induced about 10-15 days later with purified urinary follicle stimulating hormone (pFSH; Metrodin, Serono, Italy; 75 IU FSH/ampoule), 2-3 ampoules/day on day 1-5 and individualized thereafter. Follicular growth was monitored by transvaginal ultrasound examination and plasma E2 by daily measurement using a radioimmunoassay, starting on day 6 of the cycle. When at least one follicle reached > 16 mm in diameter and plasma E2 was about 200 pg/ml per follicle, hCG (Profasi, Serono, Italy), 10.000 IU, was administered. Oocyte retrieval was performed by transvaginal ultrasound-guided follicle aspiration 34-38 hours after hCG administration. 25 cycles were suspended.

Before starting the second cycle, basal plasma GH and IGF-I levels and the pituitary GH response to exogenous GRF [Geref 500 mcg, Sermorelin; Serono (GRF test = Groliberin 1 mcg/Kg/body weight as an iv bolus and blood samples at –15 minutes before and at 0, +15, +30, +45, +60, +90, +120 minutes after GRF administration)] were evaluated in all patients. During the second cycle, all patients were treated with the same scheme of GnRHa used previously and pFSH 4 ampoules/day, combined with GRF (500 mcg x 2/day s.c.) from the 1st to the last day of pFSH administration. hCG was administered as in the previous cycle. Only in one patient was the stimulation not successful. In all patients GH and IGF-I plasma levels were measured before and after GRF administration on the 1st, 4th, 6th, 8th and the day of hCG administration. Blood samples were taken at –45, –30, –15, 0, +30, +45 min with respect to sc GRF administration (GRF mini-test).

Statistical analysis Analysis of variance (repetetive sampling) and paired Student t test were used when appropriate. Results are expressed as mean ± SEM.

RESULTS

Clinical results concerning the number of ampoules used, cycles suspended, length of stimulation and plasma levels of E2 on the day of pick-up in the pFSH and pFSH+GRF cycles are reported in Table 1. We have found significant differences in both cycles in terms of number of cycles suspended and plasma E2 levels. Also the mean value of the total number of follicles recruited and of the follicles >1.6 cm on the hCG administration day in both cycles are significantly different (Table 2). The mean number of oocytes recruited, fertilized, transferred and the pregnancy rate in the first and second cycle reported in Table 3 reveals a significant difference in terms of total number of oocytes recruited and pregnancy rate. Plasma E2 levels on the 1st, 4th, 6th, 8th and hCG day (Fig. 1) were evaluated in both cycles, while the GH and IGF-I response to GRF minitest on the same days (Figs. 2, 3) was assessed only in the second one. By GRF minitest we have revealed a significant progressive increase in plasma GH and IGF-I levels, compared to basal values, at 30 and 45 minutes following sc injection on the 1st, 4th, 6th, 8th and hCG day. Moreover, long-term stimulation only in plasma GH release was observed. In fact, plasma IGF-I levels increase in the first 4-6 days of stimulation and decrease thereafter.

Table 1. *Clinical results in the pFSH and pFSH + GRF cycles. Data=mean ± SEM*

	pFSH	pFSH+GRF
N. ampoules	46.49±7.83	46.43±4.87
Day of pick-up	13.04±3.28	12.88±1.11
N. cycles suspended	25/50 *	1/50 *
Plasma E2 levels (ng/mL)	616.22±202.5 *	1130.62±384.91 *

* $p<0.01$.

Table 2. *Ovarian data in the pFSH and pFSH + GRF cycles. Data=mean ± SEM*

	pFSH	pFSH+GRF
Follicles (total number)	5.52 ± 1.96*	11.96 ± 1.89*
Diameter > 1.6 cm	1.22 ± 0.83*	4.55 ± 1.37*
Diameter 1.2-1.6 cm	2.18 ± 1.72	3.57 ± 1.14
Diameter < 1.2 cm	2.12 ± 1.54	3.84 ± 1.59

* $p<0.01$.

Table 3. *Laboratory results in pFSH and pFSH + GRF cycles. Data=mean ±SEM*

	pFSH	pFSH+GRF
Oocytes recruited	1.69 ± 1.01*	5.33 ± 1.97*
Oocytes fertilized	1.21 ± 0.82	2.24 ± 1.08
Oocytes transferred	1.12 ± 0.92	2.04 ± 1.18
Pregnancy rate (%)	0 *	24 *

* $p<0.01$.

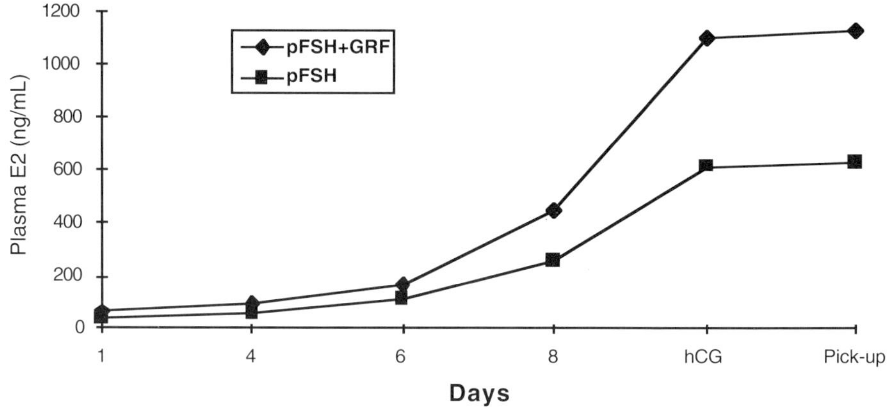

FIG. 1. Pattern of plasma E2 variations in pFSH and pFSH+GRF cycles.

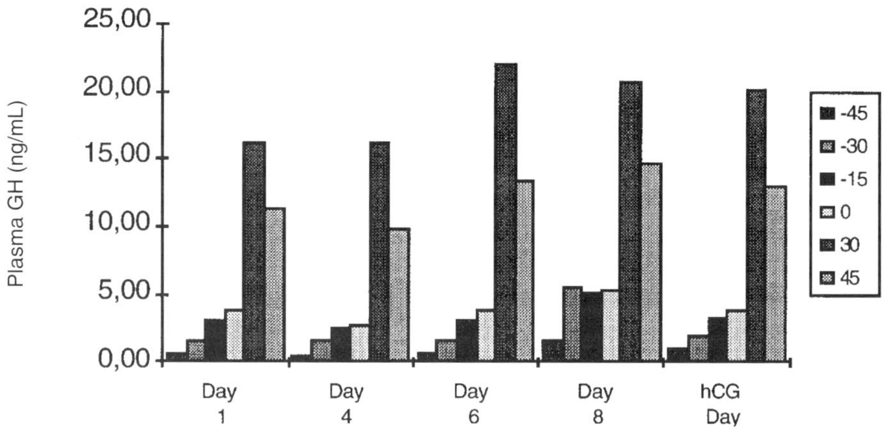

FIG. 2. Plasma GH levels in pFSH and pFSH+GRF cycles on the 1st, 4th, 6th, 8th and hCG day at –45, –30, –15, 0, +30 and +45 minutes with respect to sc GRF administration (GRF mini-test).

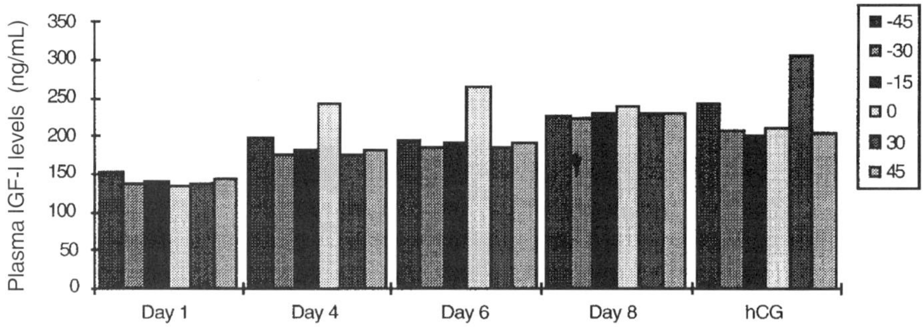

FIG. 3. Plasma IGF-I levels in pFSH and pFSH+GRF cycles on the 1st, 4th, 6th, 8th and hCG day at –45, –30, –15, 0, +30, +45 minutes with respect to sc GRF administration (GRF mini-test).

DISCUSSION

The present data show that GRF plus pFSH administration may improve the ovarian response in poor-responder patients with respect to a previous cycle of superovulation induction with only pFSH.

Our clinical results are consistent with previous reports on the effects of GH administration for induction of ovulation in patients with a normal response to Gn (16, 17). However, the improvement in the ovarian response is much more evident in the poor-responder patients. In fact, in the first cycle 25/50 patients were suspended, while in the second one only 1/50.

Moreover, in the second cycle, we have found significant differences with respect to the first one in terms of plasma E2 levels on the pick-up day, number of follicles, oocytes retrieved and pregnancy rate.

In agreement with previous reports (19), we have revealed, by means of the GRF minitest, a significant progressive increase of plasma GH and IGF-I levels, compared to basal values, at 30 and 45 minutes following sc injection on the 1st, 4th, 6th, 8th and hCG day. Therefore, the clinical effects of GRF administration might be mediated by the stimulation of the GH-IGF-I axis. In fact, in normal adults as well as in subjects with abnormalities of the GRF-GH axis, continuous infusion, or intermittent administration for a 5-day period, or bolus administration of GRF, results in an increase of integrated plasma GH and of 24-h plasma IGF-I levels (5, 10, 23). These data suggest that administration of GRF activates the entire GH-IGF-I axis. Indeed, by GRF minitest we have noticed a long-term stimulation only of plasma GH release. In fact, plasma IGF-I levels increase in the first 4-6 days of stimulation and decrease thereafter. This biphasic pattern may be explained by the opposite effects of E2 and GH on hepatic IGF-I production. As shown in *in vitro* and *in vivo* experiments (1, 6, 15), in contrast to GH, elevated E2 concentrations decrease plasma IGF-I levels and suppress hepatic IGF-I gene expression. Therefore, in the second part of superovulation induction, GH stimulating effect may be counteracted by high endogenous plasma E2 levels.

As recently shown, it is possible that GH also acts directly on the ovary (3). In fact, it has been demonstrated that the human ovary contains a substance that reacts with a specific antiserum raised against GRF (21). The presence of a GRF-like substance in the ovary suggests that GRF might represent an intra-ovarian regulatory peptide, and that the effects of GRF supplementation might be due also to a direct action of the peptide on the ovary. Moreover, we have recently shown also that IGF-I follicular fluid (FF) levels were higher in the GRF-supplemented cycle than in the previous one (24).

In spite of the fact that there is no evidence that IGF-I is synthesized in the human ovary (26) and as it has been shown that FF IGF-I levels are lower than plasma IGF-I levels (22), the increase of FF IGF-I levels in the pFSH+GRF cycle may reflect the ovarian production or, more probably, high plasma concentrations of IGF-I. Therefore, the activation of the plasma

GH-IGF-I axis and the increase of follicular fluid IGF-I levels enhance the stimulatory effect of pFSH on follicular growth in the GRF supplemented cycle.

As far as concerns the administration of GRF, the mechanism regulating GH pituitary release suggests that pulsatile infusion of GRF would be the ideal pattern (12), however, intermittent sc injection of GRF is also effective in eliciting and/or enhancing the GH-dependent functions (11, 12, 14) and appears suitable for protocols of superovulation induction.

Supplementation requires a normally responsive pituitary GH production. In fact, patients with endocrine and/or metabolic disorders, showing abnormalities of the GRF-GH axis (for instance obese and/or hypopituitary patients) may show a blunted response of pituitary GH to GRF (4, 20), while an increased GH response to provocative stimuli has been observed in patients with hypothalamic amenorrhoea (2) and in PCO patients (25).

In conclusion, administration of GRF in a protocol for a superovulation induction proved effective and resulted in enhancement of the ovarian response to Gn in poor-responder patients. These effects of GRF might be due to a possible direct action of the peptide on the ovary, or more probably be mediated by the activation of the GH-IGF-I axis, as suggested by the prompt increase of plasma GH following GRF administration and by increased follicular fluid levels of IGF-I.

REFERENCES

1. Adashi E.Y., Resnick C. E., D'Ercole A. J., Sviboda M. E. and Van Wyk J.J. (1985): Endocrin. Rev. 6: 400-420.
2. Anapliotou M.L.G., Syrigos K., Panayiotakopoulos G., Kalos A. and Batrinos M.L. (1989): Horm. Res. 31: 119-124.
3. Barreca A., Artini P.G., Del Monte P., Ponzani P., Pasquini P., Cariola G., Volpe A., Genazzani A.R., Giordano G. and Minuto F. (1993): J. Clin. Endocrinol. Metab. 77: 61-67.
4. Bing-You R.G., Bigos S.T. and Oppenheim D.S. (1993): Metabolism 42 (6): 790-794.
5. Borges J.L.C., Blizzard R.M., Evans W.S., Furlanetto R., Rogol A.D., Kaiser D.L., Rivier J., Vale W. and Thorner M.O. (1984): J. Clin. Endocrinol. Metab. 59: 1-6.
6. Coppeland K.C. (1988): J. Clin. Endocrinol. Metab. 66: 1278.
7. Daughaday W.H. and Rotwein P. (1989): Endocr. Rev. 10: 68-91.
8. Davoren J.B. and Hsueh A.J.W. (1986): Endocrinology 118: 888-890.
9. Erickson G.F., Garzo V.G. and Magoffin D. (1989): J. Clin. Endocrinol. Metab. 69: 716-724.
10. Evans W.S., Borges J.L.C., Vance M.L., Kaiser D.L., Rogol A.L., Furlanetto R., Rivier J., Vale W. and Thorner M.O. (1984): J. Clin. Endocrinol. Metab. 59: 1006-1010.
11. Evans W.S., Vance M.L., Kaiser D.L., Sellers R.P., Borges J.L., Downs T.R., Frohman L.A., Rivier J., Vale W. and Thorner M.O. (1985): J. Clin. Endocrinol. Metab. 61: 846-850.
12. Frohman L.A. and Jannson J.O. (1986): Endocr. Rev. 7: 223-253.
13. Gospodarowicz D. and Bialecki H. (1979): Endocrinology 104: 757-764.
14. Hernandez E.R., Resnick C.E., Svoboda M.E., Van Wyk J.J., Payne D.W. and Adashi E.Y. (1988): Endocrinology 122: 1603-1612.
15. Hernandez E.R., Roberts C.T., LeRoith D., Jr and Adashi E.Y. (1989): Endocrinology 125: 572.
16. Homburg R., West C., Torresani T. and Jacobs H.S. (1990a): Fertil. Steril. 53: 254-260.
17. Homburg R., West C., Torresani T. and Jacobs H.S. (1990b): Clin. Endocrinol. 32: 781-785.
18. Hugues J.N. and Torresani T. (1989): XIII World Congress on Fertility and Sterility, Marrakesh, October 1-6, Abstract n. 308.

19. Hugues J.N., Torresani T., Herve F., Martin-Pont B., Tamboise A. and Santarelli J. (1991): Fertil. Steril. 55, n. 5: 945-951.
20. Kopelman P.G., Noonan K., Gronlton R. and Forrest A.J. (1985): Clin. Endocrinol. 23: 87-94.
21. Moretti C., Fabbri A., Gnessi L., Bonifacio V., Bolotti M., Arizzi M., Nazzicone Q. and Spera G. (1990): J. Endocrinol. Invest. 13: 301-305.
22. Rabinovici J., Dandekar P., Angle M.J., Rosenthal S. and Martin M.C. (1990): Fertil. Steril. 54: 428-433.
23. Vance M.L., Kaiser D.L., Evans W.S., Furlanetto R., Vale W., Rivier J.A. and Thorner M.O. (1985): J. Clin. Endocrinol. Metab. 75: 1584-1589.
24. Volpe A., Coukos G., Barreca A., Giordano G., Artini P.G. and Genazzani A.R. (1991): Human Reprod. vol. 6, n. 9: 1228-1232.
25. Volpe A., Artini P.G., Barreca A., Minuto F., Coukos G. and Genazzani A.R. (1992): Human Reprod. vol. 7, n. 10: 1347-1352.
26. Voutilainen R. and Miller W.L. (1987): Proc. Natl. Acad. Sci. USA 84: 1590-1594.

ANDROLOGY

p. 257 - 288

SOCIETA'
ITALIANA
DI ENDOCRINOLOGIA

Frontiers in Endocrinology
Volume 9 - 1994

ITALIAN ENDOCRINE SOCIETY
1994 AWARD LECTURE

Effects of Progesterone on Human Spermatozoa: a Model for non-Genomic Actions of Steroids

G. Forti, E. Baldi, M. Luconi, Cs. Krausz, R. Casano, L. Bonaccorsi, M. Maggi, G. Finetti, M. Mancini, C. Falsetti and G. Gervasi

Andrology Unit, Department of Clinical Physiopathology, Viale Pieraccini 6, 50139 Florence, Italy

Lecture delivered at the XXV National Congress - Rome, 22-25 May 1994.

MODEL FOR NON-GENOMIC ACTIONS OF STEROIDS

Increasing evidence suggests that steroids can exert rapid, non-genomic effects in several cells: these effects, which have been recently reviewed (11), have been reported for testosterone, progesterone, glucocorticoids, estrogens, 1α, 25-$(OH)^2$ vitamin D, and, more recently, for aldosterone. The best studied non-genomic actions of steroids perhaps relate to progesterone and its ability to induce maturation of oocytes (26) and spermatozoa (8). Mature spermatozoa represent an interesting model for the study of cell-surface steroid receptors because the transcriptional activity of these cells is arrested so that the superimposition of genomic and non-genomic effects can be excluded.

The aim of the present report is to focus on some recent results obtained in our laboratory concerning:

1) the intracellular calcium accumulation and responsiveness to progesterone in human spermatozoa and their possible clinical relevance;
2) the responsiveness to progesterone of spermatozoa in oligozoospermic men;
3) the effects of progesterone on the synthesis of platelet-activating factor (PAF) by human spermatozoa;
4) the effects of PAF on motility and acrosome reaction of human spermatozoa and their possible clinical applications;
5) preliminary data related to the effects of progesterone and PAF on signal transduction in human spermatozoa.

EFFECTS OF PROGESTERONE ON CAPACITATING HUMAN SPERMATOZOA

Mammalian sperm capacitation, which physiologically occurs in the female genital tract, can also be achieved *in vitro* and is characterized by marked changes in the protein and lipid composition of the sperm plasma membrane including, in most species, an increased influx of Ca^{2+}. In a preliminary study we demonstrated, for the first time, that basal intracellular free calcium $[Ca^{2+}]i$ increases during *in vitro* capacitation of human sperm (4). We also confirmed that progesterone induces an increase in the concentration of $[Ca^{2+}]i$ in capacitated human sperm as previously reported (25, 7). Furthermore, during capacitation, we found: 1) a progressive increase of progesterone-stimulated $[Ca^{2+}]i$: this increase was dose-related and correlated (r=0.93) with basal sperm $[Ca^{2+}]i$; 2) a progressive increase of progesterone-induced acrosome reaction, an exocytotic event which is needed for sperm-oocyte fusion.

The rapidity of the effects of progesterone and the finding that the cytosolic progesterone receptor antagonist RU486 did not affect the progesterone-mediated Ca^{2+} increase suggested an interaction of progesterone with the sperm surface, which was recently confirmed by the use of progesterone conjugated to BSA (17).

As progesterone is present in high concentrations in the follicular fluid as well as in the cumulus matrix (21), we suggest that the progressive, parallel increase of [Ca^{2+}]i and response to progesterone during *in vitro* capacitation of human spermatozoa might be relevant *in vivo* during capacitation of sperm in the female genital tract.

RESPONSIVENESS TO PROGESTERONE OF SPERMATOZOA IN OLIGOZOOSPERMIC MEN

Infertility associated with oligozoospermia is likely to be due to defective sperm function rather than defective sperm number. From a functional point of view, spermatozooa from oligozoospermic patients are less responsive to stimuli that trigger the acrosome reaction *in vivo* such as follicular fluid (9) and the ionofore A23187 (1).

We then hypothesized that a decreased responsiveness to progesterone might be a biochemical feature of spermatozoa from oligozoospermic men. We evaluated the sperm [Ca^{2+}]i in response to progesterone 0.1 μg/ml in 19 normo- and 17 oligozoospermic men. The average percentage of [Ca^{2+}]i increase over the basal level was significantly lower in spermatozoa from oligozoospermic men (138.7 ± 8.22 % increase) than in spermatozoa from normozoospermic men (263.3 ± 39.7% increase, $p < 0.001$). The increase of [Ca^{2+}]i induced by progesterone was significantly correlated with sperm motility, concentration and percentage of normal forms (10). Furthermore, we found that progesterone is able to induce a significant increase in acrosome reaction in spermatozoa from normozoospermic men, whereas it has no significant effect on spermatozoa from oligozoospermic men (10).

These results, which have been recently confirmed by other authors (23, 20), indicate that spermatozoa from oligozoospermic men have a reduced ability to initiate the cascade of events that lead to the acrosome reaction in response to a physiological stimulus, such as progesterone, and might contribute to explain the reduced fertilizing capacity of these subjects.

Preliminary results obtained in our laboratory also seem to show that the human sperm responsiveness to progesterone, both in terms of [Ca^{2+}]i and acrosome reaction increase, is significantly related to the ability of human sperm to fertilize human oocytes *in vitro* (Krausz et al., unpublished observations).

EFFECTS OF PROGESTERONE ON THE SYNTHESIS OF PLATELET-ACTIVATING FACTOR (PAF) BY HUMAN SPERMATOZOA

Platelet-activating factor (PAF), a potent pro-inflammatory phospholipid with several biological effects, was recently detected by several authors (14, 15, 18) in rabbit and human washed spermatozoa, suggesting that these cells are able to synthesize this phospholipid. However, it was not known whether PAF production by spermatozoa could be enhanced by stimuli that induce Ca^{2+} entry and acrosome reaction in human sperm. Therefore we decided to investigate whether PAF synthesis and release occurs in human spermatozoa following incubation with progesterone and the ionofore A23187, two known inducers of Ca^{2+} entry and acrosome reaction in human sperm. We found that treatment with progesterone and the ionofore A23187 resulted in an increase of PAF synthesis assessed by [^{3}H] acetate incorporation into PAF (remodelling pathway). Most of the newly synthesized [^{3}H]PAF was found in the supernatant, suggesting a release from spermatozoa. PAF-like material extracted from human spermatozoa was able to induce aggregation of rabbit platelets and showed identical retention time and the same m/e values as authentic PAF when analysed with gas-chromatography mass spectrometry (5). We also found that Lyso-PAF: acetylCoA acetyltransferase activity with similar kinetic parameters to those found in other cells is present in human spermatozoa (5).

EFFECTS OF PAF ON MOTILITY AND ACROSOME REACTION OF HUMAN SPERMATOZOA

The effects of PAF on human sperm motility are controversial, as both positive (22, 12) and negative effects (3) have been reported. We designed a study to evaluate the effect of PAF on human sperm motion parameters and percent acrosome reaction in a group of men with different degrees of sperm motility. We found that incubation with 10 nM PAF for 1-4 h significantly enhanced total and progressive sperm motility in 25 subjects (13). However the increase in sperm motility, which was inversely correlated with basal motility, was present only in 16 subjects who were defined as 'responders' whereas no effect could be observed in 9 subjects, who were defined 'non responders'. In 11 samples (6 responders and 5 non responders) where incubation with PAF was prolonged overnight, a significantly higher sperm motility was maintained in all the subjects studied. An increase in the percentage acrosome-reacted sperm in response to 1 h incubation with PAF 10 nM was also present in 20 out of 26 subjects examined.

We believe that the finding of 'responder' and 'non responder' subjects to PAF probably explains the previous conflicting results present in the literature. As PAF is present in follicular fluid (2) and, presumably, in the cumulus matrix which surrounds the oocyte, a pysiological role for PAF during the fertilization process, together with progesterone, can be postulated. Furthermore our results suggest a potential use of PAF in *in vitro* fertilization techniques in cases with reduced sperm motility.

EFFECTS OF PROGESTERONE AND PAF ON SIGNAL TRANSDUCTION IN HUMAN SPERMATOZOA

It has recently been reported that tyrosine phosphorylation of proteins is increased with capacitation and in response to physiological stimulation of acrosome reaction with zona pellucida proteins in mice (16) and human (19) spermatozoa. Recently, progesterone has been shown to increase tyrosine phosphorylation of a 94 kd protein in human sperm (24). In a preliminary study, using western blotting and a polyclonal antiphosphotyrosine antibody, we found that during capacitation the level of tyrosine phosphorylation of a 97 and 75 kd protein increased as a function of capacitation time (6). In addition tyrosine phosphorylation in these two proteins in capacitated human spermatozoa was increased by treatment with progesterone (0.1-1.0 μg/ml) and PAF (100 nM) and was reduced by preincubation with the tyrosine kinase inhibitor erbstatin. As we suggest that both progesterone and PAF are probably physiologic stimulators of sperm function, we hypothesize a role for tyrosine kinase(s) in the mechanism of capacitation and activation of human spermatozoa.

ACKNOWLEDGEMENTS

This work was supported by Grants from the Università di Firenze, Ministero della Università e della Ricerca Scientifica e Tecnologica, and from Consiglio Nazionale delle Ricerche (Rome, Italy, Progetto FAT.MA, contratto 92.00097-PF41).

REFERENCES

1. Aitken R.J., Ross A., Hargreave T., Richardson D. and Best F. (1984): J. Androl. 5: 321-329.
2. Amiel M.L., Testart J. and Benveniste J. (1991): Fertil. Steril. 56: 62-65.
3. Angle M.J., Tom R., Khoo D. and McClure R.D. (1991): Fertil. Steril. 56: 314-318.
4. Baldi E., Casano R., Falsetti C., Krausz Cs., Maggi M. and Forti G. (1991): J. Androl. 12: 323-330.
5. Baldi E., Falsetti C., Krausz Cs., Gervasi G., Carloni V., Casano R. and Forti G. (1993): Biochem. J. 292: 209-216.
6. Baldi E., Luconi M., Krausz Cs., Bonaccorsi L., Mancini M., Casano R. and Forti G. (1994): 8th European Workshop on Molecular and Cellular Endocrinology of the Testis. De Panne, March 27-31, Miniposter 118.
7. Blackmore P.F., Beebe S.J., Danforth D.R. and Alexandre M. (1990): J. Biol. Chem. 265: 1376-1380.
8. Blackmore P.F., Neule J., Lattanzio F. and Beebe S.J. (1991): J. Biol. Chem. 266: 18655-18659.
9. Calvo L., Vantman D., Banks S.M., Tezon J., Koukolis G.N., Denniso, L. and Sherins R.J. (1989): Fertil. Steril. 52: 1048-1054.
10. Falsetti C., Baldi E., Krausz Cs., Casano R., Failli P. and Forti G. (1993): J. Androl. 14: 17-22.
11. Griffing G.T. (1993): J. Clin. Endocrinol. Metab. 77: 1450-1451.
12. Hellstrom W.J.G., Wang R. and Sikka S.C. (1991): Fertil. Steril. 56: 768-770.
13. Krausz Cs., Gervasi G., Forti G. and Baldi E. (1994): Hum. Reprod. 9: 471-476.
14. Kumar R., Harper M.J.K. and Hanahan D.J. (1988): Arch. Biochem. Biophys. 260: 497-502.
15. Kuzan F.B., Geissler F.T. and Henderson W.R., Jr. (1990): Prostaglandins 9: 61-74.

16. Leyton L. and Sailing P. (1989): Cell 57: 1123-1130.
17. Meizel S. and Turner K.O. (1991): Mol. Cell. Endocrinol. 11: R1-R5.
18. Minhas B.S., Kumar R., Ricker D.D., Robertson J.L. and Dodson M.G. (1991): Fertil. Steril. 55: 372-376.
19. Naz R.K., Ahmad K. and Kumar R. (1991): J. Cell. Sci. 99: 157-165.
20. Oehninger S., Blackmore P., Morshedi M., Sueldo C., Acosta A.A. and Alexander N.J. (1994): Fertil. Steril. 61: 349-354.
21. Osman R.A., Andria M.L. and Jones A.D. (1989): Biochem. Biophys. Res. Comm. 160: 828-833.
22. Ricker D.D., Minhas B.S., Kumar R., Robertson J.L. and Dodson M.G. (1989): Fertil. Steril. 52: 655-658.
23. Tesarik J. and Mendoza C. (1992): Fertil. Steril. 58: 793-797.
24. Tesarik J., Mos J. and Mendoza C. (1993): Endocrinology 133: 328-335.
25. Thomas P. and Meizel S. (1989): Biochem. J. 264: 539-546.
26. Wasserman W.J., Pinto L.H., O'Connor C.M. and Smith L.D. (1980). Proc. Natl. Acad. Sci. USA 77: 1534-1536.

Frontiers in Endocrinology
Volume 9 - 1994

Endothelin in Human Testis

M. Maggi, G. Fantoni, G. Finetti, G.B. Vannelli[1], T. Barni[1], R. Mancina, E. Macorsini and G. Forti

Department of Clinical Physiopathology, Andrology Unit, Viale Pieraccini 6, 50139 Florence; [1]Department of Human Anatomy, Viale Morgagni 85, 50134 Florence, Italy

INTRODUCTION

Testicular activity is essentially regulated by the hypophyseal hormones FSH and LH. FSH mainly coordinates the proliferation of germ cells in the tubular compartment, while LH regulates the steroidogenic activity of the interstitium. The cross-talk between the tubules and the interstitial cells is mediated by a variety of autocrine/paracrine factors, testosterone being the more relevant one. The interaction of these hormones and factors in controlling the function of each cell type and the interaction of the various cell types with each other are all necessary to create the unique environment for spermatogenesis. Recent data from our (4) and other laboratories (1-3, 15) indicate that a family of peptides termed endothelins might play an ancillary role as intratesticular regulatory factor.

ENDOTHELIN

The endothelin (ET) family includes three peptides of 21 aminoacids in length (ET-1, ET-2 and ET-3) (11). ET-1 was originally isolated from vascular endothelial cells as the most powerful constrictor of blood vessels. Multiple subtypes of ET receptors have been postulated by ligand binding and cross-linking experiments (11). So far, three isoreceptors have been cloned and termed ETA, ETB and ETC. The latter, recently identified in *Xenopus laevis* dermal melonophores, selectively binds ET-3 (5). Conversely, ETA binds with high affinity ET-1 and ET-2, while ETB shows virtually equal affinity for all the family isopeptides. Receptors and peptides are not just confined to the cardiovascular system, but are widely distributed (11). In particular, they are present in reproductive tissues (6, 8-10, 13, 14), including gonads (4).

ENDOTHELIN IN RAT TESTIS

Early on it was noticed that rat testis contains elevated concentrations of ET-1 (100 pM) (12). Since preproET-1 mRNA is expressed in rat testis (16) a local production was suggested. We originally found that Sertoli cells are the main source of testicular ET-1 (4). We indeed studied the secretion of ET-1 from immature rat Sertoli and Leydig cells in primary culture using a specific radioimmunoassay (13). We were unable to show any ET-1 immunoreactivity in the spent medium from Leydig cells, while Sertoli cells secreted ET-1 in a time- and FSH-dependent fashion. In particular, different concentrations of FSH (50 and 300 ng/ml) induced a 10-fold decrease in ET-1 secretion. This effect is apparently related to an increase in cAMP levels, since 10 μM forskolin mimicked the FSH effect. Reverse-phase high pressure liquid chromatography analysis indicated that the ET-1 produced by rat Sertoli cells corresponds to authentic ET-1 (4). Immunohistochemical studies in immature rats confirmed that ET-1 immunoreactivity was confined to the tubular compartment. In contrast, in adult rats, some positivity is also identified in the cytoplasm of the interstitial cells. Hence, the immunolocalization of ET-positive cells in rat testis is apparently developmentally regulated (4).

ETA receptors are present in peritubular myoid (3, 15) and Leydig cells (2, 4, 15). In Leydig cells ET-1 positively regulates basal and human chorionic gonadotrophin (hCG)-induced steroidogenesis (1, 2). In myoid cells, ET-1 increased inositol triphosphate and calcium mobilization (3), suggesting a role in the control of tubular motility. Since ET-1 release from Sertoli cells is negatively regulated by FSH, it is possible that the ET system in rat testis is activated in physiological conditions characterized by low levels of FSH, as in prepubertal life.

ENDOTHELIN IN HUMAN TESTIS

We therefore extended our studies from rat to human testis. Northern analysis of total RNA from adult human testis indicated the expression of specific transcript for ETA, ETB and ET-1 but not ET-3 (data not shown). Radioligand binding studies confirmed the expression of both subtypes of ET isoreceptors (Fig. 1).

ETA receptors in human testis are present in elevated concentration (700 fmoles/mg prot.) and bind with high affinity ET-1, ET-2, VIC (the mouse homologue of ET-2) and the ETA receptor antagonist BQ 123. Conversely, they show lower affinity for ET-3, sarafotoxin (SRTX) and the ETB selective agonist ALA-ET. ETB receptors are 10-fold less concentrated than ETA and binds with high affinity all the peptides tested but not BQ 123. Hence, in human testis BQ 123 is selective for the ETA receptor.

Immunohistochemical studies performed in human testis indicate that ET-1-like protein is expressed with an almost identical pattern of positivity to

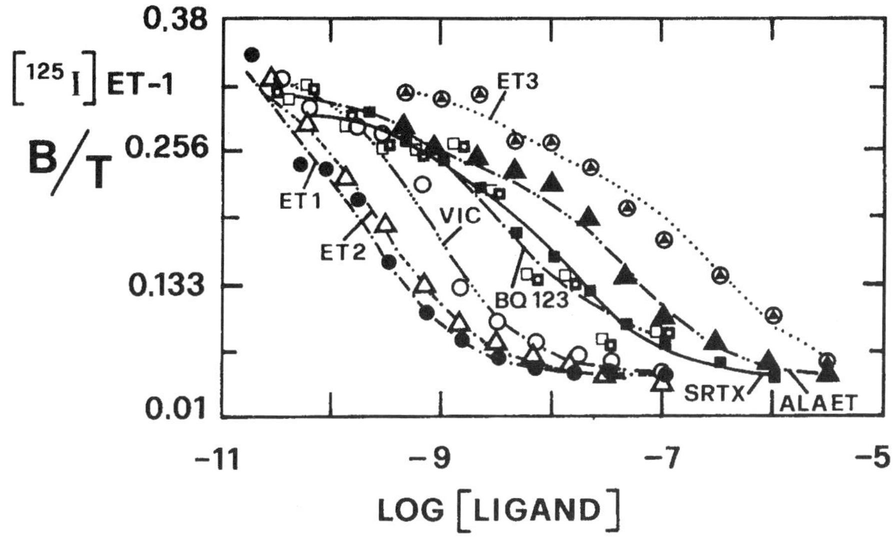

FIG. 1. Displacement of ^{125}I-ET-1 binding to pooled membranes prepared from human testis. Membranes (0.075 mg/ml) were incubated for 60 minutes at 22 C with 50 pM ^{125}I-ET-1 in the presence or absence of increasing concentration of ET-1 (closed circles), ET-2 (open triangles), VIC (open circles), BQ 123 (open boxes), SRTX (closed boxes), ALAET (closed triangles), ET-3 (triangles in circles).

that of the rat testis. Furthermore, such positivity is apparently developmentally regulated. Indeed, in fetal, neonatal and prepubertal human testis ET-1 positivity was confined to the Sertoli cells, while during reproductive life, specific staining was also detected in the interstitium. Figure 2 shows a typical staining for ET-1 in human testis.

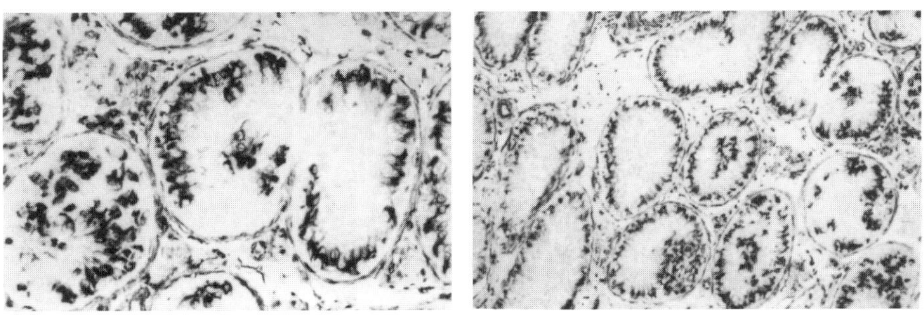

FIG. 2. Seminiferous tubules from an adult human testis immunostained with a polyclonal antibody against ET-1 as described in (4). Sertoli cells with stained cytoplasm are seen in the tubules. Some interstitial cells show also positive staining for ET-1. Note the intense positivity of the endothelial cells of the blood vessels. (Left panel: x 100; right panel: x 40).

CONCLUSIONS

ETs are produced by mammalian testis and exert biological functions. However, the precise function, if any, of ETs in the testis is still undefined. It is remarkable that in heterozygous mice deficient for ET-1, fertility was still retained (7). In homozygous mice, although not viable, major anomalies in the reproductive tract were not reported (7).

REFERENCES

1. Conte D., Questino P., Fillo S., Nordio M., Isidori A. and Romanelli F. (1993): J. Endocrinol. 136: R1-R4.
2. Ergul A., Glassberg M.K., Majercik M.H. and Puett D. (1993): Endocrinology 132: 598-603.
3. Filippini A., Tripiciano A., Palombi F., Teti A., Paniccia R., Stefanini M. and Ziparo E. (1993): Endocrinology 133: 1789-1796.
4. Fantoni G., Morris P.L., Forti G., Vannelli G.B., Orlando C., Barni T., Sestini R., Danza G. and Maggi M. (1993): Am. J. Physiol. 265: E267-E274.
5. Karne S., Jayawickreme C.K. and Lerner M.R. (1993): J. Biol. Chem. 268 : 19126-19133.
6. Kenigsberg D., Island L. and Jefferson P. (1992): J. Clin. Endocrinol. Metab. 74: 12-13.
7. Kurihara Y., Kurihara H., Suzuki H., Kodama T., Maemura K., Nagai R., Oda H., Kuwaki T., Cao W.-H., Kumada N., Jishage K., Ouchi Y., Azuma S., Toyada Y., Ishikawa T., Kumada M. and Yazaki Y. (1994): Nature 368: 703-710.
8. Maggi M., Vannelli G.B., Peri A., Brandi M.L., Fantoni G., Giannini S., Torrisi C., Guardabasso V., Barni T., Toscano V., Massi G. and Serio M. (1991): Am. J. Physiol. 260: E292-E305, 1991a.
9. Maggi M., Fantoni G., Peri A., Rossi S., Baldi E., Magini A., Massi G. and Serio M. (1993): Reg. Pept. 45: 97- 101.
10. Maggi M., Vannelli G.B., Fantoni G., Baldi E., Magini A., Peri A., Giannin S., Gloria L., Del Carlo P., Casparis D., Tomei T. and Serio M. (1994): J. Endocrinol. (in press).
11. Masaki T. (1993): Endocrine Rev. 14: 256-268.
12. Matsumoto H., Suzuki N., Onda H. and Fujino M. (1989): Biochem. Biophys. Res. Comm. 164: 74-80.
13. Orlando C., Brandi M.L., Peri A., Giannini S., Fantoni G., Calabresi E., Serio M. and Maggi M. (1990): Endocrinology 126: 1780-1783.
14. Peri A., Vannelli G.B., Fantoni C., Giannini S., Barni T., Orlando C., Serio M. and Maggi M. (1992): Am. J. Physiol. 263: E158-E167.
15. Sakaguchi H., Kozuka M., Hirose S., Ito T. and Hagiwara H. (1992): Am. J. Physiol. 263: R15-R19.
16. Sakurai T., Yanagisawa M., Inoue A., Ryant U.S., Kimura S., Mitsui Y., Goto K. and Masaki T. (1991): Biochem. Biophys. Res. Commun. 175: 44-47.

Frontiers in Endocrinology
Volume 9 - 1994

Effects of Clonidine on the Sympathoadrenal System of Patients with Hypogonadism

G. Zizzo, C. Carani, E. Toschi, R. Menozzi, F. Coletta, A. Velardo, G. Del Rio and P. Marrama

Department of Internal Medicine, Endocrine Unit, University of Modena, via del Pozzo 71, 41100 Modena, Italy

INTRODUCTION

Several studies (4, 6, 7, 9) have demonstrated that sex steroids play a regulatory role on the secretion of adrenal medulla. A sexual dimorphism in catecholamine secretion has been reported in several conditions (1, 2). Testosterone can influence catecholamine secretion (8) and it has been reported (7) to inhibit re-uptake of catecholamines.

It has been demonstrated *in vivo* that testosterone can regulate the number of adrenoceptors in male rat adipocytes (10)

Recently, Kiem et al. (5) showed that the effects of clonidine, an α2-agonist drug, on the GH release and blood pressure were lost in long-term castrated rats, but were restored by testosterone replacement in the castrates. The authors suggested that testosterone might act to maintain the sensitivity of α2-adrenoceptors to clonidine.

In order to study the relationship between testosterone, catecholamine and α2-adrenergic activity in men, we evaluated the cardiovascular and catecholamine responses to clonidine in a group of male hypogonadal subjects before and after testosterone therapy and in a group of control subjects.

MATERIAL AND METHODS

Eight male hypogonadal patients (age 32.2±5.0 years; BMI: 23.9±1.1) were studied before and after 3 months of testosterone treatment

(Testoviron depot 250 mg i.m. every 21 days). Eight normal male subjects (age 28.7±4.3 years; BMI: 22.8±2.3) constituted the control group.

Five out of eight patients were affected by hypergonadotropic hypogonadism while three patients were affected by hypogonadotropic hypogonadism.

All the subjects were disease free and did not habitually consume drugs or alcohol. They were selected on the basis of normal blood pressure (BP) (systolic BP < 140 mmHg; diastolic BP < 90 mmHg).

All subjects were hospitalized 24h before the study; at 07:00 h, after an overnight fast, an 18-gauge iv catheter was placed in an antecubital vein and a 0.9% saline infusion was started at a slow rate. Three blood samples were drawn at –30',–15', 0 for the basal determination of norepinephrine (NE) and epinephrine (E). At –30' we also measured testosterone plasma levels. At 0' a 300 μg dose of clonidine was swallowed with water. Blood samples for catecholamine determinations were drawn again at 120', 130', 140' after clonidine administration. Systolic (SBP), diastolic blood pressure (DBP) and pulse rate (PR) were measured, with an automated cuff device, every 15 minutes during the entire test.

Plasma catecholamines were determined using a reversed-phase high performance liquid chromatography method with electrochemical detection (3). The intra-assay coefficients of variation of E and NE were 4% and 3%, respectively, and the inter-assay coefficients of variation were 8.2% and 7.3%, respectively.

Conventional RIA techniques was used for plasma testosterone determination.

Results were expressed as mean ± SEM; Two-way ANOVA was used for statistical analysis. A p value less than 0.05 was considered significant.

RESULTS

In hypogonadal subjects, plasma testosterone levels were 170±50 ng/ml before therapy and 753±22 ng/ml after therapy. Basal plasma NE levels were found to be lower in hypogonadal patients before therapy than in control subjects (125±31 pg/ml vs 196±44 pg/ml, respectively; $p<0.05$). Testosterone treatment increased plasma NE levels in hypogonadal patients (185±33 pg/ml; $p<0.05$ vs before therapy). Basal plasma E levels were comparable (p=NS) in hypogonadal patients before (33±9 pg/ml), and after therapy (33±6 pg/ml) as well as in the control group (38±5 pg/ml). Clonidine administration induced a percent decrease of plasma NE levels (ANOVA $F=13$, $p<0.005$) which was of a similar magnitude both before and after therapy (46±9% vs 50±10% respectively; p=NS) and was not different to that of control subjects (42±8% p=NS).

Clonidine administration did not affect ($F=0.1$, p=NS) plasma E levels in hypogonadal subjects either before (30±8 pg/ml), or after therapy (31±7 pg/ml) or in the control group (27±2 pg/ml).

Basal SBP and DBP values in patients before therapy (SBP=117±3 mmHg, DBP=74±3 mmHg) were comparable to those after therapy (SBP=116±2 mmHg, DBP=72±2 mmHg), and to those in the control subjects (SBP=120±3 mmHg, DBP=81±2 mmHg). We observed a decrease in SBP values after clonidine ($F=12$, $p<0.001$) values being comparable in the patients before (90±2 mmHg), and after testosterone therapy (91±2 mmHg) and in the control group (110±2 mmHg). Clonidine administration induced a significant ($p<0.001$) decrease in DBP values in hypogonadal subjects both before (52±1 mmHg), and after testosterone treatment (55±2 mmHg) and in the control subjects (71±3 mmHg). This decrease was comparable in hypogonadal men and in the control group.

Basal PR values in patients before therapy (62±2 b/min), were comparable to those after therapy (61±3 b/min) and with those in the control group (67±2 b/min). Clonidine did not significantly (p=NS) affect PR values in the hypogonadal subjects either before (55±1 b/min) or after treatment (55±1 b/min) or in the control subjects (60±3 b/min).

DISCUSSION AND CONCLUSIONS

Our data provide evidence, for the first time in humans, that a decreased Sympathetic Nervous System (SNS) activity is present in male hypogonadism. Since testosterone treatment is able to restore normal plasma NE levels it seems likely to suggest a relationship between plasma NE levels and testoterone secretion. Testosterone may play an important role in the regulation of catecholamine secretion (5, 7, 8), exerting a regulatory action on the transcriptional and/or post-transcriptional levels (10). Furthermore, it has been demostrated that testosterone stimulates catecholamine-induced lipolysis *in vivo* and increases the number of β-adrenoceptors in adipose tissue (10).

An increase in the α2-adrenoceptors activity, which, in turn, is able to inhibit SNS activity, may be responsible for the low plasma NE in hypogonadal men. However the similar percent decrease of catecholamines after clonidine and the comparable cardiovascular responses observed in hypogonadal patients both before and after testosterone treatment demonstrate a normal α2-adrenergic activity. So it is feasible that sexual dimorphism demonstrated in catecholamine secretion may be dependent on the opposite regulatory effects of sex-steroids.

In conclusion, the decreased sympathoadrenergic tone observed in hypogonadal subjects, unlike previously reported findings in rats (5), does not seem to be related to alterations of α2-adrenergic activity. The normal GH response to clonidine found in hypogonadal men (data not shown) seems to lend support to the above conclusions. The exact mechanisms involved in the regulatory action of testosterone on NE secretion remains to be defined.

REFERENCES

1. Amiel S.A., Maran A., Powrie J.K., Umpleby A.M. and Macdonald I.A. (1993): Diabetologia 36: 460-464.
2. Davidson L., Vandogen R., Rouse I.L., Beilin L.J. and Tunney A. (1984): Clin. Sci. 67: 347-352.
3. Del Rio G., Velardo A., Zizzo G., Marrama P. and Della Casa L. (1993): Int. J. Obes. 17: 465- 469.
4. Gandia L., Casado L.F., Lopez M.G. and Garcia A.G. (1991): Br. J. Pharmacol. 103: 1073-1078.
5. Kiem D.T., Stark E. and Fekete M.I.K. (1990): Neuroendocrinology 51: 226- 232.
6. Lopez M.G., Abad F., Sancho C., de Pascual R., Borges R., Maroto R., Dixon W. and Garcia A.G. (1991): J. Pharmacol. Exp. Ther. 259: 279-285.
7 Salt P.J. (1972): Eur. J. Pharmacol. 20: 329-340.
8. Simpkins J.W., Kalra P.S. and Kalra S.P. (1980): Neuroendocrinology 30: 94-100.
9. Wiechman B.E. and Borowitz J.L. (1979): Pharmacology 18: 279-285.
10. Xu X., De Pergola G. and Bjorntörp P. (1991): Endocrinology 128: 379-382.

Frontiers in Endocrinology
Volume 9 - 1994

Role of P_2-Purinergic Receptors in the Acrosome Reaction of Human Sperm

M. Rossato, F. Di Virgilio[1], A. Varotto, A. Bettella and C. Foresta

Institute of Internal Medicine, University of Padova, Via Ospedale 105, 35128 Padova;
[1]Institute of General Pathology, University of Ferrara, Via Borsari 46, 44100 Ferrara, Italy

INTRODUCTION

In order to fertilize the oocyte spermatozoa need to undergo a complex series of events collectively known as capacitation and acrosome reaction (12). These processes take place in the female genital tract but the precise identity of the factors that induce sperm acrosome reaction is still unknown (11).

Recently, we demonstrated that extracellular ATP (ATP_e) is a potent inducer of sperm activation in non capacitated human sperm (5). It has long been shown that ATP_e has important effects on cellular functions (7): in the nervous system it acts as a neurotransmitter, in a variety of smooth muscle cell types it induces vasorelaxation or vasoconstriction (3). Furthermore, ATP_e plays a role in the immune system as a cytotoxic mediator (2, 4) and it has been shown to act as a secretagogue in adrenal chromaffin and insulin secreting cells (8). These different actions of ATP_e are mediated by plasma membrane receptors termed P_2-purinergic receptors inducing ion fluxes, phosphoinositide turnover and other responses (3).

The intracellular mechanisms whereby ATP_e trigger acrosome reaction in human sperm are poorly understood since a role for calcium, the best known intracellular mediator of sperm activation, in ATP_e action was ruled out under our experimental conditions (5).

The present study was undertaken to elucidate the mechanisms of ATP_e-induced sperm activation.

MATERIAL AND METHODS

Sperm collection Sperm samples were obtained from healthy sperm donors after 3 days of sexual abstinence. After liquefaction semen samples were analyzed for semen volume, pH, sperm concentration, morphology, motility and viability. Experiments were performed with spermatozoa isolated with the swim-up technique as previously described (5), centrifuged for 10 min at 800 x g and resuspended in BWW (1) at a concentration of 15×10^6/ml. In some experiments NaCl was replaced by an iso-osmotic concentration of choline, methylglucamine or sucrose.

Induction of acrosome reaction with ATP Sperm suspensions were incubated in each specific medium for 2 h at 37°C in the presence of ATP_e (2.5 mM). Aliquots were collected every 30 min for evaluation of motility, viability and acrosome reaction. Acrosome reaction was evaluated by the triple stain technique, as described by Talbot and Chacon (10).

Measurement of sperm $[Ca^{2+}]_i$ and plasma membrane potential Sperm intracellular Ca^{2+} concentration ($[Ca^{2+}]_i$) was measured utilizing the fluorescent dye fura-2/AM: sperm suspensions were incubated in BWW for 30 min at 37 °C in the presence of fura-2/AM (2 μM). $[Ca^{2+}]_i$ was evaluated as previously described (5). Sperm plasma membrane potential changes were monitored with the potential-sensitive dye bis-oxonol at the wavelength pair 540/580 nm as previously described (6).

Statistical analysis Data were analyzed with Stat View II (Abacus Concepts, Berkely, CA) statistical package.

RESULTS

Incubation with ATP_e (2.5 mM) was able to stimulate acrosome reaction in human sperm (from 3.8 ± 1.7 % to 25.9 ± 3.0 %, $p < 0.01$ vs control). Figure 1 shows that ATP is able to induce a rapid sperm plasma membrane depolarization (trace a) that was completely dependent on an influx of sodium (Na^+) from the extracellular medium since, when extracellular Na^+ was isoosmotically replaced by choline or methylglucamine, ion less permeant than Na^+ through the ATP_e-gated channel (9), the depolarizing effect was reduced (Fig. 1, trace b and c, respectively). Furthermore, Na^+ substitution with sucrose, completely impermeant through the ATP_e-gated channel (9), prevented the ATP_e induced plasma membrane depolarization (Fig. 1, trace d).

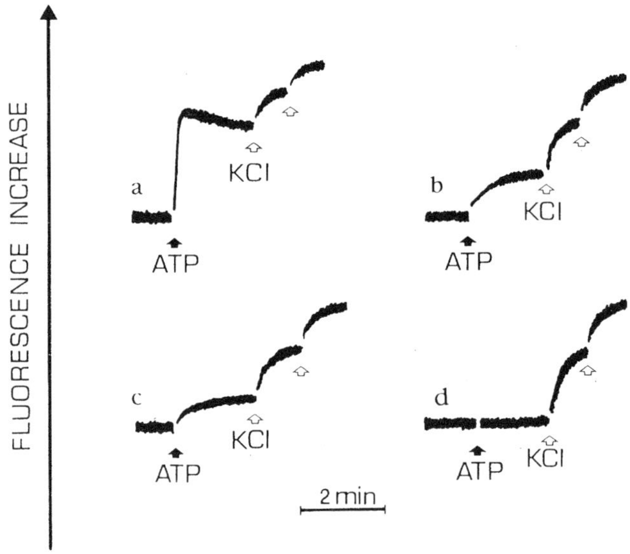

FIG. 1. Effects of ATP_e on plasma membrane potential of sperm suspended in BWW (trace a), Na-free choline supplemented (trace b), Na-free methylglucamine supplemented (trace c), Na-free sucrose supplemented saline. ATP 2.5 mM (black arrows), KCl 30 mM (white arrows).

The role of Na^+ in the induction of acrosome reaction by ATP_e is further supported by the results reported in Table 1 which demonstrate that sperm acrosome reaction was inhibited when extracellular Na^+ was omitted from the medium.

Table 1. *Effects of ATP_e on sperm acrosome reaction percentages in the presence (BWW) and in the absence (sucrose) of extracellular Na^+*

Time (minutes)	0	120
BWW	4.7 ± 1.7	5.9 ± 2.1
BWW + ATP (2.5 mM)	3.8 ± 1.7	25.9 ± 3.0*
Sucrose	4.9 ± 1.0	6.0 ± 1.8
Sucrose + ATP (2.5 mM)	3.9 ± 1.1	5.9 ± 4.8

* $p < 0.01$ vs control.

DISCUSSION

In a recent study, we demonstrated that ATP is able to induce acrosome reaction in non capacitated human spermatozoa, but we were unable to explain the underlying mechanisms (5). Our results, however, allowed us to exclude a role for Ca^{2+} in ATP_e effects since, under our experimental conditions, this nucleotide did not induce any modification of $[Ca^{2+}]_i$ and it was able to induce acrosome reaction also in the absence of Ca^{2+} in the extracellular medium. Our present study confirms that ATP_e is able to stimulate acrosome reaction in human sperm and demonstrates that ATP_e is able to induce a rapid plasma membrane depolarization due to an influx of Na^+ from the extracellular medium. This influx of Na^+ seems involved in the stimulation of the acrosome reaction since ATP_e was able to induce this effect only when Na^+ was present in the extracellular medium. ATP_e-gated Na^+-channel in human sperm share similarities with channels described only in a few other cells (3) and possess properties that could be ascribed to a novel subtype of ATP_e-activated P_2-purinergic receptor that opens a channel permeable to Na^+ but not to Ca^{2+}, in contrast to the majority of other ATP_e-gated channels which admit Na^+ together with Ca^{2+}.

REFERENCES

1. Biggers J.D., Whitten W.K. and Whittingam D.G. (1971): In: Methods in Mammalian Embryology, edited by Daniel, J.C., pp. 86-116, W.H. Freeman. San Francisco.
2. Di Virgilio F., Pizzo P., Zanovello P., Bronte V. and Collavo D. (1990): Immunol. Today 11: 274-277.
3. Dubyak G.R. and El-Moatassim C. (1993): Am. J. Physiol. 265: C577-C606.
4. Filippini A., Taffs R.E. and Sitkovsky M.V. (1991): Proc. Natl. Acad. Sci. USA 87: 8267-8271.
5. Foresta C., Rossato M. and Di Virgilio F. (1992): J. Biol. Chem. 267: 19443-19447.
6. Foresta C., Rossato M. and Di Virgilio F. (1993): Biochem. J. 294: 279-283.
7. Gordon J.L. (1986): Biochem. J. 233: 309-319.
8. Li G., Milani D., Dunne M.J., Pralong W.F., Theler J.M., Petersen O.H. and Wollheim C.B. (1991): J. Biol. Chem. 266: 3449-3457.
9. Pizzo P., Zanovello P., Bronte V. and Di Virgilio F. (1991): Biochem. J. 274: 139-144.
10. Talbot P. and Chacon R.S. (1981): J. Exp. Zool. 215: 201-208.
11. Wassarman P.M. (1987): Ann. Rev. Cell Biol. 3:109-142.
12. Yanagimachi Y. (1988): In: Physiology of Reproduction, edited by E. Knobil and D. Neils, pp. 135-185, Raven Press. New York.

Frontiers in Endocrinology
Volume 9 - 1994

Responsiveness to Progesterone of Spermatozoa is significantly related to the Fertilization Rate in IVF Cycles

Cs. Krausz, L. Bonaccorsi, M. Luconi, G. Forti, B. Fuzzi[1], L. Criscuoli[1], S. Pellegrini[1] and E. Baldi

Department of Clinical Physiopathology, Andrology Unit, Viale Pieraccini 6, 50139 Florence; [1]Department of Obstetrics and Gynaecology, Viale Morgagni 85, 50134 Florence, Italy

INTRODUCTION

Achievement of egg fertilization is one of the most important steps in the process of an *in vitro* fertilization (IVF) treatment program. A higher percentage of fertilized oocytes would increase the number of embryos available for transfer and thus ensure a higher probability of a successful pregnancy. Considering the human involvement and the high cost of IVF it would be of great value to be able to predict the fertilizing ability of sperm.

It has been reported that follicular fluid components that are released at ovulation together with the oocyte modulate different aspects of sperm function. Progesterone (P) appears to be primarily involved in the action of follicular fluid since there is evidence that P stimulates acrosome reaction (6, 1), and hyperactivation (3) of spermatozoa. A decreased sperm responsiveness to P has recently been described in oligospermic (2), as well as in some infertile patients (7), suggesting the presence of an alteration of the putative sperm membrane P receptor in some cases of male infertility. However, these studies did not directly correlate response to P with sperm fertilizing ability.

The aim of the present study was to investigate if the sperm ability to fertilize human oocytes *in vitro* was related to their responsiveness (measured as increase of intracellular free calcium concentration ([Ca 2++]i) and acrosome reaction) to P.

MATERIAL AND METHODS

Subjects The study population consisted of 22 unselected couples undergoing IVF therapy.

Sperm preparation Motile sperm were separated by the swim-up procedure in IVF medium, washed and divided into three aliqouts, one for subsequent oocyte insemination and the other two for calcium and acrosome reaction studies.

Measurement of [Ca 2++]i was carried out with a spectrofluorimetric method using FURA/2AM as Ca2++ probe (1). The acrosome reacted spermatozoa were evaluated using the fluorescent probe FITC-labeled Arachis hypogea lectin as previously described (2, 4).

RESULTS

Subjects were arbitrarily divided into two groups on the basis of percentage fertilization rate (%FR): group 1 with a FR >50% and group 2 with a FR <50% with the inclusion of 7 subjects that did not fertilize any oocytes.

Basal and post swim-up conventional parameters (number and motilty) were significantly different in the two groups of patients, however, only a weak correlation with FR was observed. Moreover, it is worthwhile noting that in 7 patients who failed to fertilize, sperm motility ranged from 5 to 50% in seminal fluid and from 50% to 90% after swim-up procedure.

There was no difference in basal sperm [Ca2++]i and in spontaneous acrosome reaction between the two groups of subjects.

As reported in Table 1 intracellular calcium increase in response to 1 ug/ml P and acrosome reaction following 4µg/ml P challenge (ARPC: P induced- spontaneous reaction) were significantly higher in subjects with FR >50% ($p<0.005$ and $p<0.05$, respectively). Furthermore, both the intracellular calcium increase and ARPC were significantly correlated with the FR ($r=0.69$, $p<0.001$ and r=0,79, $p<0.001$, respectively).

Table 1. *The % increase of [Ca++]i and the % increase of AR in response to P (ARPC) in the two groups of subjects*

	% increase [Ca++]i (n=18)	% ARPC (n=16)
FR > 50%	101.1±48.9	5.8±1.6
FR < 50%	286.6±59.0*	15.6±2.9°

p<0.005*; p<0.05°.

DISCUSSION

In the past few years, several studies have been performed in order to find a good predictive parameter of sperm fertilizing ability. As previously described by Liu and Baker (5), our study confirmed that traditional parameters of semen analysis, such as sperm concentration and motility have little or no predictive value of sperm fertilizing ability. On the other hand, it is generally believed that biochemical alterations of sperm function are responsible for defective sperm-egg interaction. Our study indicates a defective responsiveness to P in subjects with lower fertilizing ability. Moreover, we directly correlated intracellular calcium as well as the acrosome reaction increase in response to P with the rate of fertilization of human oocytes and found a highly significant correlation between responsiveness to P and FR.

These preliminary results suggest that the assessment of P-sperm responsiveness in male patients undergoing assisted reproductive techniques could be a reliable test in the prediction of fertilizing ability.

REFERENCES

1. Baldi E., Casano R., Falsetti C., Krausz Cs., Maggi M. and Forti G. (1991): J. Androl. 12, 323-330.
2. Falsetti C., Baldi E., Krausz Cs., Casano R., Failli P. and Forti G. (1993): J. Androl. 14, 17-22.
3. Fetterolf P.M., Meriano J., Choma F.P., Cooblal-Sooknaan R. (1991): In 47th Annual Meeting of the American Fertility Society, Abstracts P-0-79, s100 pp.
4. Krausz Cs., Gervasi G., Forti G. and Baldi E. (1994): Hum. Reprod. 9, 471-476.
5. Liu D.Y. and Baker H.W.G. (1992): Fertil. Steril. 58, 465-483.
6. Osman R.A., Andria M.L., Jones A.D. and Meizel S. (1989): Biochem Biophys. Res. Commun. 160, 828-833.
7. Tesarik J. and Mendoza C. (1992): Fertil. Steril. 58, 793-797.

Frontiers in Endocrinology
Volume 9 - 1994

Galanin and Testicular Steroidogenesis: *in vitro* Study

F. Romanelli, S. Fillo, P. Questino, A. Isidori and D. Conte

Chair of Andrology, Institute of Medical Clinics V,
University of Rome La Sapienza,
00161 Rome, Italy

INTRODUCTION

Galanin (GAL) is a 29-aminoacid peptide initially isolated from porcine intestine (11). Immunohistochemical studies demonstrated that this peptide is widely distributed in the central nervous system (8), and in gastrointestinal, respiratory and genitourinary tracts (1, 10).

It has been shown that GAL exerts numerous biological actions like the modulation of neurotransmitter activity, the contraction of smooth muscle (particularly of gastrointestinal tract) and the regulation of various hormonal secretions, notably at hypothalamo-pituitary and pancreatic level. On the hypothalamo-pituitary axis this peptide stimulates the secretion of GH (2), TSH (5), LH (6, 9) and prolactin (14) and inhibits ACTH (5) release. The afore-mentioned effects seem to be due to a hypothalamic and/or pituitary site of action.

GAL at pancreatic level is able to increase insulin secretion and to decrease somatostatin production (9); it exerts stimulatory effects on corticosterone and aldosterone secretion by the adrenal gland (7); it has been shown to be localized in the male genital system and particularly in the testis (12); and moreover, Ghosh et al. (4), observed that it is able to stimulate estradiol and lactic acid production *in vitro* by Sertoli cells of prepubertal rats.

In the light of these data, the present study was designed to evaluate the activity of GAL on rat testicular steroidogenesis *in vitro*. To this purpose, the effects of different doses of GAL, on basal and hCG-induced testosterone (T) production by purified Leydig cells, were examined.

MATERIAL AND METHODS

Leydig cells from ten-week-old Sprague Dawley rats were obtained after collagenase treatment and purified on Percoll gradient (3). 10^5 Leydig cells were incubated for three hours at 34°C under O_2/CO_2 (95:5) in 500 μL of medium M199 containing the different tested substances. At the end of incubation, cells were centrifuged and supernatants were stored at -70°C until assayed for T by RIA (values are expressed as ng/10^5 cells). Statistical analysis has been performed and data were analyzed by Student t test; *$p<0.01$ was considered statistically significant.

RESULTS AND DISCUSSION

Galanin concentrations ranging from 1pM to 100nM were tested, either alone or in the presence of a low effective dose of hCG (0.01ng/ml), as determined in separate experiments.

As shown in Figure 1 GAL alone did not affect basal T production (GAL 1pM: 0.55±0.07; GAL 10pM: 0.54±0.03; GAL 100pM: 0.58±0.05; GAL 1nM: 0.62±0.07; GAL 10nM: 0.61±0.06; GAL 100nM: 0.59±0.04 vs control: 0.55±0.04), while, when such peptide was added in combination with

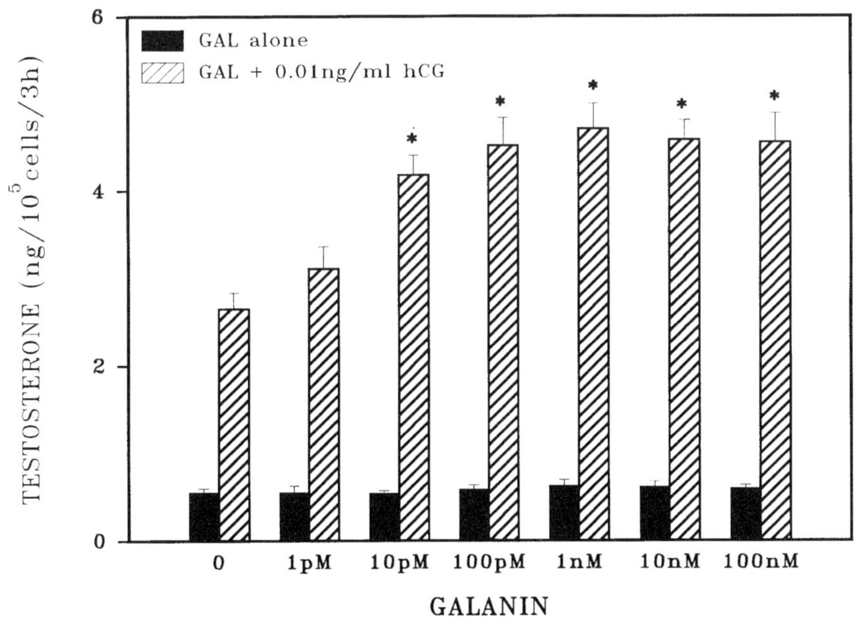

FIG.1. Effects of galanin (GAL), alone or together with a low effective dose of hCG, on testosterone secretion by rat Leydig cells in vitro. *p<0.01 GAL+hCG vs hCG.

0.01ng/ml hCG, an amplification of Leydig cells response was observed (GAL 1pM+hCG: 3.11±0.25; GAL 10pM+hCG: 4.18±0.23*; GAL 100pM+hCG: 4.52±0.32*; GAL 1nM+hCG: 4.71±0.29*; GAL 10nM+hCG: 4.59±0.22*; GAL 100nM+hCG: 4.56±0.33* vs hCG alone: 2.65±0.19).

Data obtained in the present study indicate for the first time that GAL has no effect on basal steroidogenesis indicating a lack of tonic action, while this peptide is able to enhance the acute gonadotropic stimulation of T output, probably increasing Leydig cell sensitivity to hCG.

Further studies are needed to identify the biological meaning of this secretagogue activity of galanin and to clarify its mechanism of action.

REFERENCES

1. Bauer F.E., Christofides N.D., Hacker G.W., Blank M.A., Polak J.M. and Bloom S.R. (1986a): Peptides 7: 5-10.
2. Bauer F.E., Ginsberg L., Venetikou M., Mackay D.J., Burrin J.M. and Bloom S.R. (1986b): Lancet 2: 192-5
3. Conte D., Questino P., Fillo S., Nordio M., Isidori A. and Romanelli F. (1993): J. Endocrinol. 136: R1-R4.
4. Ghosh P.K., Uzumcu M., York J.P. and Lin Y.C. (1993): The Endocrine Society 75th Annual Meeting, Abst. 206, p. 102.
5. Hooi S.C., Maiter D.M., Martin J.B. and Koenig J.I. (1990): Endocrinology 127: 2281-9.
6. Lopez F.J., Merchenthaler I., Ching M., Wisniewski M.G. and Negro-Vilar A. (1991): Proc. Natl. Acad. Sci. USA 88: 4508-12.
7. Mazzocchi G., Malendowicz L.K., Rebuffat P. and Nussdorfer G.G. (1991): Res. Exp. Med. Biol. 192: 373-381.
8. Merchenthaler I., Lopez F.J. and Negro-Vilar A. (1993): Progr. Neurobiol. 40: 711-769.
9. Sahu A., Xu B. and Karla S.P. (1994): Endocrinology 134 (2): 529-536.
10. Shew R.L., Papka R.E. and McNeill D.L. (1992): Peptides 13: 273-279.
11. Tatemoto K., Rokaeus A., Jorwall H., McDonald T.J. and Mutt V. (1983): FEBS Lett. 164: 124-128.
12. Torsello A., Vrontakis M.E., Schroedter I.C., Vuille J.C., Ikejiani C. and Friesen H.G. (1992): Endocrinology 130:3301-6.
13. Vrontakis M.E., Torsello A. and Friesen H.G. (1991): J. Endocrinol. Invest. 14: 785-794.
14. Wynick D., Hammond P.J., Akinsanja K.O. and Bloom S.R. (1993): Nature 365 (6437): 529-532.

Frontiers in Endocrinology
Volume 9 - 1994

Autocrine Growth Regulation of Human Prostatic Cancer Cells: Role of the EGF/TGFα System

P. Limonta, D. Dondi, M. Montagnani Marelli, R.M. Moretti and M. Motta

Center for Endocrinological Oncology, Department of Endocrinology
Via Balzaretti 9, 20133 Milan, Italy

INTRODUCTION

The androgen-dependence of prostatic carcinoma has been widely demonstrated (6, 12, 16). However, it is becoming increasingly clear that also locally produced growth modulatory factors play a crucial rôle in the control of prostatic tumor growth (4, 7, 9, 11, 14, 17). These growth factors seem to regulate cell proliferation by acting in an autocrine way through the binding to specific cell surface receptors.

The human androgen-responsive prostate cancer cell line LNCaP (Lymph Node Carcinoma of the Prostate) provides a very useful *in vitro* system for the elucidation of these mechanisms (8). LNCaP cells have been reported to produce EGF and TGFα polypeptides (3). Moreover, these cells express receptors for EGF, and respond to EGF with a significantly increased growth rate (10, 15).

Taken together, these data seem to suggest that an EGF/TGFα growth modulatory system might be expressed in this cell line and might participate in the autocrine regulation of cell proliferation. The present experiments have been performed to verify this hypothesis.

RESULTS AND DISCUSSION

Effect of EGF on the expression of the c-fos protooncogene in LNCaP cells
The *c-fos* protooncogene is believed to act as an intracellular signal

mediating the mitogenic action of EGF (5, 13). It has been shown that the activation of the EGF receptor is followed by an increased expression of this gene in a variety of cell lines.To verify whether the activation of the EGF receptor is followed by a modification of the expression of the *c-fos* gene also in prostatic tumor cells, LNCaP cells were maintained in a quiescent state (RPMI-1640 supplemented with 0.5% FCS) for 24 hours, and then treated with EGF (5 ng/ml) for 15, 30 and 60 minutes. After this period, total cellular RNA was isolated (2), fractionated by electrophoresis and blotted onto a nylon membrane. The membrane was then hybridized with a specific ^{32}P-labeled *c-fos* cDNA probe. The results obtained show that EGF induces a significant increase of *c-fos* mRNA levels, which peak at 30 minutes.

These data indicate that the intracellular mechanisms usually associated with the activation of the EGF receptor are functional in LNCaP cells. Moreover, these results suggest that, also in prostatic tumor cells, the mitogenic action of EGF may be mediated by the activation of the *c-fos* protooncogene.

Effect of a monoclonal antibody against the EGF receptor on LNCaP cell proliferation To verify whether the activation of the EGF receptor may be involved in the autocrine regulation of prostatic tumor cell proliferation, the effects of a monoclonal antibody against this receptor (Ab225, kindly provided by Dr. J. Mendelshon, Memorial Sloan-Kettering Cancer Center, NY) have been analyzed on LNCaP cell proliferation. Cells were cultured in serum-free conditions (RPMI-1640 containing 6.25 μg/ml of insulin and transferrin, 6.25 ng/ml of selenous acid, 1.25 mg/ml of bovine serum albumin) and treated for 4 days with Ab225 (1 μg/ml) either in the absence or in the presence of exogenous EGF. The treatment with Ab225 resulted in a significant decrease of LNCaP cell proliferation; this effect was completely reversed by the addition to the culture medium of EGF at the dose of 0.5 μg/ml.

These data suggest that, in the absence of all exogenous growth factors, the specific activation of the EGF receptor plays a crucial role in the autocrine regulation of LNCaP cell proliferation.

Effect of immunoneutralizing antibodies against either EGF or TGFα on LNCaP cell proliferation It is well known that both EGF and TGFα stimulate cell proliferation by binding to a common cell surface receptor (1).

To establish which one of the two peptides might be responsible for the autocrine activation of the EGF receptor which participates in the control of prostatic tumor growth, the effects of immunoneutralizing antibodies against either EGF or TGFα have been studied on LNCaP cell proliferation. Cells have been cultured in serum-free conditions (as described above), and treated for 4 days with either the anti-human EGF or the anti-human TGFα neutralizing antibody in the dose of 5 μg/ml.

The results obtained show that the treatment with either anti-EGF or anti-TGFα antibodies significantly inhibits cell proliferation (59.4% and 58.8% inhibition of cell growth for the EGF and the TGFα antibody, respectively) (Table 1).

Table 1. *Effect of both anti-EGF and anti-TGFα antibodies on LNCaP cell proliferation*[a]

Groups	Vehicle	Anti-EGF	Anti-TGFα
Cells/well x 10^{-4}	27.29 ± 1.51	11.07 ± 1.22*	11.22 ± 0.31*

[a]Values are expressed as mean cell number ± SE; * $p < 0.05$ vs vehicle treated cells.

These data suggest that both EGF and TGFα, secreted by LNCaP cells, are involved in the local mechanisms regulating prostatic tumor cell proliferation.

These observations are in line with those recently reported for the human androgen-independent prostate cancer cell lines DU 145 and PC3 (4, 7).

CONCLUSIONS

The present data suggest that: a) a functional EGF receptor is present in LNCaP cells; b) this receptor plays a crucial role in the autocrine regulation of LNCaP cell proliferation; c) both EGF and TGFα seem to be involved in these mechanisms; d) in addition to androgens, also specific growth factors seem to participate in the control of cell proliferation in prostatic tumors.

ACKNOWLEDGEMENTS

This study was supported by A.I.R.C., by Consiglio Nazionale delle Ricerche through the special projects 'B.T.B.S.' contract n. 93.01103.PF70, 'A.C.R.O.' contract n. 93.01200.PF39, 'Aging' contract n. 93.00438.PF40, 'FATMA' contract n. 93.007008.PF41 and by MURST

REFERENCES

1. Carpenter G., Stoscheck C.M., Preston Y.A. and De Larco J.E. (1983): Proc. Natl. Acad. Sci. USA 80: 5627-5630.
2. Chirgwin J., Aeyble A., McDonald R. and Rutter W. (1979): Biochemistry 18: 5294-5299.
3. Connolly J.M. and Rose D.P. (1990): Prostate 16: 209-218.
4. Connolly J.M. and Rose D.P. (1991): Prostate 19: 173-180.
5. Hauguel-DeMouzon S., Csermely P., Zoppini G. and Kahn C.R. (1992): J. Cell Physiol. 150: 180-187.
6. Hodges C.V. (1979): In: Endocrinology of Cancer, edited by D.P. Rose, pp. 57-67. C.R.C. Press. Boca Raton.

7. Hofer D.R., Sherwood E.R., Bromberg W.D., Mendelshon J., Lee C. and Kozlowski J.M. (1991): Cancer Res. 51: 2780-2785.
8. Horoszewicz J.S., Leong S.S., Kawinski E., Karr J.P., Rosenthal H., Ming Chu T., Mirand E.A. and Murphy G.P. (1983): Cancer Res. 43: 1809-1818.
9. Knabbe C., Kellner U., Schmahl M. and Voigt K.D. (1991): J. Steroid Biochem. Molec. Biol. 40: 185-192.
10. MacDonald A. and Habib F.K. (1992): Br. J. Cancer 65: 177-182.
11. MacGrogan D., Saint-Andre J.P. and Dicou E. (1992): J. Neurochem. 59: 1381-1391.
12. Motta M., and Serio M. editors (1988): Hormonal Therapy of Prostatic Diseases: Basic and Clinical Aspects. Medicom Europe. Amsterdam.
13. Muller R., Bravo R., Burkhardt S. and Curran T. (1984): Nature 312: 716-720.
14. Mydlo J.H., Michaeli J., Heston W.D.W. and Fair W.R. (1988): Prostate 13: 241-247.
15. Schuurmans A.L.G., Bolt J., Veldscholte J. and Mulder E. (1991): J. Steroid Biochem. Molec. Biol. 40: 193-197.
16. Wilding G. (1992): Cancer Surv. 14P: 113-130.
17. Yang Y., Chisholm G.D. and Habib F.K. (1993): Br. J. Cancer 67: 152-155.

FEMALE REPRODUCTIVE SYSTEM

p. 289 - 322

SOCIETA'
ITALIANA
DI ENDOCRINOLOGIA

Frontiers in Endocrinology
Volume 9 - 1994

Effect of IGFBP-3 on Basal and Stimulated Estradiol (E2) Production by Granulosa Cells (GC) in Culture

A. Barreca, P.G. Artini[1], A. Cesarone, M. Arvigo, A.R. Genazzani[1], G. Giordano and F. Minuto

Department of Endocrinology and Metabolism, DiSEM, University of Genova, Viale Benedetto XV 6, 16132 Genova; [1]Department of Obstetrics and Gynecology, University of Modena, Italy

INTRODUCTION

A novel role attributed to somatomedin peptides is related to their capacity to act, on some occasions, more as differentiating rather than mitogenic factors. Regarding the ovary, several experimental data have indicated that the IGF-I can act by paracrine or autocrine mechanisms (1). Indeed, its synthesis and the presence of its specific receptors have been demonstrated in the follicular cells which, in turn, appear to be sensitive to the actions of IGF-I in a dose-dependent manner. In particular, immunoreactive and bioactive IGF-I is present in medium conditioned by porcine granulosa cells (GC). Its production in the rat ovary has been further confirmed by the presence of high levels of IGF-I mRNA, which imply its gene expression, in GC, notably GC of developing follicles. Ovarian IGF-I synthesis appears to be dependent on GH, gonadotropins (Gn) and estradiol (E2), EGF and TGF-alpha. As for GH, it is well known that treatment with GH induces an increase in the intraovarian content of IGF-I in hypophysectomized estrogen-treated rats, increases ovarian progesterone (PG) production in response to Gn, and enhances *in vitro* the rat GC response to Gn stimulation (5).

Recently, it has been hypothesized that IGFBPs may play a role in regulating the local action of the IGFs in the ovary. It has been demonstrated, particularly in rat and porcine species, that both IGFs and their specific binding proteins are synthetized in the ovary (3, 4, 8, 11, 12).

The fact that, using an "in situ" hybridization technique, the mRNA for IGFBP-2, -3 and -4 have been localized in the rat interstitial cells, corpora lutea, and atretic GC, respectively, hints at a different regulation for each of these IGFBP, which may have a role as autocrine/paracrine factors in regulating the local actions of the IGFs in the ovary (9).

We have therefore studied the production of some IGFBPs by human granulosa cells and its regulation by FSH. We have also investigated the effect of increasing concentrations of recombinant deglycosylated IGFBP-3 on IGF-I and FSH stimulated estradiol release by human GC *in vitro*.

MATERIAL AND METHODS

12 patients, aged 27-36 years, with spontaneous ovulatory cycles and infertility due to mono- or bilateral tubal impatency or male factor were studied. Superovulation for *in vitro* fertilization/embryo transfer (IVF/ET program) was induced with a gonadotropin-releasing hormone analog, purified urinary follicle stimulating hormone, and human menopausal gonadotropin. Follicular aspiration for oocyte retrieval was performed by laparoscopy, under general anesthesia, 34-38 h after hCG administration.

Granulosa cells from patients undergoing laparoscopy were resuspended with 1 ml medium M 199 and pools were prepared from each individual patient. Granulosa cells of individual patients were plated (1x106 cells) in multiwell dishes in 2 ml of serum-free medium for 24 h and, subsequently submitted to 0, 2, 4, 8 nM of IGFBP-3 (kindly provided by Dr. A. Sommer, Celtrix , Santa Clara, CA) for 48 h, in presence or absence of increasing concentrations (2-8 nM) of IGF-I, Des (1-3) IGF-I - a truncated analog of human IGF-I with markedly reduced binding ability to IGFBPs - and FSH (5-20 mU/ml).

The conditioned medium of granulosa cells was acidified with 0.5 M acetic acid-0.15 M NaCl (pH of the mixture was <3), and gel-filtered on Sephadex G-50 column (1x40 cm) equilibrated with 0.1 M acetic acid-0.15 M NaCl, pH 2.75. Fractions corresponding to 0-0.20, 0.21-0.40, 0.41-0.70, 0.71-0.90, and 0.91-1 Kav were pooled, lyophilized, reconstituted in phosphate buffered saline and analysed for IGF and IGF specific binding.

The production of IGFBPs was evaluated in the medium conditioned by GC by SDS-PAGE and ligand blot, after gel-filtration in acidic conditions to remove the IGF peptides. The fraction containing IGF binding sites was incubated overnight at 4 C with approximately 100,000 cpm of 125I-IGF-I in 0.1 M Na phosphate buffer, pH 7.4, with or without 1µg of unlabeled IGF-I or Des (1-3)IGF-I. The cross-linking agent disuccinimidyl suberate (DSS) was then added to a final concentration of 0.5 mM and the samples were incubated for 20 min at room temperature. The reaction was stopped by adding 62.5 mM Tris-HCl, pH 6.8, and the samples were denatured by boiling for 5 min in 3X sample buffer (end concentration: 55.5 mmol/L Tris, pH 6.8, 1.33% SDS, 11.11% glycerol). The proteins were separated by 12.5% SDS-PAGE, according to the Laemmli method. The air-dried gel was applied to sensitive film and developed after 2-4 days of exposure in order to generate autoradiograms.

For ligand blotting samples were denatured and fractionated under nonreducing conditions on 12.5% SDS-PAGE, then transferred electrophoretically to PolyScreenTM PVDF membranes. After transfer, membranes were dried and then washed consecutively in a 0.01 M Tris HCl, 0.15 M NaCl, 0.05% Na azide (saline solution) containing 3% Nonidet P40 (buffer A), 1% BSA (buffer B), 0.1 % Tween 20 (buffer C) and, finally, with 50 mL of buffer containing 1% BSA, 0.1% Tween 20 and 40,000 CPM/mL of 125I-IGF-I. After incubation with labeled IGF-I for 48 h at 4 C, membranes were washed twice with buffer C and three times with saline solution, dried and subjected to autoradiography.

We have determined IGFBP-3 and IGFBP-1 concentrations both in GC conditioned media and in pools of follicular fluids by specific radioimmunoassay (IGFBP-3; Immunodiagnostik GmbH, Germany) or by immunoenzymatic assay (IGFBP-1; Immunodiagnostik GmbH, Germany).

Estradiol was assayed, using commercially available kits, by RIA: (DPC, Los Angeles, CA).

RESULTS

Analysis of GC conditioned medium by ligand blot has demonstrated the presence of three bands of specific binding to radioiodinated IGF-I, which, on the basis of their molecular weight, can be attributed to IGFBP-3, IGFBP-2 and the third band to IGFBP-1 and/or IGFBP-4.

The IGFBPs present in GC-conditioned medium are able to form specific complexes with radioiodinated IGF-I. The binding is inhibited by an excess of cold IGF-I, but not by the same amount of Des-IGF-I, confirming that this IGF analog has markedly reduced binding ability to IGFBPs (Fig. 1).

An inhibitory action of FSH on IGFBP-1 has been shown in a pool of media conditioned by GC treated with increasing concentrations of FSH. This effect appears to be dose-dependent (Table 1).

Table 1. *Effect of FSH and GH on IGFBP-1 production by granulosa cells in vitro*

	0	5	10	20
FSH (mIU/ml)	60.0	25.2	13.6	8.05
	33.6		19.4	
GH (ng/ml)	33.6		4.0	

Also growth hormone, at a dose of 10 ng/ml medium, is able to reduce IGFBP-1 secretion by GC. This inhibitory effect seems to be more evident than that obtained by 10 mU/ml of FSH (Table 1).

In agreement with the data observed *in vitro*, in the follicular fluids (FF) of women treated with gonadotropins plus GH we found lower levels of IGFBP-1 (36.6 ng/ml) than those observed in FF of women treated with gonadotropins alone (54.9 ng/ml).

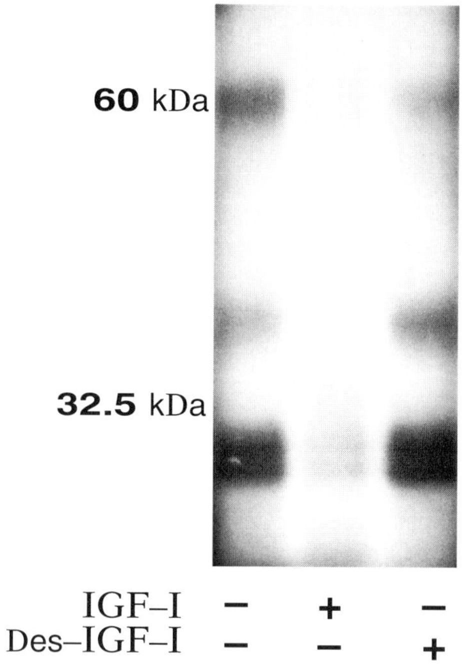

FIG. 1. Autoradiogram of radioiodinated IGF-I cross-linked to IGFBPs present in GC conditioned medium.

FSH is also able to reduce IGFBP-3 levels in GC-conditioned medium (from 464 to 116.5 ng/ml).

Preincubation for 2 h at 22°C with IGFBP-3, to allow the formation of the IGF-IGFBP complex, significantly reduces the stimulatory effect of IGF-I, but not of Des-IGF-I, on estradiol production by GC (Table 2).

IGFBP-3 is also able to drastically inhibit the stimulatory effect of FSH on estradiol release by GC.

Table 2. *Effect of IGFBP-3 on estradiol production (nmol/l) by human granulosa cells in culture with increasing concentrations of IGF-I, Des (1-3) IGF-I or FSH (± SEM)*

IGFBP-3 (nM)					
	0	**2**	**4**	**8**	**IGF-I (nM)**
0	4.31 ± 0.90	9.34 ± 2.70	14.64 ± 4.10	19.22 ± 4.58	
2		6.63 ± 1.15			
4			7.76 ± 0.23		
8				7.69 ± 0.42	
	0	**2**	**4**	**8**	**Des(1-3)IGF-I (nM)**
0	5.24 ± 1.04	9.33 ± 0.71	8.81 ± 1.53	12.14 ± 1.19	
2		7.40 ± 2.30			
4			9.9 ± 0.45		
8				10.06 ± 0.21	
	0	**5**	**10**	**20**	**FSH (mU/ml)**
0	7.89 ± 1.33	13.72 ± 4.13	16.10 ± 3.41	18.14 ± 3.50	
2		8.14 ± 1.20			
4			8.65 ± 1.45		
8				7.31 ± 0.73	

CONCLUSIONS

In the last few years a number of data have revealed an important role of the IGFs which - through the interaction with their specific cell surface receptors and with the modulatory effect of IGFBPs - regulate the development and function of the ovarian follicle. In the murine and porcine species the synthesis of all components of the system has been demonstrated, so that IGFs and IGFBPs can act by autocrine/paracrine mechanism in addition to the classic endocrine action (5).

As far as the human species is concerned our study, in agreement with others (6), showed that the IGF prevalently expressed by granulosa cells is IGF-II (2), the synthesis of which could be stimulated by GH, by FSH or by prolactin (10). IGF-I seems to be prevalently expressed in theca cells (6).

Analysis of conditioned medium could reveal that human granulosa cells release IGFBP-1, -2, -3, into culture and, possibly, IGFBP-4. These binding proteins are able to form, with labeled IGF-I, complexes of about 60 kDa (IGF-IGFBP-3), 38 kDa (IGF-IGFBP-2), and 31 kDa (IGF-IGFBP-1, IGF-IGFBP-4). The formation of radioactive complexes is inhibited by addition of excess amount of cold IGF-I, but not by Des(1-3)IGF-I (Fig.1), an analog known to have greatly reduced binding activity to IGFBPs, but not to IGF receptors.

A dose-dependent inhibitory effect of FSH on IGFBP-1 production has been demonstrated in our study (Table 1). This inhibitory effect was even more pronounced by incubation of cells with 10 ng/mgl of GH. The fact that the follicular fluids of patients treated with GH and gonadotropins combination contain a lower concentration of IGFBP-1 than the follicular fluids of patients treated with gonadotropins alone support *in vivo* the inhibitory effect of GH observed *in vitro*. Since IGFBP-1 has an inhibitory effect on the IGF biological activity, this finding explains, at least in part, the amplifying effect of GH shown in previous studies (2) on IGFs action.

FSH also revealed a potent inhibitory action on IGFBP-3 secretion. IGFBP-3 has an inhibitory action on the biological activity of IGF-I but has no effect on Des(1-3)IGF-I, therefore the IGFs lose their effect when bound to IGFBPs, and this loss of activity is due to the binding of IGFBP with the IGF and not to an effect of IGFBP at the receptor or post receptor level. It is likely that the binding of the IGFBP to IGF competes with the binding of the peptide to its receptor.

IGFBP-3 also showed an inhibitory effect on FSH action on estradiol production by granulosa cell. Since we already demonstrated that the IGFBP-3 inhibitory effect is exerted through the binding to IGF, this is indirect evidence of the amplifying action of the IGF(-II) produced by the granulosa cells in culture on the FSH action.

FSH, on the one hand, stimulates the ovarian synthesis of IGFs (7, 10), on the other (as shown before) inhibits the local synthesis of the IGFBPs which, in turn, have an inhibitory effect on IGF biological activity. The consequence is a great enhancement of its own biological effect on follicular maturation. Therefore, from these data it appears that IGFs and IGFBPs have an important, if not critical, role on the development of the ovarian follicle.

In conclusion, these data demonstrate that the stimulatory effect of IGF peptides on ovarian function can be modulated by the presence of their specific binding proteins. IGFs and IGFBPs in the ovary are important modulators of gonadotropin actions, so that together they contribute to the normal growth and maturation of ovarian follicles.

REFERENCES

1. Adashi E.Y., Resnick C.E., D'Ercole A.J., Svoboda M.E. and Van Wyk J.J. (1985): Endocrine Reviews 6: 400-420.
2. Barreca A., Artini P.G., Del Monte P., Ponzani P., Pasquini P., Cariola G., Volpe A., Genazzani A.R., Giordano G. and Minuto F. (1993): J. Clin. Endocrinol. Metab. 77: 61-67.
3. Erickson G.F., Nakatani A., Ling N. and Shimasaki S. (1992): Endocrinology 130: 625-36.
4. Erickson G.F., Nakatani A., Ling N. and Shimasaki S. (1992): Endocrinology 130: 1867-78.
5. Giordano G., Barreca A. and Minuto F. (1992): J. Endocrinol. Invest. 15: 689-707.
6. Hernandez E.R., Hurwitz A., Vera A., Pellicer A., Adashi E.Y., LeRoith D. and Roberts C.T. (1992): J. Clin. Endocrinol. Metab. 74: 419-425.
7. Hsu C.J. and Hammond J.M. (1987): Endocrinology 120: 198-207.
8. Mondschein J.S., Etherton T.D. and Hammond J.M. (1991): Biol. Reprod. 44: 315-19.
9. Nakatani A., Shimasaki S., Erickson G.F. and Ling N. (1991): Endocrinology 129: 1521-29.
10. Ramasharma K. and Li C.H. (1987): Proc. Natl. Acad. Sci. USA 84: 2643-47.
11. Ricciarelli E., Hernandez E.R., Hurwitz A., Kokia E., Rosenfeld R.G., Schwander J. and Adashi E.Y. (1991): Endocrinology 129: 2266-68.
12. Ricciarelli E., Hernandez E.R., Tedeschi C., Botero L.F., Kokia E., Rohan R. M., Rosenfeld R.G., Albiston A.L., Herington A.C. and Adashi E.Y. (1992): Endocrinology 130: 3092-94.

Frontiers in Endocrinology
Volume 9 - 1994

Estrogen Regulation of Blood Coagulation Factor XII Gene Expression

A. Farsetti[1], S. Misiti[2], F. Moretti[1], M. Andreoli[2] and A. Pontecorvi[3]

[1]Laboratory of Molecular Oncogenesis, Regina Elena Cancer Institute; [2]2nd Chair of Endocrinology, University of Rome La Sapienza, Viale Regina Elena 324, 00161 Rome; [3]Institute of Medical Pathology, Catholic University, Rome, Italy

INTRODUCTION

Blood coagulation is a host defense system against injury and infection. Once clotting begins, the sequential activation of certain plasma proenzymes to their active enzyme forms proceeds through either the intrinsic or the extrinsic pathway of blood coagulation (4) (Fig. 1).

In recent years, new techniques in molecular biology have made it possible to isolate, characterize, and identify the chromosomal location of the genes for most of the proteins known to participate in the coagulation process (4). Abnormalities in nearly every coagulation protein have been identified by DNA sequence analysis of the genes from patients with various coagulation disorders (4).

Interestingly, mutations have also been observed in the regulatory region of these genes (5). In fact, a series of mutations identified in the promoter region of the factor IX (FIX) gene have been demonstrated to impair factor IX transcriptional activity by preventing the binding of a liver-enriched nuclear protein, known as LFA1/HNF4, to the FIX gene promoter (16). These alterations are responsible for the inherited, X-linked, bleeding disorder Hemophilia B Leyden (16), characterized by a clinical phenotype which gradually improves after puberty, plasma factor IX concentrations reaching up to 60% of normal. An especially interesting mutation, identified at position -26 of the factor IX promoter, also disrupts an Androgen Response Element (ARE) which overlaps the LFA1/HNF4 binding site (3). This alteration causes

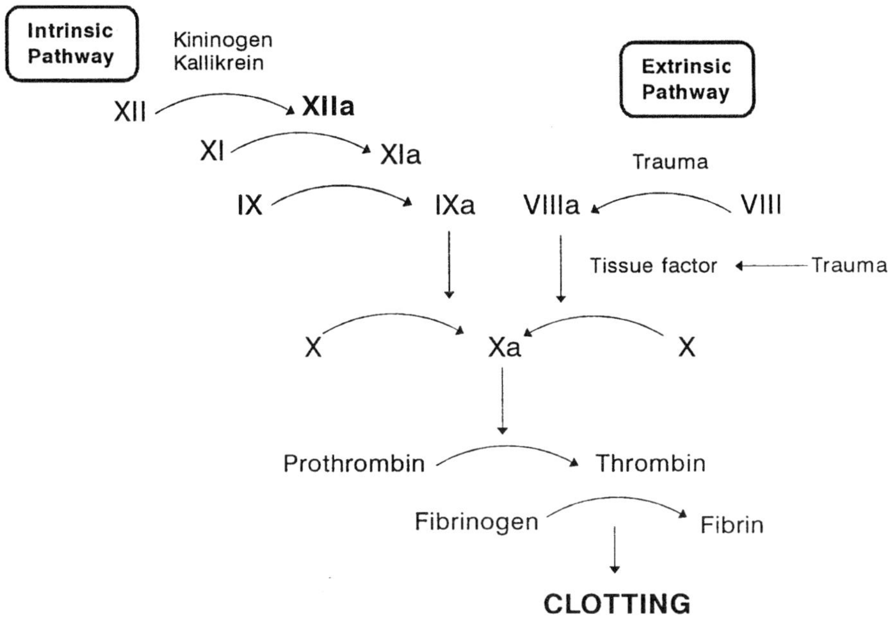

FIG. 1. The blood coagulation cascade. The cascade reactions culminate in the conversion of fibrinogen to fibrin and the formation of a fibrin clot. Numbered factors are abbreviated FXII, FXI, etc.

the severe form of Hemophilia B Brandenburg characterized by failure in post-puberal recovery of FIX plasma concentration (Fig. 2).

This recent discovery emphasizes the role of hormones in the regulation of blood coagulation genes *in vivo*. Identification of other hormone response elements within the regulatory regions of this class of genes and further insight into their physiological role may lead to a better understanding of the mechanism by which hormones and hormone receptors can modulate the clotting factor gene expression.

In this regard we are investigating the estrogen regulation of factor XII (FXII), formerly known as Hageman factor, gene expression. FXII is the primary activator of the intrinsic pathway of blood coagulation, also known as the "contact activation system". This system is also responsible for the activation of the fibrinolytic and complement cascades (10). Human coagulation FXII is a glycoprotein that circulates in plasma as an inert zymogen and is converted from a single-chain zymogen (M_r 80,000) into the enzyme factor XIIa, a two chain disulfide-linked enzyme, which then displays serine-protease activity (10). Although it was discovered on account of its procoagulant activity *in vitro*, the structure of FXII closely resembles that of fibrinolytic proteins, in particular the fast-acting inhibitor of tissue-type plasminogen activator, rather than that of

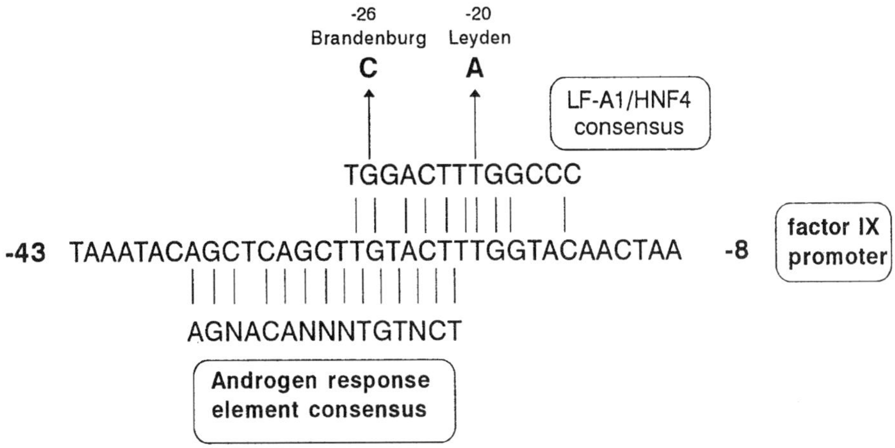

FIG. 2. Sequence of overlapping ARE and LF-A1/HNF4 binding site in the factor IX promoter. Residues matching the LF-A1/HNF4 consensus above and the ARE consensus below are aligned.

coagulation factors (10). Moreover, the ability of the contact system to release the potent vasodilating agent bradykinin is in keeping with a fibrinolytic role for FXII *in vivo* (Fig. 3); inhibition of FXII may indeed alter the balance between pro- and anticoagulant mechanisms to promote a procoagulant state. This is the case of the Hageman trait, the hereditary deficiency of Hageman FXII, which produces a thrombophilic state, clinically characterized by venous thrombosis, due to insufficient contact activation-dependent fibrinolysis (15).

The influence of estrogen on the coagulation system is a complex and, as yet, controversial issue. It is well known that the use of oral contraceptive agents containing synthetic estrogens, is associated with an increased risk of developing hemostatic and thromboembolic abnormalities (11). These coagulation defects have been attributed to an increased synthesis of clotting factors VIII, IX and XII (6) as well as to decreased antithrombin activity (13). In contrast, the recent introduction of postmenopausal low-dose estrogen replacement therapy has been associated with a marked decrease in the frequency of cardiovascular diseases (17). Thus, the hemostatic abnormalities appear to be strictly related to dose and estrogen strength (1). A shift in the balance between circulating procoagulant and pro-fibrinolytic factors, particularly in response to a dose- and potency-dependent effect of estrogens, may be responsible, therefore, for the contrasting effects on hemostasis observed when estrogens are used as oral contraceptives or as replacement therapy in post-menopausal women (14). A significant rise in Hageman factor titer has been reported in plasma of women using oral contraceptives (5). Moreover, studies in rats have demonstrated that estrogen treatment induces a dramatic increase in the Hageman factor protein and mRNA levels (7, 9).

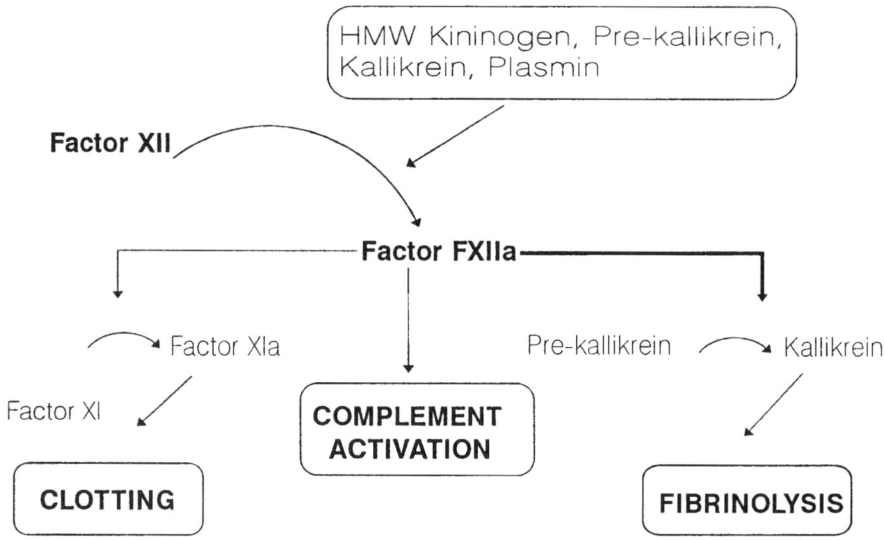

FIG. 3. Coagulation factor XII physiology. FXII activation and its metabolic pathways.

In this regard data indicate that estrogens directly enhance the Hageman factor gene expression either at transcriptional and/or post-transcriptional level. Whether this effect contributes to the thrombotic tendency of oral contraceptive users is uncertain. In this context, FXII appears to be highly sensitive to estrogen treatment, since only with this procoagulant are plasma levels seen to be modified even at low estrogen dosages, such as those commonly used in post-menopausal replacement therapy (8, 12). The mechanism by which estrogens regulate FXII gene expression is, therefore, crucial in understanding the pathogenesis of estrogen-induced alterations of hemostasis.

Computer-assisted analysis of the recently cloned human genomic fragment containing the FXII 5' flanking region (2), from nucleotide sequences at position -3076 to +51 relative to the first transcription start site, showed the presence of transcription regulatory elements typical of liver-specific and estrogen-modulated genes. In particular, we found two LFA1 core sequences, TGGACC, homologous to that observed in the Factor IX promoter; a 13 basepair palindromic sequence for the estrogen receptor binding, the Estrogen Response Element (ERE), GGGCAnnnTGACC, localized at positions from -44 to -31 relative to the start codon and four additional half-motifs 5'-TGACC-3', localized far upstream to this element (Fig. 4). The presence of this ERE in the regulatory region of the FXII gene strongly supports the observation of FXII gene modulation by estrogens.

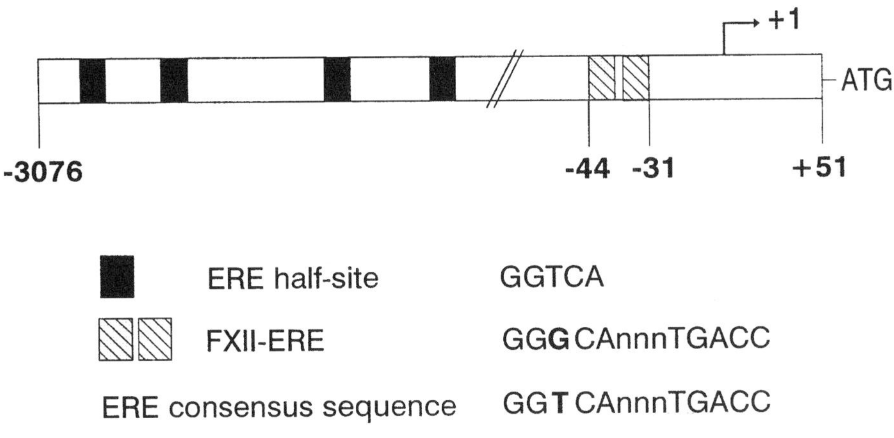

FIG. 4. Structure of FXII gene promoter with putative ERE sites. Location of palindromic ERE (*striped* boxes) and four half-palindromic 5'-GGTCA-3' motifs (*black* boxes) on the 5' flanking region of FXII gene. The transcription initiation site (+1) and translation start codon ATG (+50), are indicated.

Further investigations are in progress in the attempt to demonstrate, at molecular level, the regulation of a blood coagulation gene by estrogens and to characterize the function of the estrogen response element identified in the FXII gene promoter.

In conclusion, a better understanding of the molecular basis of blood coagulation will provide further insight into the mechanisms by which this class of genes are regulated by hormones.

REFERENCES

1. Bottiger L.E., Boman G., Eklund G. and Westerholm B. (1980): Lancet 24: 1097-1101.
2. Citarella F., Misiti S., Felici A., Aiuti A., La Porta C. and Fantoni A. (1993): Biochim. Biophys. Acta 1172: 197-199.
3. Crossley M., Ludwig M., Stowell K.M., De Vos P., Olek K. and Brownlee G.G. (1992): Science 257: 377-379
4. Furie B. and Furie B.C. (1988): Cell 53: 505-518.
5. Giannelli F., Green P.M., High K.A., Sommer S., Lillicrap D.P., Ludwig M., Olek K. and Reitsma P. H. (1991): Nucleic Acids Res. 19: 2193-2219.
6. Gordon E.M., Ratnoff O.D., Saito H., Donaldson V.H., Pensky J. and Jones P.K. (1980): J. Lab. Clin. Med. 96: 762-769.
7. Gordon E.M., Douglas J.G., Ratnoff O.D. and Arafah B.U.M. (1985): Blood 66: 602-605.
8. Gordon E.M., Williams S.R., Frenchek B., Mazur C.A. and Speroff L. (1988): J. Lab. Clin. Med. 111: 52-56.
9. Gordon E.M., Johnson T.R., Ramos L.P. and Schmeidler-Sapiro K.T. (1991): J. Lab. Clin. Med. 117: 353-358.
10. Hack C.E. and Dors D. (1992): Current Opinion in Investigational Drugs. November/December 1992: 95-110.
11. Inman W.H.W., Vessey M.P., Westerholm B. and Engelund A. (1970): Br. Med. J. 2: 203-209.

12. Jespersen J. and Kluft C. (1985): Thromb. Haemost. 54: 454-459.
13. Kobaiashi N. and Takeda Y. (1977): Eur. J. Clin. Invest. 7: 373-381.
14. Lobo R.A. (1992): Am. J. Med. 92: 283-285.
15. Ratnoff O.D. (1991): J. Lab. Clin. Med. 117: 343.
16. Reijen M.J., Sladek F.M., Bertina R.M. and Reitsma P.H. (1992): Proc. Natl. Acad. Sci. 89: 6300-6303.
17. Stampfer M.J., Colditz G.A., Willett W.C., Manson J.E., Rosner B., Speizer F.E. and Hennekens C.H. (1991): New Engl. J. Med. 325: 756-762.

Frontiers in Endocrinology
Volume 9 - 1994

Tyrosine Kinase-Inhibiting Phytoestrogens and their Synthetic Derivatives produce Cell Cycle Arrests and Apoptosis in *in vitro* Cultured Human Tumor Cells

M.C. Pagliacci, F. Spinozzi, G. Migliorati[1], F. Grignani, C. Riccardi[1] and I. Nicoletti

Institutes of Internal Medicine and Oncological Sciences;
[1]Medical Pharmacology, University of Perugia, 06122 Perugia, Italy

INTRODUCTION

Cell growth is controlled, to a large degree, by extracellular signals which bind to specific receptors on the surface of cells (4). A number of these receptors, including EGF-receptor, PDGF-receptor, and receptors for insulin and insulin-like growth factors (IGFs) have intrinsic tyrosine-kinase (TK) activity (12). Tyrosine protein kinases play a key role in tumorigenesis, and many proto-oncogenes (src, yes, fgr, fps/fes, abl/bcr-abl, ros erbB2/neu, fms, met, trk, ret and others) encode for receptor and non-receptor protein tyrosine kinases (3). Ligand-dependent activation of receptor-associated TK or unregulated synthesis of TK oncoproteins result in tyrosine phosphorylation of cellular substrates which have a critical role in the control of mitogenesis, cell-cycle regulation, cell survival and cell transformation (10).

Tyrosine-kinase inhibitors are a useful tool for investigating the role of TK-dependent cellular pathways in tumor cell growth and might represent a new class of antitumor agents (11). Isoflavonoid (genistein) and flavonol (quercetin) phytoestrogens are strong *in vitro* inhibitors of TK (7). They are abundant in vegetal foods, are efficiently absorbed by the gastrointestinal tract and reach measurable levels in the plasma and urine (1). A series of synthetic TK inhibitors (tyrphostins) have recently been generated and tested as novel antiproliferative agents and dissectors of signal transduction

These compounds compete with the substrate subsite of the enzyme with minimal influence on ATP binding, exert weak or no inhibition on ser/thr kinases and display some specificity for distinct TK (5).

MATERIAL AND METHODS

We analysed the effect of genistein, quercetin and a panel of tyrphostins (1, 25, and B56) on the *in vitro* growth of human ER+ breast tumor cell line (MCF-7) and in Jurkat cells, a human T-cell leukemia line which displays a constitutively increased protein tyrosine phosphorylation pattern. The effects of these substances on cell growth, cell-cycle progression, apoptotic death and tyrosine-phosphorylation of cellular proteins were investigated using the previously described procedures (8).

RESULTS AND DISCUSSION

Genistein and quercetin exerted a strong dose-dependent inhibition of MCF-7 and Jurkat cell growth (Fig. 1). Flow-cytometric cell cycle analysis of Jurkat cells treated with 100 μM genistein showed a progressive accumulation of cells in the G_2 phase of the cell cycle indicating an arrest in the G_2/M transition. The same dose of quercetin produced an increase in the percentage of G_0/G_1 cells with a corresponding reduction in S-phase cells. This is the hallmark of the G_1-S block. At a later time, cells with reduced DNA content (hypodiploid peak corresponding to the apoptotic nuclei) were clearly evident in cultures treated with either genistein or quercetin (Fig. 2). Thus, the growth inhibiting effects of the two natural phytoestrogens on *in vitro* tumor cell growth is the sum of cytostatic and apoptotic effects. The results were similar in MCF-7 breast cancer cells, and, also in this case, apoptosis followed the cell-cycle block. In MCF-7 cell line, however, genistein produced also an evident G_1-S arrest. Furthermore, it almost entirely abolished the S-phase entry produced by insulin and/or IGF-I in serum-free precultured cells. Immunofluorescence analysis with a FITC-conjugated anti-phosphotyrosine antibody (PY-20, ICN) revealed a strong increase in MCF-7 cell staining after insulin stimulation, but not when genistein was added to insulin.

A number of synthetic tyrosine-kinase inhibitors (tyrphostins), based on the structure of the smallest natural TK blocker (erbstatin), have recently been generated (5). Certain of these compounds can discriminate between receptor and nonreceptor TK and possess different substrate specificities and/or affinities toward intracellular targets. We tested a panel of these molecules on growth and cell-cycle parameters of MCF-7

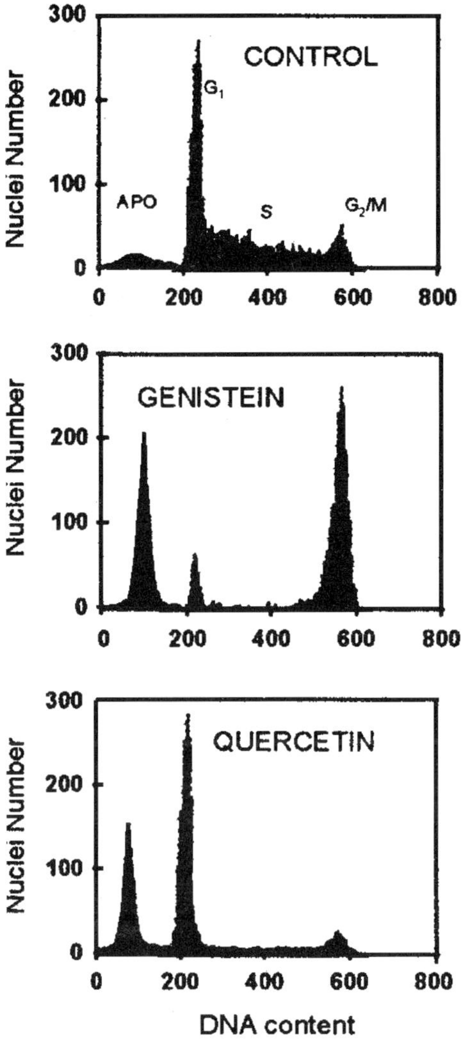

FIG. 1. Effect of different concentrations of genistein and quercetin on growth of Jurkat and MCF-7 tumor cell lines. Cells were cultured for 72 h and viable cells counted with a hemocytometer. Results (mean±SD) are the percentage of viable cells with respect to controls incubated n the same conditions.

and Jurkat cells cultured *in vitro*. Whilst tyrphostin-1, which is a weak TK inhibitor, did not exert any noteworthy effect on cell number, the more potent TK blockers tyrphostin-25 and B56 produced a strong, dose-dependent inhibition of tumor cell growth (Fig. 3). Cell cycle analysis

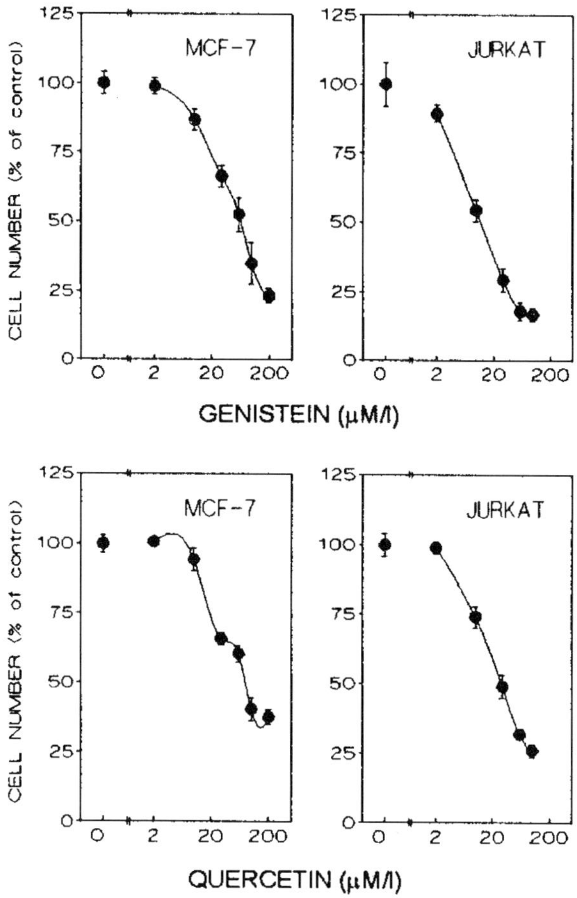

FIG. 2. DNA-fluorescence histogram of Jukat cell nuclei after a 48h treatment with 100 μM genistein or quercetin in a representative experiment. Genistein-treated cells show a marked increase in the G_2/M peak whilst quercetin-treated cultures display a clear reduction in S-phase. In both cases there is an evident hypodiploid DNA peak which corresponds to the apoptotic nuclei.

revealed a striking G_1-S block in cultures treated with the latter two compounds which was followed by apoptotic death. Despite the powerful inhibition of G_1-S transition in MCF-7 cells cultured in 10% FCS, tyrphostins did not inhibit the S-phase entry produced by insulin in serum-free precultured MCF-7 cells nor abolished the insulin-induced increase in tyrosine phosphorylated proteins. This shows that also in live cells tyrphostins can easily discriminate between the insulin receptor kinase and other receptor-linked or oncogenic TK (5). Finally, Western blot analysis of tumor cell lysates with a specific antiphosphotyrosine Ab showed that the different TK inhibitors reduced the tyrosine

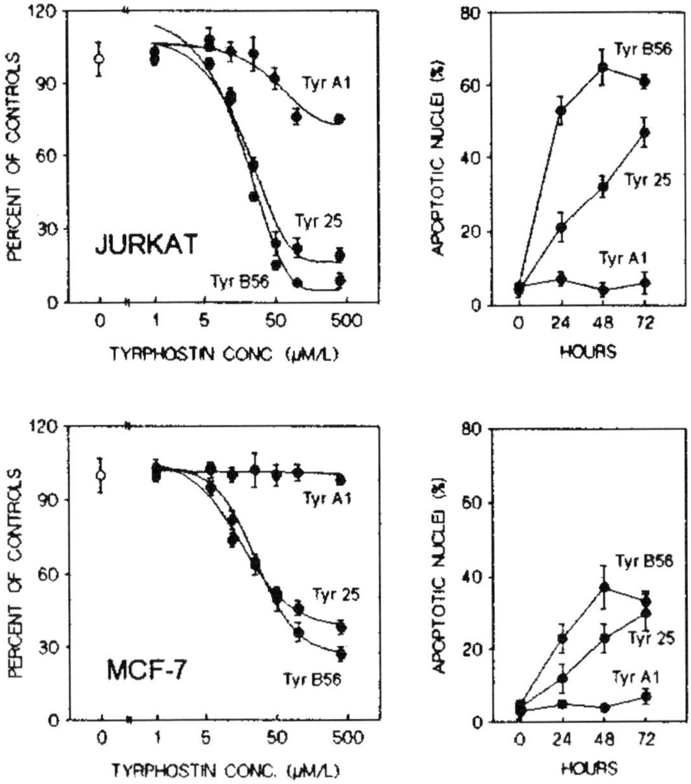

FIG. 3. Dose-dependent effects of tyrphostin-1, tyrphostin-25 and tyrphostin B56 on growth and apoptotic death of Jurkat and MCF-7 tumor cells cultures *in vitro*. For growth analysis, cells were counted with a hemocytometer. Results (mean±SD) are the percentage of viable cells with respect to controls incubated in the same conditions. Apoptosis was measured by flow-cytometry as described (8).

phosphorylation of distinct protein bands. This confirms that the different biological effects of the various TK inhibitors are actually due to activities on distinct cell targets.

Our results demonstrate that TK inhibitors, both natural and synthetic, inhibit tumor cell growth *in vitro* through arrests in the "critical check points" of cell cycle control (6) and induction of apoptotic cell death (9). That phytoestrogens and the synthetic TK inhibitors tyrphostins exert a cytostatic effect is not an unexpected finding, since the two key events in cell-cycle control, namely S-phase entry and transition form G_2 to mitosis are both regulated by phosphorylation and dephosphorylation of $pp34^{cdc2}$ protein kinase (6), and a finely tuned balance between TKs and phosphatases is essential for normal cell-cycle progression. A series of recent reports demonstrate that both receptor-linked and oncogenic TKs are able to promote cell growth through inhibition of apoptotic cell death. PDGF and IGF-I protect oligodendrocytes from apoptosis during optic nerve development (2) and tumor cells that overexpress either pp^{185} Her2/neu or v-abl oncogenic TKs are resistant to the apoptosis produced by TNF-α and cytotoxic T-cells (9). It can, therefore, be hypothesized that both natural and synthetic TK inhibitors exert their antitumor effect through a negative interference with survival signals; the resulting effect being the induction of apoptosis. These data indicate that phytoestrogens and tyrphostins can be promising molecules in cancer chemoprevention and treatment.

ACKNOWLEDGEMENTS

This work was supported by the Italian Association for Cancer Research (AIRC), MURST, and P.F. ACRO, CNR, Italy.

REFERENCES

1. Aldercreutz H., Markkanen H. and Watanabe S. (1993): Lancet 342: 1209-1210.
2. Barres B.A., Hart I.K., Coles H.S.R., Burne J.F., Voyvodic J.T., Richardson W.D. and Raff M.C. (1992): Cell 70: 31-46.
3. Cantley L.C., Auger K.R., Carpenter C., Duckwoth B., Graziani A., Kaeller R. and Soltoff S. (1991): Cell 64: 281-302.
4. Cross M. and Dexter M.T. (1991): Cell 64: 2171-280.
5. Levitzki A. (1992): FASEB J. 6: 3275-3282.
6. Murra A.W. (1992): Nature 359, 599-604.
7. Ogawara H., Akiyama T., Ishida J., Watanabe S. and Suzuki K. (1986): J. Antibiot. 39: 606-608.
8. Pagliacci M.C., Tognellini R., Grignani F. and Nicoletti I. (1991): Endocrinology 129: 2555-2562.
9. Smith C.A., Grimes E.A., McCarthy N.J. and Williams G.T. (1994): In: Apoptosis II: The Molecular Basis of Apoptosis in Disease, edited by L.D. Tomei and F.O. Cope, pp. 43-88. CSHL Press. New York.
10. Ullrich A. and Schlessinger J. (1990): Cell 61: 203-212.
11. Workman P. (1992): Am. Oncol. 3: 527-531.
12. Yarden Y. and Ullrich A. (1988): Annu. Rev. Biochem. 57: 443-478.

Frontiers in Endocrinology
Volume 9 - 1994

Polycystic Ovary Syndrome in the Rat and Ovarian Receptors for Epidermal Growth Factor and Luteinizing Hormone Releasing Hormone

R.M. Moretti, D. Dondi, M. Milani and L. Domingues

Department of Endocrinology, University of Milan,
Via G. Balzaretti, 9, 20133 Milan, Italy

INTRODUCTION

Epidermal Growth Factor (EGF) and luteinizing hormone releasing hormone (LHRH) are produced locally in the ovary (1) and influence many aspects of the ovarian function. In particular, it has been reported that, in many species, EGF is a potent stimulator of mitogenesis in follicular granulosa cells (4), but decreases the gonadotropin-induced synthesis of estrogens by inhibiting the aromatization of androgens (7). LHRH has been reported to interfere with many intrafollicular processes activated by the gonadotropins; the peptide inhibits granulosa cell differentiation, the formation of LH receptors induced by FSH, the aromatization of androgens, etc. (7).

On the basis of these data, it was deemed of interest to analyze whether EGF and LHRH receptors undergo some modifications when the polycystic ovary syndrome (PCO) is induced in female rats.

METHODS AND RESULTS

PCO was induced in young adult female rats (70 days of age) exhibiting at least three consecutive regular 4-day estrous cycles by two approaches:

a) by exposing the animals to constant illumination for 90 days (LC animals);

b) by injecting a single dose of 2 mg/rat of estradiol valerate (EV).

At the end of the period of constant illumination or 70 days after EV administration, the animals showing clear signs of constant estrus, as evaluated by daily vaginal smears, were sacrificed by decapitation; adult female rats with a regular 4-day estrous cycle were also killed in the phase of estrus to be used as controls. At sacrifice, the ovaries of the experimental and control animals were collected, weighed and submitted to different evaluation procedures:

1) histological examination;

2) study of the binding characteristics (Bmax as an index of the number of receptors; Kd as an index of their affinity for the ligands utilized) of the LHRH and EGF receptors, utilizing specific radioreceptor assays;

3) analysis of the distribution of EGF receptors by immunohistochemistry. At sacrifice, blood was collected from the trunk vessels for the measurement of serum levels of LH and FSH by radioimmunoasay. The weights of the ovaries of the LC and EV animals were significantly lower than those recorded for the ovaries collected from the controls. The histological examination showed that, in the ovaries of the experimental groups, large mature follicles were present in a significantly higher number than that observed in controls. In LC and EV animals, the theca externa and interna of the large follicles was hyperplastic, and the granulosa layers were atrophic.

In LC and EV animals, serum LH levels were significantly higher and serum FSH titers significantly lower than those recorded in the controls. The analysis of the binding characteristics of LHRH receptors present in the ovaries of LC and EV animals and of controls showed that the number and the affinity of these receptors for their ligand remained in the same range. On the contrary, the number of ovarian EGF receptors was significantly lower in LC and EV animals than in controls. This fall in the number of EGF receptors in experimental animals took place without any significant variation of the Kd. The immunohistochemical analysis of the distribution of EGF receptors in the follicles of control and experimental animals has indicated that, in control follicles, these receptors are present in all the layers of granulosa cells. On the contrary, in LC and EV ovaries the few receptors still detectable were confined only on the cells facing the follicular cavity.

DISCUSSION AND CONCLUSIONS

The present data indicate, first of all, that the two procedures adopted are able to induce an experimental PCO syndrome in the treated animals. The results also show that the two manipulations adopted, even if extremely different in nature, induce a remarkably similar effect on ovarian histology and on the serum profile of the two gonadotropins (a significant increase of serum levels of LH and a significant decrease of serum titers of FSH) (8).

Finally, the data reported confirm the presence of LHRH and EGF receptors on rat granulosa cells (2, 6, 7) and show a specific decline of the EGF receptors in the ovaries of the animals exhibiting either form of PCO syndrome. It is possible that the observed reduction in the number of EGF receptors in PCO animals might be a consequence of the alteration of the circulating levels of the gonadotropins induced by the two treatments. It has been reported that FSH and LH up- and down-regulate, respectively, the number of EGF receptors in rat granulosa cells (2). It remains for further studies to clarify whether the gonadotropins affect EGF receptor density in the granulosa cells of PCO animals by acting directly on the cellular events leading to the synthesis and/or degradation of the EGF receptors, or whether this effect is secondary to a local stimulation of the synthesis and/or release of EGF which is known to down-regulate its own receptors (9). This possibility finds support in the recent reports showing that PCO is characterized by a significant increase of EGF in the follicular fluid (of sows and women) (3, 5). The present data have also shown that the two models of PCO do not modify the number and the binding characteristics of the LHRH receptor in the granulosa cells. This suggests that PCO, obtained in the female rat through the procedures adopted in this laboratory, does not seem to exert a particular impact on this ovarian component. Obviously, human studies are needed to confirm the role of the modifications in ovarian EGF receptors here reported in the pathogenesis of this clinical syndrome.

ACKNOWLEDGEMENTS

Supported by C.N.R. through the Projects Aging (93.00438PF40) FATMA (93.00700PF41) ACRO (93.02197PF39) and by funds from MURST.

REFERENCES

1. Adashi E.Y. and Roha, R.M. (1992): Trends Endocr. Met. 3: 243-248.
2. Feng P., Knecht M. and Catt K. (1987): Endocrinology 120: 1121-1126.
3. Genazzani A.R., Bencini S., Battaglia C., D'Ambrogio G. and Artini P.G. (1994): In: La Medicina della Riproduzione. edited by C. Foresta, A. Isidori and C. Scandellari, pp. 115-118. Panda Edizioni. Padova.
4. Gospodarowicz D. and Bialecki H. (1979): Endocrinology 104: 757-764.
5. Hsu C.J., Holmes S.D. and Hammond J.M. (1987): Biochem. Biophys. Res. Commun. 147: 242-247.
6. Hsueh A.J.W. and Jones P.B.C. (1981): Endocr. Rev. 2: 437-461.
7. Hsueh A.J.W., Adashi E.Y., Jones P.B.C. and Welsh T.H., Jr. (1984): Endocr. Rev. 5: 76-127.
8. Mahajan D.K. (1988): Endocr. Met. Clin. North Amer. 17: 705-732.
9. Vlodavsky I., Brown K.D. and Gospodarowicz D. (1978): J. Biol. Chem. 253: 3744-3750.

Frontiers in Endocrinology
Volume 9 - 1994

Expression of the Growth Hormone Releasing Hormone Receptor (GHRH-R)/Vasoactive Intestinal Peptide Receptor (VIP-R)-like Genes in the Rat Ovary

C. Moretti, M.L. Scaldaferri, S. Rossi, G. Frajese jr. and G. Frajese

Department of Internal Medicine, Chair of Andrology, University of Rome Tor Vergata, Via di Tor Vergata 135, 00133 Rome, Italy

INTRODUCTION

Ovarian folliculogenesis is a dynamic process characterized by the proliferation and differentiation of the somatic and germ cell elements of the follicle. The action of FSH on this process depends, firstly, on the dose of bioactive FSH reaching the follicle and, secondly, on the paracrine modulation of the FSH signal by intragonadal factors. Several substances have been identified as intraovarian regulators considering the possibility of their local production, reception and action. Among these, the 43 aminoacid peptide Growth Hormone Releasing Hormone (GHRH), the major regulator of GH synthesis and secretion in the anterior pituitary gland (6), seems to play a positive modulatory role *in vivo* and *in vitro*, amplifying the stimulatory action of FSH on granulosa cell function (15).

GHRH is believed to belong to a Glucagon/Vasoactive Intestinal Peptide (VIP) superfamily of peptides, due to evident sequence homology and cross-reactivities in various bioassay systems (17). In particular, the GHRH family included VIP, PHI/PHM (intestinal peptides arising from the same precursor peptide of VIP), Secretin and the Pituitary Adenylcyclase Activating Polypeptide (PACAP) (14, 4). Considering the GHRH sequence, PHM/PHI and PACAP-related peptides (PRP) display the greatest sequence identity (37-63%; 35-55%, respectively), followed by VIP (25-43%), Glucagon (21-35%), Secretin (22-37%) and Gastric Inhibitory Peptide (5-19%) (4).

Multiple receptors for peptides of the VIP-family The tissue distribution of the peptides of VIP-family and their biological effects have been extensively investigated. They act both on specific and on structurally related receptor proteins that are present in several target tissues (17), coupling to regulatory proteins belonging to the cyclic AMP system (Table 1). GHRH realizes its main physiological effect, the positive regulation of GH synthesis and secretion in the anterior pituitary, acting through its own specific receptor (13) but it is also potentially able to recognize other receptors of the VIP family in different tissues (11). VIP, PACAP and GHRH are structurally related and capable of activating adenylate cyclase after binding to their specific cell-surface receptors (4, 1). In the ovary, we have demonstrated that VIP and GHRH bind a common receptor present on rat granulosa cells (16). Binding has been characterized using $[^{125}I]$VIP and the VIP/GHRH analog [His1, Nle27]hGRF(1-32)NH2. The specificity was indicated by the competitive inhibition by VIP, GHRH and PHI, but not by glucagon and unrelated peptides. The Scatchard analysis of the saturation isotherm showed a high affinity binding site with dissociation constant of 0.16 nM and binding capacity of 0.58 fmol per 106 cells, and an additional low affinity site with Kd of 15 nM and binding capacity of 87 fmol/106. It has also been demonstrated that treatment with increasing concentrations (50-500 ng/ml) of FSH causes a dose dependent increase in the expression of the binding sites with no change in binding affinity (2). FSH was then able to raise the receptor number by 160% compared to the control value (12,000 GHRH-like receptors after FSH treatment vs 4,600 in untreated cells).

Table 1. *The VIP family of receptors belonging to the Gs protein receptor superfamily*

- VIP-R
- VIP_2-R
- $PACAP_1$-R (A/B)
- $PACAP_2$-R
- Secretin-R
- GHRH-R
- Glucagon-R
- Glucagon-like peptide 1-R
- Calcitonin-R
- PTH-R
- PTH-P-R

Thus, several types of receptors can interact with VIP, GHRH and PACAP (12). Using ^{125}I-PACAP27 as tracer, it is possible to characterize several classes of receptors (1). One class of receptor, which binds VIP, PACAP1-27 and PACAP1-38 with very similar affinities is present in brain and in a variety of peripheral tissues including liver, lung, spleen and intestine (8). A second class of receptors, which is highly specific for PACAP, has been hypothesized to exist in brain, pituitary, testis and adrenal medulla (9). This receptor (PACAP type I), has been further subdivided into two subtypes on the basis of binding data: PACAP1A receptors bind PACAP1-27 with slightly higher affinity than PACAP1-38 whilst PACAP1B receptors bind PACAP1-38 with high affinity and PACAP1-27 with low affinity (14).

The recent reports describing the cloning of PACAP and VIP receptors demonstrate that PACAP1A and PACAP1B receptors may correspond to different states of a single receptor protein and that at least two different VIP receptors, with different distribution, exist (TIPS). VIP receptors have recently been cloned from rat lung (10), pituitary gland (12), HT-29 cells (18) and human intestine (5). The VIP receptors contain seven transmembrane domains and are markedly homologous to the Secretin, PACAP, Calcitonin and Parathyroid Hormone receptors, constituting a subfamily of the Gs protein receptor superfamily. The specific receptor for GHRH, cloned from rat pituitary gland belongs to the same family (14).

Expression of VIP-R and GHRH-R-like genes in the rat ovary Using the pituitary GHRH-R and the rat lung VIP-R as probes in a Northern blot, the mRNA transcripts are not detectable in the rat ovary but only, in pituitary and lung, respectively (10, 14). This evidence is due to the possibility that additional receptor forms might mediate the VIP/GHRH action at this level or, alternatively, the same receptors could be expressed in the gonads at very low level, not being easily detectable by RNA blot analysis. For this reason, we have used RT-PCR and colony-hybridization protocols in order to detect lower signals and amplify their sequence. The expression of the GHRH-R-like gene has been studied, using a rat pituitary GHRH-R probe, through the PCR analysis of a rat ovarian cDNA library in lambda gt11. Amplification studies, using different sense (93rd to 109th, 282nd to 303rd) and antisense (913th to 932nd, 1054th to 1070th) primers, revealed products of the predicted size. Figure 1 shows the Southern blot analysis of the PCR-amplified products with the GHRH-R probe in which a sequence of ~ 900 nt is specific for the GHRH-R. Considering the failure to detect a GHRH-R mRNA transcript in the rat ovary using GHRH-R cDNA as probe, it is possible that the sequence amplified is related to a different receptor form existing in the ovarian tissue. Unlike several other genes encoding G protein-coupled receptors, which lack introns within their coding sequence, the rat GHRH receptor gene is quite large and is interrupted by numerous introns within the coding region (14). Thus, alternative RNA processing might be used to generate isoforms of the GHRH receptor, expressed in the ovary at very low levels.

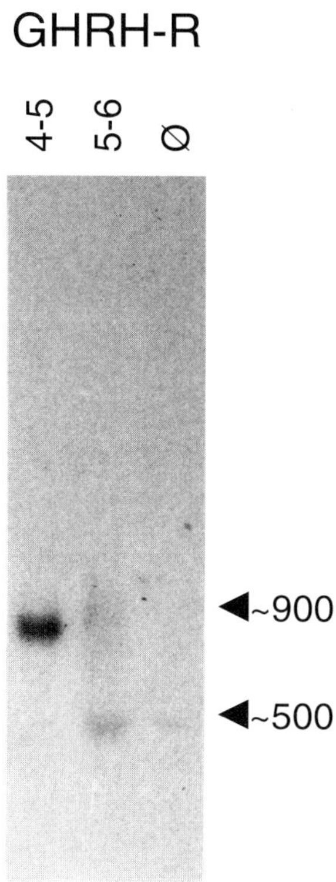

FIG. 1. Amplification studies by RT-PCR of a rat ovarian cDNA library cloned in λ gt11 and Southern blot analysis of the PCR-amplified products. It can be sean that a sequence of ~900 nucleotides is specific for the GHRH-R

To evaluate the VIP-R expression in the ovary, an amplified rat ovarian cDNA library was screened, using as probe, sequences from the 4th and 5th transmembrane regions of the lung VIP receptor. Twelve clones were isolated and purified through three successive rounds of plaque hybridization. A PCR was performed on positive clones showing products of ~ 800 nt that hybridized with the sequence of the lung VIP-R used as probe. Figure 2 shows amplified products of plaques from the 3rd screening of the rat ovarian cDNA library, suggesting the expression of a VIP-like receptor gene in the rat ovary. The VIP receptor from the rat lung cDNA library has been cloned using low-stringency screening conditions (10). This receptor, known as VIP1 receptor, is also present in liver, intestine and certain regions of the brain, such as the cortex, hippocampus and olfactory bulb. The human homologue of this receptor has been cloned from human colon carcinoma cells and is also present in lung and kidney (18). A second VIP receptor, named VIP2 receptor, has also been recently isolated from the rat pituitary and olfactory bulb (12)

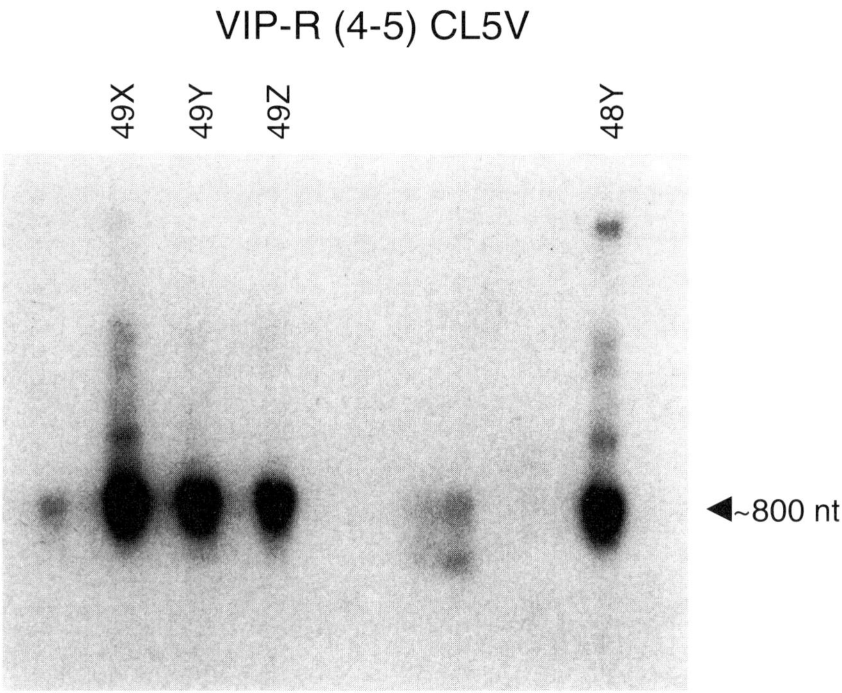

FIG. 2. Amplification studies and Southern blotting on different plaques from the screening of a rat ovarian cDNA library. The products are homologous to the sequence of the VIP-R in the region of 4th-5th transmembrane loop.

and has been found in the CNS (thalamus, hippocampus, suprachiasmatic nucleus and hypothalamus). Autoradiographic studies indicate a combined distribution of the two receptor binding sites in several tissues. Our finding of PCR products, positive for sequences from a region with high level of homology for VIP1 and VIP2 receptors, appears to suggest that the rat ovary can express genes for multiple VIP receptor subtypes.

CONCLUSIONS

The optimal gonadotropin function is dependent upon the action of tissue-specific intraovarian factors. In this regard, gonadotropins are only the initiators of a cascade of events mediated through interaction with putative intragonadal regulators. The present study provides evidence for the expression of GHRH-R and VIP-R-like genes in the rat ovary. This observation can be related to the finding that the ovary is a site of GHRH-like peptide production, reception and action (16, 2).

Both pharmacological and molecular biological approaches will be needed to establish what kind of receptor subtypes account for all of the known actions of GHRH and VIP at gonadal level.

REFERENCES

1. Arimura A. (1992): Trends. Endocrinol. Metab. 3: 288-294.
2. Bagnato A., Moretti C., Frajese G. and Catt K.J. (1991): Endocrinology 128: 2889-2894.
3. Campbell R.M. and Scanes C.G. (1992): Growth Regulation 2: 175-191.
4. Christophe J., Svoboda M., Dehaye J.P., Winand J., Vandermeers-Pire M.C., Vandermeers A., Cauvin A., Gourlet P. and Robberecht P. (1989): In: Peptides Hormones as Prohormones: Processing, Biological Activity, Pharmacology, edited by Martinez, J. pp. 211-242. Halsted Press. New York.
5. Couvineau A., Rouyer-Fessard C., Darmoul D., Maoret J.J., Carrero I., Ogier-Denis E. and Laburthe M. (1994): BRC 200: 769-776.
6. Guillemin R., Brazeau P., Bohlen P., Esch F., Ling N. and Wehremberg W.B. (1982): Science 218: 585-587.
7. Harmar T. and Lutz E. (1994): Trends in Pharmacological Science 15: 97-99.
8. Hashimoto H., Ishihara T., Shigemoto R., Mori K. and Shigekazu N. (1993): Neuron 11: 333-342.
9. Hosoya M., Onda H., Ogi K., Masuda Y., Miyamoto Y., Ohtaki T., Okazaki H., Arimura A. and Fujino M. (1993): Biochem. Biophys. Res. Comm. 1: 133-143.
10. Ishihara T., Shigemoto R., Mori K., Takahashi K., Negata S. (1992): Neuron 8: 811-819.
11. Laburther M., Amiranoff B., Boige N., Rouyer-Fessard C., Tatemoto K. and Moroder L. (1976): FEBS Lett. 1559: 89-92.
12. Lutz E.M., Sheward W.J., West K.M., Morrow J.A., Fink G. and Harmar A.J. (1993): FEBS Lett. 1: 3-8.
13. Mayo K.E. (1992): Mol. Endocrinol. 6: 1734-1744.
14. Miyata A., Arimura A., Dahi R.R., Minamino N., Uehara A., Jiang L., Culler M.D. and Coy D.H., (1989): Biochem. Biophys. Res. Comm. 164: 175-191.
15. Moretti C., Fabbri A., Gnessi L., Forni L., Fraioli F. and Frajese G. (1989): In: Reproductive Medicine: Medical Therapy, edited by Frajese, G., Steinberger, E., Rodriguez- Rigau, L.J. n. 875, pp 103-112. Elsevier Science Publishers. New York.
16. Moretti C., Bagnato A., Solan N., Frajese G. and Catt K.J. (1990): Endocrinology 127: 2117-2126.
17. Rosselin G. (1986): Peptides 7 (Supp 1): 89-100.
18. Shreedharan S.P., Robichon A., Peterson K.E. and Goetzl E.J. (1991): Proc. Natl. Acad. Sci. USA 88: 4986-4990.

Frontiers in Endocrinology
Volume 9 - 1994

Transient Developmental Exposure of Female Mice to Diethylstilbestrol affects Adult Bone Density

S. Migliaccio[1,2], R.R. Newbold[1], M. Centanni[2], J.A. McLachlan[1], M. Andreoli[2] and K.S. Korach[1]

[1] *Laboratory of Reproductive and Developmental Toxicology, National Institute of Environmental Health Sciences, Research Triangle Park, NC, USA;*
[2] *II Division of Endocrinology, Department of Experimental Medicine, University of Rome La Sapienza, Viale Regina Elena 324, 00161 Rome, Italy*

INTRODUCTION

Osteoporosis, a disease of world-wide proportions, is characterized by a decrease in bone tissue, with a consequent increase in spontaneous fractures (1, 15, 16). The incidence is particularly high in women during the immediate post menopause years. It is believed that the sharp decrease in estrogen levels following the onset of menopause is one of the factors playing an important role in the pathogenesis of this disease (1, 15, 16).

Furthermore, estrogens dramatically affect bone tissue turnover (1, 2, 8, 15-17) and it is well known that estrogen replacement therapy (ERT) can block the loss of bone tissue both in post menopausal women (2, 17) and in ovariectomized animals (1, 3, 15, 16). While the effects of estrogens on bone tissue were believed to be indirect, the presence of estrogen receptor (ER) has been described in bone cells, strongly suggesting that these steroids have a direct effect on bone tissue (5, 10, 17, 18). *In vitro* studies have also demonstrated that estrogens can modulate osteoblast-like cell activity (7) by a direct ER-mediated mechanism (6, 12). Although it is now well known that estrogens can modulate bone turnover after menopause, little is known about the effects that these hormones may have before the climacteric period, for instance during the development of skeletal tissue (3, 9, 13).

The aim of our recent investigations was to evaluate the effects of changing estrogen levels, during early phases of development, on the peak bone density in adulthood (11).

MATERIAL AND METHODS

In order to evaluate whether transient modifications in estrogen levels during development can affect bone density in adulthood, female mice were injected with 2 μg/pup/day of the synthetic analog diethylstilbestrol (DES) dissolved in corn oil, from day 1 through 5 after birth. Control (CTL) mice were treated with corn oil alone. Following this transient treatment, both control and treated mice were weaned when 25 days old, kept in controlled temperature and light conditions and fed ad libitum until adulthood. Animals were evaluated between 7 and 14 months of age. Right femurs and lumbar vertebrae were collected and fixed in 10% neutral buffered formalin, decalcified, embedded in paraffin and sectioned at 6 μm. Tissue sections were stained with hematoxylin and eosin (H & E) and evaluated using a light microscope (11).

The same tissue sections prepared for histological analysis from control and DES-treated animals were evaluated for histomorphometric measurements using a SMI-Microcomp image analysis system (Southern Micro Instruments, Inc., Atlanta, GA) interfaced with an IBM computer and an Olympus BH-2 microscope. Areas of interest were selectively traced and the areas bounded by tracing were automatically calculated by the computer software.

RESULTS AND DISCUSSION

Animals were evaluated in different periods to establish whether this transient modification in estrogen levels soon after birth might have any effects on physical and biochemical characteristics of the skeleton in adulthood. Body weight of DES-exposed mice showed no significant differences compared to vehicle-treated control animals (Table 1) at the different ages considered. Interestingly, however, in DES-treated mice the length of long bones, such as the femurs, was decreased as compared to control animals (Table 1). Furthermore, since it is well known that estrogens can affect bone density at vertebral sites, lumbar vertebrae of these DES-treated animals were analyzed to evaluate the presence of any potential change in bone mass in adulthood. Cross sections of lumbar vertebrae of control and neonatally DES-exposed animals were evaluated by histological analysis. The evaluation of the histological specimens showed that this transient treatment with estrogen could significantly increase bone mass in these animals in adulthood (Table 1). Moreover, the biochemical analysis of the calcium concentration in the femur, used as a marker of the skeleton mineralization (4, 14), showed no statistical difference when normalized with femur length (data not shown). These data strongly suggest a normal mineralization of the skeleton in the DES-treated mice, indicating that the increase in bone mass seems to be due to increased bone matrix formation rather than a difference in the mineralization process (11).

Table 1. *Comparison of body weight, femur length and bone mass between control and DES-treated mice at different ages*

	Body weight (g)	Femur length (mm)	Bone mass (µm)2
7-9 months			
CTL (15)	49.13 ± 1.97	15.74 ± 0.22	0.59 ± 0.05
DES (10)	47.10 ± 2.48	14.76 ± 0.11	0.85 ± 0.09*
12-14 months			
CTL (4)	48.53 ± 3.21	15.86 ± 0.33	0.67 ± 0.03
DES (7)	54.02 ± 3.21	14.92 ± 0.04*	0.92 ± 0.07*

CTL: control group; DES: diethylstilbestrol-treated group. Data are expressed as mean ± SEM. Nos. in brackets = no. animals in each group; * $p < 0.5$ vs control. Part of the data taken from reference 11.

Interestingly, the results of the present studies demonstrate that alterations in estrogen levels during the early phases of development can dramatically influence the skeletal tissue in adulthood, since both trabecular and compact bone compartments were augmented following the transient estrogen treatment of the growing animals.

Finally, a significant increase in the peak bone mass was observed in these animals when they reached adulthood. Likewise, these data suggest that alterations in estrogen levels during early phases of development may play a fundamental role in the determination of the final peak bone mass in adult life.

REFERENCES

1. Albright F., Bloomberg F. and Smith P.H. (1940): Trans. Assoc. Am. Physician. 55: 298-305.
2. Balfour J.A. and McTavish D. (1992): Drugs and Aging 2: 487-507.
3. Bonjour J.P., Theintz G., Buchs B., Slosman D. and Rizzoli R. (1991): J. Clin. Endocrinol. Metab. 73: 555-563.
4. Cox A.C., and Balloun S.L. (1971): Poultry Sci. 50: 186-194.
5. Eriksen E.F., Colvard D.S., Berg N.J., Graham M.L., Mann K.G., Spelsberg T.C. and Riggs B.L. (1988): Science 241: 84-86.
6. Ernst M., Parker M.G. and Rodan G.A. (1992): Mol. Endocrinol. 5: 1597-1606.
7. Gray T.K., Flynn T.C., Gray K.M. and Nabell L.M. (1987): Proc. Natl. Acad. Sci. USA 84: 6267-6271.
8. Komm B.S., Terpening C.M., Benz D.J., Graeme K.A., Gallegos A., Kore M., Greene G.L., O'Malley B.W. and Haussler M.R. (1988): Science 241: 81-84.
9. Lindsay R., Hart D.M., Aikken J.M., McDonald E.B., Anderson J.B. and Clark A.C. (1976): Lancet 1: 1038-1040.
10. Lloyd T., Rollings N., Andon M.B., Deners L.M., Eggli D.F., Kieselhorst K., Kulin H., Landis J.R., Marte J.K., Orr G. and Smith P. (1992): J. Clin. Endocrinol. Metab. 75: 383-7.

11. Migliaccio S., Newbold R.R., Bullock B.C., McLachlan J.A. and Korach K.S. (1992): Endocrinology 130: 1756-1758.
12. Migliaccio S., Davis V.L., Gibson M.K., Gray K.T. and Korach K.S. (1992): Endocrinology 130: 2617-2624.
13. Ott S.M. (1990): J. Clin. Endocrinol. Metab. 71: 1082-1084.
14. Peng T.C., Garner S.C., Hirsch P.F. and Posillico J.T. (1986): J. Bone Mineral Res. 1: 351-357.
15. Riggs B.L. and Melton L.J. III (1986): N. Eng. J. Med. 314: 1676-1786.
16. Riggs B.L. and Melton L.J. III (1988): New York. Raven Press 25: 345-356.
17. Wronsky T.J., Cintron M., Doherty A.L. and Dann L.M. (1988): Endocrinology 123: 681-686.
18. Yamamoto T.T. and Rodan G.A. (1991): Proc. Natl. Acad. Sci. USA 87: 2172-2176.

HORMONAL CONTRACEPTION

p. 323 - 350

SOCIETA'
ITALIANA
DI ENDOCRINOLOGIA

Frontiers in Endocrinology
Volume 9 - 1994

INTRODUCTORY REMARKS

Hormonal Contraception in the Woman

P.G. Crosignani

I Department of Obstetrics and Gynecology, University of Milan,
Via Commenda 12, 20122 Milan, Italy

EFFICACY

Oral contraceptives are the most effective form of reversible contraception.

Efficacy is usually referred to as method or use effectiveness and many factors of patient compliance may influence it. When used properly, contraceptive use effectiveness can approach the theoretical method effectiveness.

From a study on a very motivated population, Vessey et al. in 1989 (3) reported a failure rate of 0.3 per 100 women years. In another study, Grady et al. in 1986 (1) found failure rates per 100 women years to be 2.9 for the pill, 6.0 for IUD, 14.1 for condom, 17.2 for the diaphragm, and 16.1 for the rhythm method.

ADVERSE EFFECTS

1. Postmarketing surveillance studies have produced important indications for intervention and prevention of vascular side effects.
2. Epidemiological evidence is remarkably consistent, in relation to female genital tract neoplasms: increased risk for cervical cancer, protection against endometrial and ovarian cancers.

For breast cancer, overall evidence is consistent in showing slightly increased risks in long-term users below age 35, but no association in middle age women as reported by Vessey et al. in 1989 (3). In another quite reasurring study, La Vecchia et al. in 1989 (2) reported that the relative risk for ever vs never users was 1.3 (95% c.i. 1.0-1.7 and that risk was not related to the duration of use.

REFERENCES

1. Gray W.R., Hayward M.D. and Yagi J. (1986): Fam. Plann. Prospect. 18, 200-203.
2. La Vecchia C., Parazzini F., Negri E., Boyle P., Gentile A., Decarli A. and Franceschi S. (1989): Eur. J. Cancer Oncol. 25: 1613-1618.
3. Vessey M.P., Villard-Mackintosh L., McPherson K. and Yeates D. (1989): Br. Med. J. 299, 1487-1491.

From: JEI, Vol. 17, suppl. 2 to n. 3, 1994, p.7.
Abstracts of the XXV National Congress of the Italian Endocrine Society.

Frontiers in Endocrinology
Volume 9 - 1994

Risks and Benefits of Oral Contraceptives in Italy

C. La Vecchia[1,2], F. Parazzini[1,3], E. Negri[1] and R. Bortolus[1]

[1]Istituto di Ricerche Farmacologiche "Mario Negri", via Eritrea, 62, 20157 Milan; [2]Istituto di Biometria e Statistica Medica, University of Milan, via Venezian, 1, 20133 Milan; [3]I Clinica Ostetrico Ginecologica, University of Milan via Commenda 12, 20122 Milan, Italy

INTRODUCTION

Most evidence on risks and benefits of oral contraceptives (OCs) is based on studies conducted in North America and Northern Europe (4, 13). Although, on aetiological and epidemiological grounds, it is conceivable that the impact of OCs on the relative risk (RR) of various diseases is similar in various populations, there are at least two reasons for producing epidemiological data specifically focused on the Italian population. First, the incidence of several diseases, including myocardial infarction and most female hormone-related neoplasms, is different in Italy and, more important, the prevalence and pattern of contraceptive use has been substantially different in Italy as compared to most other developed countries (9).

On the basis of these considerations, since the early 1980's an integrated series of case-control studies has been conducted in Italy to quantify the role of OCs on the risk of myocardial infarction, gallbladder disease, breast cancer, hepatocellular carcinoma and several benign and malignant female-genital tract tumours. For the sake of simplicity, in this review, reference will be made essentially to the original published from this dataset, where reference to other work can be obtained.

MATERIAL AND METHODS

An integrated series of case-control studies ("case-control surveillance") has been conducted since the early 1980's on acute myocardial infarction, gallbladder disease, benign and malignant breast and female genital tract tumours and liver cancer, based on a network of cooperating hospitals in the Greater Milan area, Northern Italy. The general design of this investigation has previously been described (2, 4-6, 8-12, 15, 16). Briefly, trained interviewers identified and questioned cases and controls using a standard questionnaire, including a detailed history of lifetime use of OCs and other types of contraception. Less than 5% of subjects approached for interview (cases and controls) refused to participate. The data here reported were collected before the end of 1992.

Cases were women under 60 years of age with acute myocardial infarction (n= 251), gallstone disease undergoing surgery (n= 155), uterine fibromyomas (n= 390), benign breast disease (n= 288), benign ovarian cysts (n= 202), and histologically confirmed incident cancers of the breast (n= 2309), endometrium (n= 170), ovary (epithelial, n= 406), borderline ovarian tumours (n= 91), pre-invasive (n= 362) and invasive cervical neoplasms (n= 367), and primary liver cancer (n= 43). In the overall dataset, over 2,500 controls were available, admitted to hospital for acute, non neoplastic, non gynaecological, non hormone-related diseases.

Statistical analysis was based on standard methods for case-control studies, including multivariate odds ratios, as estimators of RR, and the corresponding 95% confidence intervals (CI) (1).

RESULTS

Acute myocardial infarction (AMI) In this study (5), current OC users were 2.8% of cases vs 1.3% of controls, and past users 17.1% vs 9.7%. The multivariate RRs were 2.0 for current and 1.8 for past users. The risk of AMI decreased with increasing time since last use, although it was still elevated, but not significantly, 2 or more years since last use (Table 1).

Table 1. *Relative risk of acute myocardial infarction (AMI) in relation to various measure of oral contraceptive use. Italy, 1983-1992 (5)*

	AMI	Controls	Relative risk estimates (95% CI)[a]
Oral contraceptive use			
Never users	201	423	1[b]
Ever users	50	52	1.7 (1.1-3.1)
Current users	7	6	2.0 (0.6-6.7)
Past users	43	46	1.8 (1.0-3.2)
Duration of use			
≤ 2 years	23	25	2.1 (1.0-4.4)
> 2 years	27	27	1.5 (0.7-2.9)
Time since last use			
≤ 2 years	8	6	2.8 (0.8-9.3)
> 2 years	35	40	1.7 (0.9-3.0)

[a]Estimates from multiple logistic regression equations including terms for area of residence, smoking habits, body mass index, history of angina, diabetes, hypertension and hyperlipidemia.
[b]Reference category.

With reference to the combined effect of OCs and other major covariates, compared to nonsmokers nonusers of OCs, the RR of AMI for smokers, OC users, was 6.1 (95% CI 3.4 - 11.0). Compared to never OC users normotensive women, the RR was 28.4 (95% CI 6.7-120.1) for hypertensive women ever OC users (17 cases and 2 controls). In hyperlipidemic women ever OC users the RR was 4.4 (95% CI 1.3-15.3), compared to normolipidemic never user women.

Thus, this study confirms the substantially elevated risk in women exposed to both OC use and smoking, and suggests an action of both risk factors on similar aspects of the pathogenic process. From a public health viewpoint, however, only about 1% of myocardial infarctions in this population was attributable to OC use, in strong contrast with the approximate 50% of AMI attributable to smoking among Italian women. The association between OC use and AMI is, therefore, of modest importance on a public health level in this population.

Gallstone disease Gallstone disease requiring surgery is considered in Table 2 (6). Twenty seven (17%) cases vs 48 (15%) controls aged less than 60 years had ever used combination oral contraceptives: the corresponding age-adjusted RR was 0.8, with 95% CI 0.4 to 1.5. No trend in risk was observed with duration of use, the point estimates being 1.0 for less than two and 0.5 for two or more years of use. The risk was above unity, though not significantly (RR 1.7, 95% CI 0.6 - 4.7), for women who had last used the pill less than five years before diagnosis, but decreased to 0.4 (95% CI 0.2 - 1.0) in those who had stopped use five or more years earlier. None of the RRs was appreciably modified by allowance for several identified confounding variables using multiple logistic regression.

Table 2. *Relative risk of gallstone disease requiring surgery in relation to various measures of oral contraceptive use. Milan, Italy, 1987-1990 (6)*

	Gallstone disease	Controls	Relative risk estimates (95% CI)[a]
Oral contraceptive use			
Never users	128	274	1[b]
Ever users	27	48	0.8 (0.4-1.5)
Duration of use			
<2 years	13	19	1.0 (0.4-2.3)
≥2 years	11	27	0.5 (0.2-1.2)
Unknown	3	2	-
Time since last use			
< 5 years	15	10	1.7 (0.6-4.7)
≥ 5 years	9	35	0.4 (0.2-1.0)
Unknown	3	3	-

[a]Estimates from multiple logistic regression equations including terms for age, education, area of residence, body mass index and parity. [b]Reference category.

Thus, although the prevalence and duration of OC use in Italy are lower than in the United States, Britain, or Australia, where studies have been published, our results are in general agreement with previous reports, and confirm that the incidence of clinically relevant gallstones is not materially influenced by the use of OCs.

The point estimates for any use and for long-term use were below unity, and the only RR above unity (though not significantly) was for current or recent use. This is consistent with the findings of two British cohort studies (7, 14), which suggested that OCs may simply accelerate the appearance of symptoms or hasten the diagnosis of cholelithiasis, but do not result in a long-term increase in risk.

Uterine fibromyoma Table 3 shows the relation of various measures of OC use to the risk of uterine fibromyomas (11). A total of 78 cases (20%) and 200 controls (18%) reported ever OC use: compared with never-users, the multivariate RR for ever use was 1.0. No direct relationship emerged with duration of use: the estimated RR was 1.3 in ever users for less than 3 years and 0.8 in users for 3 years or more. The risk of fibroids was apparently, though not significantly, greater with longer more recent use: the estimated RRs were 0.9 and 1.5, respectively, in women reporting last OC use less than 10 years and 10 or more years before diagnosis of the disease. No relationship emerged with latency of use.

Thus, this study, as well as previous available evidence, did not show any consistent association between OC use and risk of fibromyomas. In a public health and clinical perspective, this indicates that the risk of developing fibromyomas should not be considered a contraindication to the use of OCs.

Table 3. *Relative risk of uterine fibromyoma in relation to various measures of oral contraceptive use. Milan, Italy, 1986-1990 (11)*

	Cases	Controls	Relative risk estimates (95% CI)[a]
Oral contraceptive use			
Never users	312	936	1[b]
Ever users	78	200	1.0 (0.8-1.5)
Duration of use[c]			
3 years	52	108	1.3 (0.9-2.0)
≥ 3 years	26	89	0.8 (0.5-1.3)
Time since last use[c]			
<10 years	44	132	0.9 (0.6-1.3)
≥ 10 years	33	62	1.5 (0.9-2.5)
Time since first use[c]			
< 15 years	56	142	1.2 (0.8-1.0)
≥ 15 years	22	56	1.0 (0.6-1.8)

[a]Estimates from multiple logistic regression equations including terms for age, education, marital status, parity, number of spontaneous and induced abortions and menopausal status. [b]Reference category. [c]Sum does not add up to total due to missing values.

Ovarian cysts The RR of ovarian cysts for ever use of OCs was 0.8 (8). This finding, although not significant, is consistent with the hypothesis that pill-induced anovulation may reduce the risk not only of malignant, but also of benign ovarian tumours. The data were, however, too scanty for any more precise or definite inference.

Benign breast disease (BBD) Compared to women who had never used OCs, the RR of histologically-confirmed BBD for OC users was 1.0 (95% CI 0.6 - 1.5) (2). There was no significant association with duration of use; however, a significantly reduced risk was found in women using OCs during the year before breast biopsy (RR 0.4, 95% CI 0.2 - 0.8). The protection in current users increased with increasing duration of use. In spite of this finding, the overall results of the present study do not support the hypothesis that OC use protects against development of histologically confirmed and clinically relevant BBD.

The lack of association between OCs and breast cancer, despite the evidence of a negative association between OCs and BBD, has long been considered hard to explain. Possible explanations for this conondrum are the too easy inclusion as BBD of often transient breast lesions presumably unrelated to malignant transformation, and the greater likelihood of progression into breast cancer of lesions that persist during use of OCs.

Breast cancer The relation between OCs and breast cancer risk in this study is considered in Table 4 (15).

Ever OC use was reported by 16% of cases and 14% of controls; the corresponding RR estimate was 1.2 (95% CI 1.0 - 1.4). However, there was no direct relation with duration of use, and short-term users (<24 months) had the highest risk (RR = 1.5); the RR decreased to 0.8 for use lasting 5 years or longer. In relation to time since first or last OC use, the risk was highest among women with the shortest intervals since first (RR = 1.5) and last use (RR= 1.3).

Thus, this study indicates that in women under 60 years of age there is no relationship between duration of OC use and breast cancer risk and, indeed, the risk was apparently lower for longer than for shorter exposure.

The low prevalence of OC use in this Italian population severely hampered analysis, and particularly inference on subgroups, time factors, dose, or type of preparation. Nevertheless, the large size of the dataset, the originality of the population, in terms of baseline breast cancer incidence and patterns of hormone use, and the consistency of the results with the overall evidence from other studies, add useful information to a better understanding of one of the major public health problems. The indications emerging from this study on the use of OCs and the risk of breast cancer are reassuring and should help to better assess the pattern of breast cancer risk for various time-related factors of OC use in a southern European population.

Table 4. *Relative risk of breast cancer in relation to various measures of oral contraceptive use. Milan, Italy, 1983-1991 (15)*[a]

	Breast cancer	Controls	Relative risk estimates (95% CI)[b]
Oral contraceptive use			
Never users	1938	1663	1[c]
Ever users	371	265	1.2 (1.0-1.4)
Duration of use			
<2 years	185	109	1.5 (1.2-2.0)
2-4 years	103	70	1.3 (0.9-1.8)
≥ 5 years	82	84	0.8 (0.5-1.0)
Time since first use			
<10 years	125	95	1.5 (1.1-2.0)
10-14 years	106	84	1.0 (0.7-1.4)
≥ 15 years	140	85	1.2 (0.9-1.6)

[a]For some variables the sum of strata does not add up to the total because of some missing values. [b]Estimates from multiple logistic regression equations, including terms for age, education, marital status, family history of breast cancer, age at menarche and menopause, parity and age at first birth. [c]Reference category.

Ovarian and endometrial cancers With reference to borderline ovarian cancer, 10% of cases vs 25% of controls, reported ever OC use (3). Compared to never users, the RRs were 0.3 for ever users, and 0.2 for users of 2 years or more (Table 5). Thus, in this study, OC users had about 70% lower risk of borderline ovarian tumours. These findings confirm the protective effect of OCs on the whole spectrum of ovarian tumours.

Table 5. *Relative risk of borderline ovarian cancer in relation to various measures of oral contraceptive use. Milan, Italy, 1983-1990 (12)*

	Cases	Controls	Relative risk estimates (95% CI)[a]
Oral contraceptive use			
Never users	82	205	1[b]
Ever users	9	68	0.3 (0.2-0.6)
Duration of use			
<2 years	5	30	0.3 (0.1-0.4)
≥ 2 years	4	38	0.2 (0.1-0.6)

[a]Estimates from multiple logistic regression equations, including terms for age, education, parity, age at menopause and oral contraceptive use. [b]Reference category.

With reference to invasive epithelial ovarian cancer and endometrial cancer, the RRs for ever use were 0.7 and 0.5, respectively, and for ovarian cancer there was a significant trend of decreasing risk with increasing duration of use (Table 6). Thus, this study confirmed, in an Italian population, the consistent protection of OCs on the risk of these cancer sites.

Table 6. *Relative risk of endometrial and ovarian cancer with reference to oral contraceptive use. Milan, Italy, 1983-1986 (3)*

	Endometrial cancer	Ovarian cancer	Controls	Relative risk estimates (95% CI)[a] Endometrial cancer	Relative risk estimates (95% CI)[a] Ovarian cancer
Oral contraceptive use					
Never users	163	367	1104	1[b]	1[b]
Ever users	7	39	178	0.5 (0.2-1.1)	0.7 (0.5-1.0)

[a]Estimates adjusted for quinquennia of age. [b]Reference category.

Cervical cancer With reference to invasive cervical cancer (Table 7) (10), patients had used OCs more frequently than controls, the RR for ever use being 1.9. This increased to 2.5 for use over 2 years.

Table 7. *Relative risk of invasive cervical cancer in relation to various measures of oral contraceptive use. Milan, Italy, 1983-1990 (10)*

	Cervical cancer	Controls	Relative risk estimates (95% CI)[a]
Oral contraceptive use			
Never users	298	276	1[b]
Ever users	69	47	1.9 (1.0-3.1)
Duration of use			
≤ 2 years	36	27	1.1 (0.8-3.2)
>2 years	33	20	2.5 (1.2-5.1)

[a]Estimates from multiple logistic regression equations including terms for age, marital status, education, parity, number of sexual partners, age at first intercourse, cigarette smoking, history of pap smears and use of barrier methods of contraception. [b]Reference category.

Thus, this study confirms the presence of a positive association between cervical cancer and OCs. Although published data are not totally consistent, the overall available evidence indicates an approximately 50% higher risk of invasive cervical cancer among long-term OC users, which was not explained by potential confounding effects of major covariates, including indicators of sexual habits (4, 13).

Interpretation of these findings in biological terms is largely tentative. There is some suggestion, in the present as well as in previous work, that the

RR is higher in the short term, and decreases with time since first and last use. In this study, however, no association was observed between OCs and the risk of intra-epithelial cervical neoplasia. This observation, if confirmed, has potentially interesting pathogenic correlates, since it would suggest a role of OCs on one of the later stages of the process of cervical carcinogenesis (3).

Liver cancer The relationship between OCs and primary liver cancer is considered in Table 8 (16). A total of nine (21%) cases and 21 (11%) controls had ever used the pill. The corresponding RR was 2.6 (95% CI 1.0-7.0). The risk increased with duration, with RRs of 1.5 for a use of ≤5 years and 3.9 for longer use. The RR was 1.1 in women who had stopped OC use 10 years or less earlier, but was significantly elevated for those who had stopped more than 10 years earlier (RR 4.3, 95% CI 1.0-18.1).

Thus, the results of this study confirm an increased risk of primary liver cancer in OC users (4, 13), and, more importantly, indicate that the risk persists for 10 or more years after stopping treatment. The indication emerging from this study of a long-lasting increase in the risk of hepatocellular carcinoma in OC users is of interest to quantify the ultimate risks and benefits of OC use.

Table 8. *Relative risk of hepatocellular carcinoma in relation to various measures of oral contraceptive use. Milan, Italy, 1984-1992 (16)*

	Hepatocellular carcinoma	Controls	Relative risk estimates (95% CI)a
Oral contraceptive use			
Never users	34	173	1b
Ever users	9	21	2.6 (1.0-7.0)
Duration of usec			
≤ 5 years	5	17	1.5 (0.5-5.0)
> 5 years	2	4	3.9 (0.6-24.5)
Time since last usec			
≤ 10 years	3	12	1.1 (0.3-4.6)
> 10 years	4	6	4.3 (1.0-18.1)

[a]Estimates from multiple logistic regression equations, including terms for age, education and parity. [b]Reference category. [c]The sum does not add up to the total of users on account of some missing values.

DISCUSSION

The results of this integrated series of Italian studies are, in general, in agreement with available evidence on the relationship between OCs and cancer risk (4, 13), and offer useful quantitative information on the impact of OCs at a public health level in this population.

It is clear, therefore, that the impact of OC on acute myocardial infarction in young women in this population, if any, is negligible, and restricted to a few points percent, as compared to an attributable risk of about 50% for cigarette smoking.

More complex is the population attributable risk estimate on neoplastic diseases. It is possible, in fact, that OCs (particularly current or recent use) are associated in a few dozen cases per year of breast and cervical cancer, and also a few cases of primary liver cancer. The protection on endometrial and, mostly, ovarian cancer, is however much more important, and may imply, even with a limited prevalence of use, avoiding a few hundred cases per year in the whole of Italy.

Finally, the absence of a relationship between OC use and uterine fibromyomas and gallstone disease is clearly reassuring, on account of the high prevalence of these diseases in the population, and their consequent major importance with on a public health level.

ACKNOWLEDGEMENTS

This work was conducted within the framework of the CNR (Italian National Research Council) Applied Project "Risk Factors for Disease" and "Clinical Application of Oncological Research" (Contracts No. 93.00779.PF41 and 93.02360.PF39), and with the contributions of the Italian Association for Cancer Research, and the Italian League Against Tumours, Milan. The Authors thank Mrs Judy Baggott, Mrs Ivana Garimoldi and the G.A. Pfeiffer Memorial Library for editorial assistance.

REFERENCES

1. Breslow N.E. and Day N.E. (1980): IARC Sci. Publ. 32.
2. Franceschi S., La Vecchia C., Parazzini F., Fasoli M., Regallo M., Decarli A., Gallus G. and Tognoni G. (1984): Am. J. Obstet. Gynecol. 149: 602-606.
3. La Vecchia C., Decarli A., Fasoli M., Franceschi S., Gentile A., Negri E., Parazzini F. and Tognoni G. (1986): Br. J. Cancer 54: 311-317.
4. La Vecchia C., Franceschi S., Bruzzi P., Parazzini F. and Boyle P. (1990): Drug Saf. 5: 436-446.
5. La Vecchia C., Franceschi S., Decarli A., Pampallona S. and Tognoni G. (1987): Am. J. Epidemiol. 125: 832-843.
6. La Vecchia C., Negri E., D'Avanzo B., Parazzini F., Gentile A. and Franceschi S. (1992): J. Epidemiol. Community Health 46: 234-236.
7. Layde P.M., Vessey M.P. and Yeates D. (1982): J. Epidemiol. Community Health 36: 274-278.
8. Parazzini F., La Vecchia C., Franceschi S., Negri E. and Cecchetti G. (1989): Int. J. Epidemiol. 18: 108-112.
9. Parazzini F., La Vecchia C. and Negri E. (1991): Ann. Ostet. Ginecol. Med. Perinat. 112: 368-375.
10. Parazzini F., La Vecchia C., Negri E. and Maggi R. (1990): Int. J. Epidemiol. 19: 259-263.
11. Parazzini F., Negri E., La Vecchia C., Fedele L., Rabaiotti M. and Luchini L. (1992): Obstet. Gynecol. 79: 430-433.

12. Parazzini F., Restelli C., La Vecchia C., Negri E., Chiari S., Maggi R. and Mangioni C. (1991): Int. J. Epidemiol. 20: 871-877.
13. Prentice R.L. and Thomas D.B. (1987): Adv. Cancer Res. 49: 285-401.
14. Royal College of General Practitioners (1982): Lancet 2: 957-959.
15. Tavani A., Negri E., Franceschi S., Parazzini F. and La Vecchia C. (1993): Br. J. Cancer 68: 568-571.
16. Tavani A., Negri E., Parazzini F., Franceschi S. and La Vecchia C. (1993): Br. J. Cancer 67: 635-637.

Frontiers in Endocrinology
Volume 9 - 1994

Non-Contraceptive Benefits of Oral Contraceptive Use

P.G. Crosignani, P. Maggioni, G. Testa and W. Vegetti

1st Department of Obstetrics and Gynecology, University of Milan, Via Commenda 12, 20122 Milan, Italy

There are considerable non-contraceptive health benefits, associated with oral contraceptive use, that are not well known to either the consumers or contraceptive counselors.

BENEFITS DUE TO INHIBITION OF OVULATION

Inhibition of ovulation by contraceptives lowers the incidence of functional ovarian cysts, ovarian cancer, benign breast disease, dysmenorrhea and premenstrual syndrome.

Ovarian cancer Epidemiological evidence regarding the relationship of oral contraceptives to ovarian cancer is as clear and convincing as that for endometrial cancer. The overall protection is estimated as approximately 40% and a strong inverse relationship, with duration of use, has also been observed in most studies (3).

For ovarian cancer, protection has been shown to persist for some time (at least ten years) after use of the pill has ceased (1). Ovario-stasis, induced by oral contraceptives, as well as by pregnancy and menopause, precludes exposure of the ovarian epithelium to recurrent trauma and contact with follicular fluid.

Since the incidence of ovarian cancer, unlike that of endometrial cancer, is already appreciable in middle age, and survival is substantially worse, protection obtained from oral contraceptive use prevents a far from negligible number of deaths.

Benign breast disease Several studies (4, 10, 11) have shown that oral contraceptive use is associated with a significantly decreased risk of benign breast neoplasia, while other studies have found no association between oral contraceptive use and prevalence of benign breast disease (5).

BENEFITS DUE TO INHIBITION OF ESTROGEN SYNTHESIS

Inhibition of the synthesis of estrogen receptors by the synthetic progestin reduces the incidence of endometrial cancer and regulates menstrual blood loss.

Endometrial Cancer Results of several studies (2, 7, 14, 15) have demonstrated, with remarkably consistent estimates, that oral contraceptive use is associated with significant protection against endometrial cancer. All the relative risks, in these studies, were close to their overall average of 0.5, indicating that, on the whole, the risk of developing endometrial cancer, is reduced by 50% in oral contraceptive users.

This protection increases with increasing duration of use, emphasizing that the treatment is indeed the cause of the reduced risk and appears to remain for up to 10-15 years after stopping use. Since continuous influence of estrogenic substances unopposed by progesterone is firmly recognized, at present, to be a major determinant of endometrial cancer (6), the protective effect of combined oral contraceptives was predictable in theory. There is almost no endometrial mitotic activity, during which DNA copying errors are likely to occur, in women taking combined oral contraceptives (6).

Endometrial cancer, nevertheless, is a rare disease in young and middle-aged women. Thus, without direct information about whether or not protection persists in older ages, its proven impact should be considered, on a public health scale, to be relatively limited.

BENEFITS DUE TO HORMONAL SUPPRESSION

The hirsutism commonly associated with polycystic ovarian syndrome is consistently improved by the use of oral contraceptives, since they lower ovarian activity and increase plasma SHBG concentrations.

Combination oral contraceptives are the most common treatment for hirsutism. Their popularity and effectiveness result from the many benefits they offer the hirsute woman. Oral contraceptives suppress luteinizing hormone secretion, decrease testosterone and dehydroepiandrosterone sulfate concentrations (16) and increase sex hormone-binding globulin concentrations. Together, these effects lower the levels of androgen both from ovarian and adrenal sources and increase the proportion of serum androgen bound to sex hormone-binding globulin. The marked decrease in biologically active serum androgen (not bound to sex hormone-binding globulin) results in reduced androgenic stimulation of hair growth. In addition to inducing contraception, this hormonal therapy controls dysfunctional uterine bleeding and prevents endometrial hyperplasia often found in these patients.

The ideal oral contraceptive for treating hirsutism should be estrogen dominant and contain a progestin with minimal androgenic activity, such as ethinodiol diacetate. Low-dose oral contraceptives (30-35 μg of ethinyl estradiol) decrease serum androgen concentrations and increase sex hormone-binding globulin (9). Oral contraceptives containing norgestrel result in less marked increases in sex hormone-binding globulin and may be less effective than those containing norethindrone or ethinodiol diacetate (11). Despite the apparently increased androgenic activity of norgestrel, use of a triphasic preparation, containing low doses of norgestrel, result in decreased hyperandrogenic activity in patients with acne and hirsutism (8).

OTHER BENEFITS OF ORAL CONTRACEPTION

Another non-contraceptive health benefit to be gained from birth control pill use is a 50% decrease in the risk of acute salpyngitis, as compared with a control group not using pharmacological methods of contraception (3). This protective effect is related to the changes in the cervical mucus induced by oral contraceptives. Oral contraceptive use also protects against ectopic pregnancy (3).

A study on seven monophasic or triphasic OCs with the same EE content has been carried out by Van der Vange et al. (12). The various combinations with norethindrone, levonorgestrel, desogestrel, gestodene and cyproterone acetate resulted in distinct differences in SHBG and absolute free testosterone values. However, total and free testosterone values decreased with all seven formulations, except for total testosterone during use of the cyproterone acetate OC. However, in 6-month studies (13) both 35 µg EE/cyproterone acetate 2 mg OCs produced an impressive decrease in plasma free testosterone levels and urinary excretion of androstanediol glucuronide, the metabolite of 5 alpha-dihydrotestosterone. OC-induced changes in plasma levels return to baseline within a month of withdrawal.

REFERENCES

1. Casagrande J.T., Louie E.W., Pike M.C., Roy S. and Ross R.K. (1979): Lancet ii: 170-172.
2. C.A.S.H. The Cancer and Steroid Hormone Study of the Centers for Disease Control and the National Institute of Child Health and Human Development. (1987): JAMA 257: 796-800.
3. Crosignani P.G. and La Vecchia C. (1994): In: Understanding Common Disorders in Reproductive Endocrinology, edited by M.M. Dooley and M.P. Brincat, pp.123-143. John Wiley & Sons Ltd. Chichester.
4. Fasal E. and Paffenbarger R.S. Jr. (1975): J. Natl. Cancer Inst. 55: 767.
5. Franceschi S., La Vecchia C., Parazzini F., Fasoli M., Regallo M., Decarli A., Gallus G. and Tognoni G. (1984): Am. J. Obstet. Gynecol. 149: 602-606.
6. Kay T.J.A. and Pike M.C. (1988): Br. J. Cancer 57: 205-212.
7. La Vecchia C., Decarli A., Fasoli M., Franceschi S. and Gentile A. (1986): Br. J. Cancer 54: 311-317.
8. Lemay A., Dewailly S.D., Grenier R. and Huard J. (1990): J. Clin. Endocrinol. Metab. 70: 8-14.
9. Murphy A.A., Cropp C.S., Smith B.S., Burkman R.T. and Zacur H.A. (1990): Fertil. Steril. 53: 35-39.
10. Ory H., Cole P., MacMahon B. and Hoover R. (1976): N. Engl. J. Med. 294: 419.

11. Pang S. (1990): J. Clin. Endocrinol. Metab. 71: 5-7.
12. Van der Vange N., Blankenstein M.A. and Kloosterboer H.J. et al. (1990): Contraception 41: 345-352.
13. Vermeulen A. and Rubens R. (1988): Contraception 38: 419-428.
14. Vessey M.P., Doll R., Peto R., Johnson B. and Wiggins P. (1976): J. Biosoc. Sci. 8: 375.
15. WHO Collaborative Study of Neoplasia and Steroid Contraceptives. (1988): Int. J. Epidemiol. 17: 263-269.
16. Wiebe R.H. and Morris C.V. (1984): Obstet. Gynecol. 63: 12-14.

Frontiers in Endocrinology
Volume 9 - 1994

Hormonal Male Contraception: Present and Perspectives

G. Forti

Andrology Unit, Department of Clinical Physiopathology, Viale Pieraccini 6, 50139 Florence, Italy

INTRODUCTION

The present world population, which is approaching 5.5 billion, has doubled since 1950 and is increasing by about 90 milion/year, that is three/second. It is roughly estimated that about 50% of conceptions are unplanned and 25% definitely unwanted, and, in fact, the number of abortions each year worldwide is estimated to be between 35-50 million. At present, the most prevalent form of contraception is female sterilization by tubal ligation, with an incidence of 26%, followed by the intrauterine device (19%) and the pill (15%). Vasectomy and use of the condom account for 10% each, whereas withdrawal, vaginal barrier, rhythm and other methods account for the remaining 20% (9). These data clearly show that, at present, the major burden of fertility regulation is carried by women. There is, however, an increasing demand that men should share also the burden of contraception. Even if vasectomy and the condom, the most widely used male methods, present the problem of irreversibility and a high failure rate, respectively, these two methods are becoming increasingly popular, indicating that the demand for male methods and the willingness of men to accept them are increasing.

New methods for male contraception should be effective, safe, and fully reversible. This area of medical research has often taken advantage of side effects of drugs long in use, such as the antifertility effects of sulfasalazine (5) or the traditonal chinese drug made from Tripterygium wilfordii (12). Other approaches such as immunological methods (1) and interference with epididymal function (4) are still in a preliminary phase of experimentation and far from clinical application. On the other hand, as the endocrine mechanisms controlling spermatogenesis are well understood, hormonal methods based upon suppression of spermatogenesis are closer to clinical application.

PRINCIPLES OF HORMONAL MALE CONTRACEPTION

The testis has two main functions: the production of androgens and of spermatozoa, which are closely related. The aim of endocrine regulation of male fertility is the suppression of spermatogenesis without affecting androgen production in order to maintain libido, potency, male sex characteristics, hematopoiesis and bone structure. Unfortunately, the suppression of pituitary secretion of FSH and LH, which results in cessation of spermatogenesis, is accompanied also by depletion of intratesticular testosterone: therefore, with the exception of the endocrine approach with high doses of testosterone, agents suppressing the pituitary secretion of gonadotropins must be used in combination with androgens.

The following hormonal approaches have been attempted in order to achieve suppression of spermatogenesis: 1) testosterone alone; 2) progestins combined with testosterone; 3) GnRH agonists combined with testosterone; 4) GnRH antagonists combined with testosterone.

Testosterone alone Testosterone has the unique advantage of providing simultaneously gonadotropin suppression and androgen replacement, and a number of clinical trials have been performed in the past. A recent multicenter WHO study demonstrated, for the first time, the efficacy of the weekly administration of 200 mg testosterone enanthate by intramuscular injection (15). However, in this study, ethnic differences were observed as Asian men showed a higher rate of azoospermia than Caucasians. The weekly administration, a major drawback of this approach, is due to the pharmacokinetics of testosterone enanthate, characterized by a high initial serum peak and, thereafter, by a rapid decline. For this reason, longer acting androgens are required, in the near future, such as 19-nortestosterone hexyloxyphenylpropionate and testosterone buciclate which have been reported to be effective when given at three-week (8) and three-month (2) intervals, respectively. Furthermore, long-term testosterone administration will require surveillance for potential side effects on body weight, prostatic size and levels of prostatic-specific antigen, lipid profile, and hemoglobin levels.

Progestins combined with testosterone Several clinical trials have been performed by WHO (14) with different progestins (norethindrone, megestrol acetate, 17-hydroxyprogesterone capronate, and medroxyprogesterone acetate) combined with physiological doses of testosterone. The monthly administration of 200 mg medroxyprogesterone acetate (MPA) combined with 200 mg testosterone enanthate or cypionate was able to induce azoospermia in nearly all Asian men and in about 60% of European men, without effects on libido and potency (6). The major consistent metabolic effect of progestin-androgen combination is lowering of HDL cholesterol, while total cholesterol, LDL and triglycerides remain unchanged. Even if these combination regimens seem to be effective and new generation depot progestins are in development (such as levonorgestrel butanoate and non-biodegradable implants of norgestrel), the theoretical benefits in safety and efficacy of progestin-androgen combinations vs androgens alone await further confirmation.

GnRH agonists combined with testosterone The results of 12 trials (including 104 fertile male volunteers) for male fertility regulation in which different GnRH agonists (decapeptyl, buserelin, nafarelin) were administered daily, alone or in combination with testosterone, showed that azoospermia could be obtained only in a few men, whereas sperm counts were reduced below 5 millions/ml in 30% of subjects and below 30 million/ml in another 30%. In the remaining volunteers, the sperm number was only slightly reduced or unaffected (10). These disappointing results were confirmed also when a depot GnRH was used instead of the daily administration (3).

GnRH antagonists combined with testosterone Clinical trials with GnRH antagonists for male contraception started only 4 years ago because most of these compounds produced skin reactions in the injection site (7). The subcutaneous administration of a daily dose of 7.5-10 mg of the GnRH antagonist Nal-Glu combined with delayed testosterone administration was able to induce azoospermia in 14/16 volunteers (11, 13). The better effects of GnRH antagonists may reflect the greater depletion of intratesticular testosterone compared with GnRH agonists which always retain a partial agonist effect. Depot formulations of antagonists and testosterone could, therefore, be a promising hormonal male contraceptive regimen. The main drawback might be the high costs of the GnRH antagonists and of the depot formulations.

CONCLUSIONS

Although reversible vas occlusion and chemical and immunological methods inhibiting sperm function are in development, hormonal contraception seems at present to be the approach closest to clinical application in the male. The effects of all the four different hormonal methods, we have briefly described, are quite reversible. However, other problems need to be solved before these methods can be accepted for widespread use: 1) as azoospermia is obtained in many but not all volunteers, further studies are required to quantitate the contraceptive efficacy of severe oligozoospermia; 2) since all hormonal methods, in males, are based on, or include, testosterone, possible side-effects of testosterone (on blood lipid profile and prostate) must be carefully evaluated. Even if, in the reported short-term clinical trials, testosterone did not alter HDL cholesterol levels, only long-term surveillance will clarify the potential risks for the cardiovascular system. Furthermore, as testosterone may enhance the growth of existing prostate cancer, men over the age of 45-50 years should be excluded from hormonal contraception. In addition, the size and the morphology of the prostate should be carefully monitored in long-term clinical trials.

In conclusion, the results of research on hormonal male contraception are promising: and, if the reluctancy of pharmaceutical companies and of governments to consider investments in this area are overcome, further and faster development will occur in this area of reproductive medicine.

ACKNOWLEDGEMENTS

This work was supported by a Grant from the University of Florence.

REFERENCES

1. Aitken R.J., Paterson M. and Koothan P.T. (1992): In: Spermatogenesis-Fertilization-Contraception: Molecular, Cellular and Endocrine Events in Male Reproduction, edited by E. Nieschlag and U.F. Habenicht, pp 461-475. Springer Verlag. Heidelberg.
2. Behre H.M. and Nieschlag E. (1992): J. Clin. Endocrinol. Metab. 74: 1204-1210.
3. Behre H.M., Nashan D., Hubert W. and Nieschlag E. (1992): J. Clin. Endocrinol. Metab. 74: 84-90.
4. Cooper T.G. (1992): In: Spermatogenesis-Fertilization-Contraception: Molecular, Cellular and Endocrine Events in Male Reproduction, edited by E. Nieschlag and U.F. Habenicht, p. 420-460. Springer Verlag. Heidelberg.
5. Giwercman A. and Skakkebaek N.E. (1986): Int. J. Androl. 9: 28-52.
6. Handelsman D.J. (1993). In: Current Topics in Andrology, edited by H. Oshima and H. Burger, pp 306-312. Japan Society of Andrology and Toyo Shobou Co. Ltd. Tokyo.
7. Karten M.J., Joeger C.A., Hook W.A., Lindberg M.C. and Naqvi R.H. (1990): In: Recent Progress on GnRH and Gonadal Peptides, edited by P. Bouchard, F. Haour, P. Franchimont and B. Schatz, p. 147-158. Elsevier. Paris.
8. Knuth U.A., Behre H.M., Belkien L., Bents H. and Nieschlag E. (1985): Fertil. Steril. 44: 814-821.
9. Leese H.J. (1992): Hum. Reprod. 7: 1183-1184.
10. Nieschlag E., Behre H.B. and Weimbauer G.F (1992): In: Spermatogenesis Fertilization-Contraception: Molecular, Cellular and Endocrine Events in Male Reproduction, edited by E. Nieschlag and U.F. Habenicht, pp 477-501. Springer Verlag. Heidelberg.
11. Pavlou S.N., Brewer K., Farley M.G., Lindner J., Bastias M.C., Rogers B.J., Swift L.L., Rivier J.E., Vale W.W., Conn M. and Herbert CM. (1991): J. Clin. Endocrinol. Metab. 73: 1360-1369.
12. Quian S.Z. (1987): In: Fertility Regulation Today and Tomorrow, edited by E. Diczfalusy and M. Bydgema, p. 217-232. Raven Press. New York.
13. Tom L., Salameh W., Bhasin S., Steiner B., Peterson M. and Swerdloff R.S. (1992): J. Clin. Endocrinol. Metab. 75: 476-483.
14. World Health Organization (1972-1983): Special Programme of Research Development and Research Training in Human Reproduction: Annual Reports, Geneva.
15. World Health Organization Task Force on Methods for Regulation of Male Fertility (1990): Lancet 336: 955-959.

Frontiers in Endocrinology
Volume 9 - 1994

Hormonal Methods for Male Contraception: Recent Progress

H.M. Behre, M. Simoni, G.F. Weinbauer and E. Nieschlag

Institute of Reproductive Medicine of the University
(WHO Collaborating Center for Research in Human Reproduction)
Steinfurterstr. 107, D - 48149 Münster, Germany

INTRODUCTION

Since family planning constitutes both an essential step towards progress in developing regions and a measure necessary to maintain welfare in developed countries, contraception is increasingly encouraged and promoted by individual states and international organizations. However, the large majority of the contraceptive methods available rely on the woman, the only possibility for the man being condoms or vasectomy. The success of the existing male methods is rather limited, due to the high failure rate of condoms and to the irreversibility of vasectomy, so that these methods account for only 20% of all the contraceptive procedures adopted worldwide. Effective, reliable, safe and reversible male methods would also relieve many women of the full responsibility in fertility regulation. At the moment, hormonal methods for male contraception are being actively pursued and tested in many centers and are very close to practical clinical application. In this chapter we will briefly review the state of the art of hormonal male contraception.

HORMONAL METHODS FOR MALE CONTRACEPTION

The principle Spermatogenesis in primates depends both upon testosterone and FSH, acting synergistically upon the Sertoli cell to stimulate, maintain and reinitiate sperm maturation (15). The hormonal approach to suppression of spermatogenesis is, therefore, based on elimination of FSH and LH, the latter leading to suppression of testosterone production. However, since this steroid has essential metabolic and behavioural effects, testosterone must be replaced in order to avoid symptoms of androgen deficiency. "The" male contraceptive, therefore, must suppress gonadotropins and intratesticular testosterone, but at the same time provide adequate androgen substitution. This goal can be achieved with testosterone, or androgens, alone or in combination with gestagens or GnRH analogs (10, 12).

Testosterone alone It has been known for a long time that testosterone suppresses pituitary gonadotropins, thereby inhibiting spermatogenesis, and a number of studies based on androgens alone have been performed in the past. The first efficacy trial on testosterone-induced azoospermia was completed in 1990 in ten centers in seven countries under the auspices of WHO (18). The study involved 271 healthy fertile men, each receiving 200 mg testosterone enanthate (TE) im at weekly intervals. After 6 months, 157 men became azoospermic and entered a 12-month efficacy phase. During this period only one pregnancy occurred, corresponding to a Pearl index of 0.8 conceptions per 100 person-years. This trial demonstrated, for the first time, that testosterone-induced azoospermia is sufficient for male contraception, is reliable and is reversible. However, only 65% of the men developed azoospermia, with important differences occurring between various countries (Fig. 1). In particular, it was shown that in China the prevalence of azoospermia was 93%, whereas rates of about 60% were obtained among Caucasian men. The reasons for this different sensitivity to hormone-induced suppression of spermatogenesis are not known. An ongoing WHO multicenter study is aimed at determining whether azoospermia is necessary for reliable contraception, or whether severe oligozoospermia (< 3 millions/ml) is also sufficient.

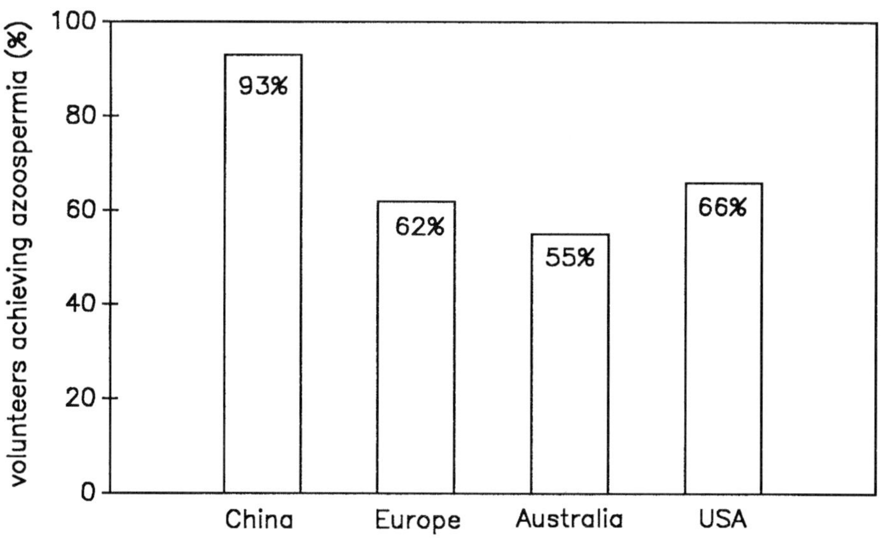

FIG. 1. Percentage of volunteers achieving azoospermia after 6 months of treatment with testosterone enanthate, 200 mg im at weekly intervals (data obtained from ref. 18).

Although testosterone is effective, the regimen of androgen administration adopted by the WHO (18) and in other contraceptive trials cannot be immediately transferred to the general population. In fact, the weekly frequency of im injections and the long time (4-6 months) required to reach azoospermia render this approach far from ideal. Moreover, the dose of TE used is relatively high and results in undesirable supraphysiological serum levels (7) and in relatively high risks of androgenic side-effects.

Some long-acting androgen preparations show more convenient pharmacokinetics. Among them, 19-nortestosterone-hexyloxyphenyl-propionate needs to be injected at 3-week intervals, whereas testosterone buciclate provides physiological testosterone levels for 3 months (Fig. 2) (2). Interestin alternatives are subdermal testosterone implants allowing normal serum levels for up to 6 months (9) and showing the same efficacy in producing azoospermia as weekly injections of TE (11), or testosterone microspheres (8).

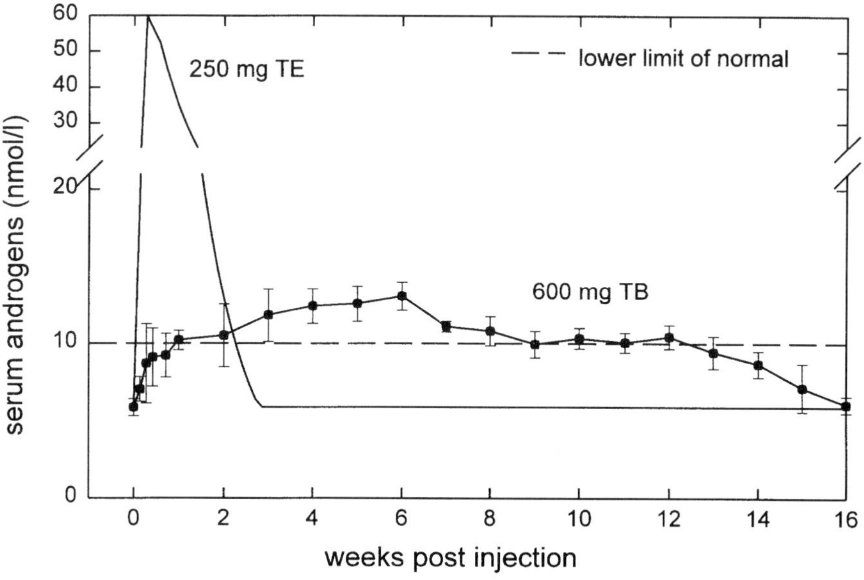

FIG. 2. Comparative pharmacokinetics of testosterone enanthate (TE) and testosterone buciclate (TB) in hypogonadal men with a mean basal serum testosterone level of 6 nmol/l.

An initial contraceptive trial with testosterone buciclate has provided promising results, showing that azoospermia can be achieved within 10 weeks of a single 1200 mg im administration in a proportion of volunteers

SOCIETA'
ITALIANA
DI ENDOCRINOLOGIA

Although testosterone is effective, the regimen of androgen administration adopted by the WHO (18) and in other contraceptive trials cannot be immediately transferred to the general population. In fact, the weekly frequency of im injections and the long time (4-6 months) required to reach azoospermia render this approach far from ideal. Moreover, the dose of TE used is relatively high and results in undesirable supraphysiological serum levels (7) and in relatively high risks of androgenic side-effects.

Some long-acting androgen preparations show more convenient pharmacokinetics. Among them, 19-nortestosterone-hexyloxyphenyl-propionate needs to be injected at 3-week intervals, whereas testosterone buciclate provides physiological testosterone levels for 3 months (Fig. 2) (2). Interestin alternatives are subdermal testosterone implants allowing normal serum levels for up to 6 months (9) and showing the same efficacy in producing azoospermia as weekly injections of TE (11), or testosterone microspheres (8).

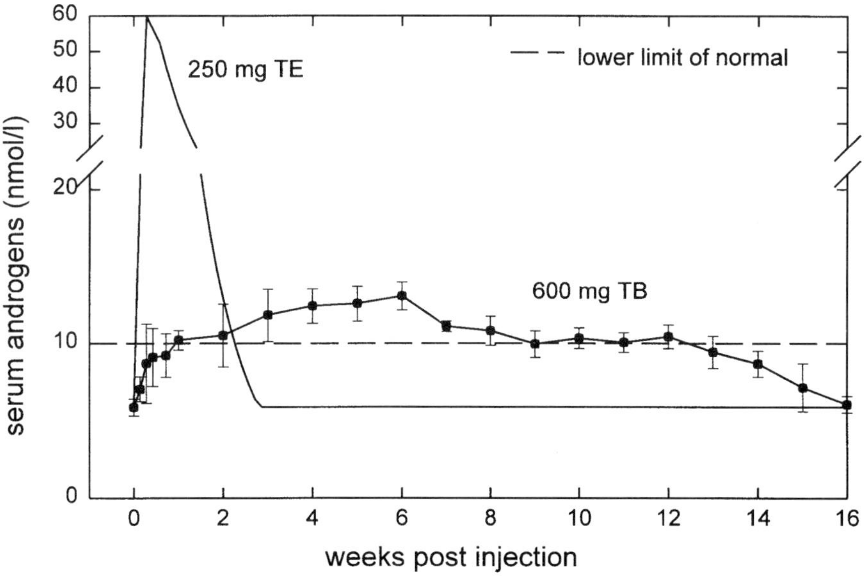

FIG. 2. Comparative pharmacokinetics of testosterone enanthate (TE) and testosterone buciclate (TB) in hypogonadal men with a mean basal serum testosterone level of 6 nmol/l.

An initial contraceptive trial with testosterone buciclate has provided promising results, showing that azoospermia can be achieved within 10 weeks of a single 1200 mg im administration in a proportion of volunteers

(Behre et al., in preparation). This study showed also that gonadotropins suppressed to a greater extent in those volunteers achieving azoospermia. The analysis of FSH and LH microheterogeneity by Concanavalin-A chromatography in these subjects, however, did not demonstrate clearcut differences in the type of gonadotropins secreted between responders and non-responders (Simoni et al., in preparation).

Testsosterone plus gestagens Since progesterone possesses very strong gonadotropin-suppressing activity, several studies were carried out to determine whether the combination of androgens and gestagens can provide a higher rate of azoospermia. TE or 19-nortestosterone used in various combinations with danazol or depot medroxyprogestrone acetate (DMPA), however, did not result in a higher success rate in Caucasian men (reviewed in 12). A recent WHO multicenter trial in Indonesia demonstrates that the combination of DMPA and TE or 19-nortestosterone is highly effective in sperm suppression, with azoospermia achieved in 96.7% of the cases, without differences between the two androgens (19). Once again, these data highlight the differences between populations in contraceptive efficacy of androgens.

Testosterone plus GnRH analogs As GnRH controls gonadotropin secretion, inhibition of GnRH action could be of help to depress LH and FSH secretion. GnRH agonists have been tested, alone or in combination with androgens, in 12 clinical trials for male contraception, giving rather disappointing results (reviewed in 12). Overall, only 21 out of 104 volunteers reached azoospermia and it was shown that the effects of androgens and GnRH agonists tend to counteract each other (6). Therefore, this approach has been abandoned.

On the contrary, GnRH antagonists are much more effective, showing a fairly rapid action, resulting in azoospermia within 6-12 weeks of treatment when testosterone substitution is delayed by two weeks after the start of the GnRH antagonist (13, 14). As already observed in the non-human primate model (16) and for unclear reasons, testosterone prevents the induction of azoospermia when administered concomitantly, from the beginning of the GnRH antagonist treatment (1). Recent studies in the preclinical monkey model have shown that the suppression of spermatogenesis achieved by GnRH antagonists can be maintained by testosterone alone (17), suggesting the possibility of curtailing GnRH antagonist administration after a few weeks.

The clinical trials carried out so far have employed the GnRH antagonist Nal-Glu. We have recently shown that the new compound Cetrorelix displays the same antigonadotropic potency as Nal-Glu, but produces far fewer side-effects (3, 4). Moreover, low doses of Cetrorelix are sufficient to maintain an effective suppression of gonadotropins and testosterone achieved by an initial high daily loading-dose (5). These data show that long-acting or depot formulations of GnRH antagonists could be very helpful in gonadotropin suppression.

CONCLUSIONS AND PERSPECTIVES

The current state of research encourages optimistic expectations of an effective male hormonal contraceptive in the next few years. Should the ongoing WHO trial demonstrate that severe oligozoospermia is also compatible with transient male infertility, one can envisage a protocol where oligo/azoospermia is achieved rapidly with a GnRH antagonist, possibly administered only once as a depot preparation, and maintained with periodical injections, say every 2-3 months, of long-acting testosterone esters. In addition to the convenience of this administration scheme, which would make it acceptable to the majority of men wishing contraception, the side-effects of testosterone are not serious. Of these, the effects on serum lipids should be given consideration.

From the experience accumulated until now, it appears that long-acting testosterone preparations are associated with a lower frequency of acne and very marginal modifications of the main hematological metabolic parameters (11). Moreover, the initial hypogonadal phase induced by GnRH antagonists resulted in an increase of HDL cholesterol, an effect that could protect against the inhibiting effect of testosterone (3). It is clear, however, that the real prevalence of side-effects can be accurately estimated only after prolonged observation.

REFERENCES

1. Bagatell C.J., Matsumoto A.M., Christensen R.B., Rivier J.E. and Bremner W.J. (1993): J. Clin. Endocrnol. Metab. 77: 427-432.
2. Behre H.M. and Nieschlag E. (1992): J. Clin. Endocrinol. Metab. 75: 1204-1210.
3. Behre H.M., Böckers A., Schlingheider A. and Nieschlag E. (1994): Clin. Endocrinol. 40: 241-248.
4. Behre H.M., Klein B., Steinmeyer E., McGregor G.P., Voigt K. and Nieschlag E. (1992). J. Clin. Endocrinol. Metab. 75: 393-398.
5. Behre H.M., Kliesch S., Pühse G. and Nieschlag E. (1994): Exp. Clin. Endocrinol. 102(Suppl. 1): 53 (Abstract).
6. Behre H.M., Nashan D., Hubert W. and Nieschlag E. (1992): J. Clin. Endocrinol. Metab. 74: 84-90.
7. Behre H.M., Oberpenning F. and Nieschlag E. (1990): In: Testosterone: Action, Deficiency, Substitution, edited by E. Nieschlag and H.M. Behre, pp. 115-135. Springer-Verlag. Heidelberg.
8. Bhasin S., Swerdloff R.S., Steiner B., Peterson M.A., Meridores T., Galmirini M., Pandian M.R., Goldberg R. and Berman N. (1992): J. Clin. Endocrinol. Metab. 74: 75-83.
9. Handelsman D.J. (1990): In: Testosterone: Action, Deficiency, Substitution, edited by E. Nieschlag and H.M. Behre, pp. 136-154. Springer-Verlag. Heidelberg.
10. Handelsman D.J. (1993): In: Current Topics in Andrology 1993, edited by H. Oshima and H.G. Burger, pp. 306-312. Japan Society of Andrology, Tokyo.
11. Handelsman D.J., Conway A.J. and Boylan L.M. (1992): J. Clin. Endocrinol. Metab. 175: 1326-1332.
12. Nieschlag E., Behre H.M. and Weinbauer G.F. (1992): In: Spermatogenesis, Fertilization, Contraception, edited by E. Nieschlag and U.F. Habenicht, pp. 477-501. Springer-Verlag. Berlin, Heidelberg, New York, London, Paris, Tokyo, Hong Kong, Barcelona.

13. Pavlou S.N., Brewer K., Farley G., Lindner J., Bastias M.C., Rogers B.J., Swift L.L., Rivier J.E., Vale W.W., Conn P.M. and Herbert C.M. (1991): J. Clin. Endocrinol. Metab. 73: 1360-1369.
14. Tom L., Bhasin S., Salameh W., Steiner B., Peterson M., Sokol R.Z., Rivier J., Vale W. and Swerdloff R.S. (1992): J. Clin. Endocrinol. Metab. 75: 476-483.
15. Weinbauer G.F. and Nieschlag E (1993): In: Molecular Biology of the Male Reproductive System, edited by D.M. De Kretser, pp. 99-142. Academic Press. New York.
16. Weinbauer G.F., Göckeler E. and Nieschlag E. (1988): J. Clin. Endocrinol. Metab. 67: 284-290.
17. Weinbauer G.F., Limberger A., Behre H.M. and Nieschlag E. (1994): J. Endocrinol. 142: 485-495.
18. World Health Organization (1990): Lancet 336: 955-959.
19. World Health Organization (1993): Fertil. Steril. 60: 1062-1068.

DIABETES - ENDOCRINE PANCREAS - METABOLISM - GROWTH FACTORS

p. 351 - 396

SOCIETA'
ITALIANA
DI ENDOCRINOLOGIA

Frontiers in Endocrinology
Volume 9 - 1994

Insulin Receptor Overexpression in CHO Cells activates Cell Replication and c-*fos* Expression

D. Maggi, C. Laurino, G. Andraghetti and R. Cordera

Department of Endocrinology and Metabolism (Di.S.E.M.),
University of Genova,
Viale Benedetto XV, 6, 16132 Genova, Italy

INTRODUCTION

Insulin and IGF-1 are progression factors in the cell cycle (1). The ligands and their receptors (IR and IGF-1R) share a high degree of homology and the very early steps of intracellular signal transduction. Both receptors are tyrosine kinases and become autophosphorylated upon ligand binding (8). These processes are believed to be essential for their biological activity (6, 3). When these receptors are tyrosine phopshorylated they become physically associated with an intracellular protein: the Insulin Receptor Substrate 1 (IRS-1). This docking protein is the juxtamembrane initial step of a complex framework that, through a cascade of phosphorylation and dephosphorylation reactions, leads to the biological effects of insulin and IGF-1 (7, 9).

Insulin is considered as a major metabolic regulator, while IGF-1 acts as a growth regulator. Expression of "primary response genes" (5) can be considered as a marker of activation of cell proliferation. Among others, c-fos expression is regulated by insulin and IGF-1.

Aim of this study was to investigate the mechanisms of specificity of signal transduction of these two hormones. Here we report experimental evidence suggesting that the amount of IRs and IGF-1Rs expressed by cells is a critical determinant of the cellular responsiveness to these two ligands. We propose that the metabolic or mitogenic effects of Insulin and IGF-1 are determined by the specific cellular expression of these two receptors and of the specialized machinery involved in peculiar biological responses.

MATERIAL AND METHODS

Cells and plasmids CHO-K1 cells were transfected with a cDNA coding for human IR. A clone (CHO-IR) overexpressing IR was selected by binding studies. A CHO-K1 clone transfected with a neomycin resistant plasmid was used as negative control (CHO-neo).

Quantitative determination of c-fos mRNA by PCR mRNA was quantified by reverse transcriptase, followed by radioactive PCR amplification. In the same reaction β actin mRNA was measured and used as an internal control.

^{3}H-thymidine incorporation Confluent cells in 24-well plates were starved for 2 hours, then incubated with different concentrations of insulin or IGF-1, for 4 hours, followed by a pulse with methyl-^{3}H-thymidine (1mC/well). Cells were then fixed by TCA 10%, solubilized and counted for radioactivity.

Insulin binding ^{125}I-insulin and IGF-1 bindings were measured as described (2).

Immunoprecipitation and western blotting After solubilization, immunoprecipitation experiments were performed with antibodies against IR or P-Tyr. The immunoprecipitates were electrophoretically transferred onto a nitrocellulose filter and probed with antibodies against IRS 1, IR or P-Tyr, using standard methodology (4).

RESULTS AND DISCUSSION

CHO-IR express about $2x10^5$ IRs/cell, while CHO-neo express only $1.8x10^3$. The binding competition curves and their Scatchard analyses show that insulin binds to transfected IR with the same affinity as the wild type cells. Competition studies with IGF-1 indicate that transfected IRs have the same kinetic parameters as the wild type cells and more important no hybrid receptors (Insulin and IGF-1) seem to be functionally present.

^{125}IIGF-1 binding was the same in CHO-IR and CHO-neo. IRs in transfected cells are autophosphorylated both *in vivo* and *in vitro* and phosphorylate IRS-1, after hormone binding. Thus CHO-IR and CHO-neo possess the same amount of IGF-1Rs while expressing a different number of functional IRs. Next the effects of insulin and IGF-1 on c-fos expression was investigated. As shown in Figure 1, CHO-IR are more responsive to insulin than the CHO-neo.

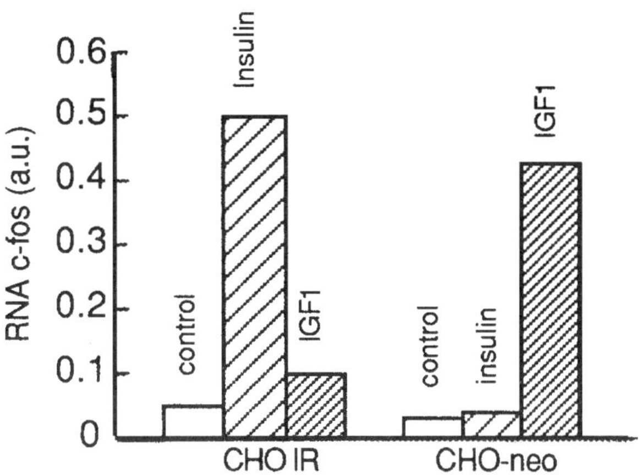

FIG. 1. Effects of insulin (100ng/ml) and IGF1 (100ng/ml) on c-fos expression in CHO-neo and IR.

This finding suggests that the expression of functional IRs is sufficient to make cells responsive to insulin. Interestingly in CHO-IR the IGF-1 effect on c-fos expression is less marked compared to that of insulin. The data is confirmed by thymidine incorporation in CHO-IR and CHO-neo: in the former, the mitogen effect of insulin is higher than in the latter where IGF-1 action is blunted. To investigate the mechanism underlying these findings, we measured the amount of tyrosine phosphorylation of IRS-1 stimulated by insulin and IGF-1. After 2 h of FCS deprivation, cells were incubated for 10' at 37°C in the presence of insulin or IGF-1 (100 ng/ml). Cells were then solubilized and immunoprecipitated by an anti IRS-1 antibody, followed by antiphosphotyrosine immunoblotting. IRS-1 is phosphorylated more by insulin than by IGF-1 in CHO-IR. Opposite results were observed in CHO-neo. These findings suggest that IRS-1 phosphorylation parallels c-fos expression, after insulin and IGF-1 stimulation. We conclude, therefore, that: i) CHO cells can be made insulin sensitive by increasing the expression of IRs; ii) IRS-1 could represent a limiting step in insulin and IGF-1 signal transduction.

REFERENCES

1. Aaronson S.A. (1991): Science 254: 1146-1153.
2. Cordera R. et al. (1990): Endocrinology 126: 2177-2183.
3. Gronborg M. and Gammeltoft S. et al. (1993): J. Biol. Chem. 268: 23435-23440.
4. Harlow E. and Lane D. (1988): Antibodies.Cold Spring Harbour Lab.
5. Herschman H.R. (1991): Annu. Rev. Biochem. 60: 281-319.
6. Rosen O.M. (1987): Science 237: 1452-1458.
7. Sun X.J. and Rothemberg P. et al. (1991): Nature 352: 73-77.
8. Ullrich A. and Gray A., et al. (1986): EMBO L5: 2503-2512.
9. White M. and Kahn C.R. (1994): J. Biol. Chem. 269: 1-4.

Frontiers in Endocrinology
Volume 9 - 1994

A Sensitive and Specific Peptide-Based Radioimmunoassay for the Two Isoforms of the Human Insulin Receptor: Applicability to Insulin-Resistant States

G. Sesti, R. D'Alfonso, M.D. Vargas Punti, P. Borboni, A. Montemurro and R. Lauro

Department of Internal Medicine, University of Rome Tor Vergata, Via Orazio Raimondo 1, 00173 Rome, Italy

INTRODUCTION

The insulin receptor is expressed in two isoforms differing by the absence (HIR-A) or presence (HIR-B) of 12 amino acids at the COOH-terminus of the α-subunit as a consequence of tissue-specific alternative splicing of the 36-basepair exon 11 (2, 11). There is evidence indicating that the two receptor species are functionally and immunologically distinct (4, 5, 9). It was shown that the binding affinity for insulin of the HIR-A form is ~2-fold higher than that of the HIR-B isoform. This difference is parallelled by a different sensitivity for both anabolic and metabolic effects of insulin (4). It has been speculated that modifications in the relative expression of the two isoforms may contribute to *in vivo* insulin resistance, a characteristic feature of obesity and non insulin-dependent diabetes mellitus (NIDDM). Data collected are at present controversial (1, 3, 6, 7). It has been reported by some (6, 7), but not all authors (1), that both diabetic and nondiabetic insulin-resistant subjects are characterized by an increased expression of the HIR-B mRNA in skeletal muscle compared with insulin sensitive controls. However, a few studies have addressed the question of whether the relative abundance of the two isoforms is altered in major target tissues of insulin action from obese and NIDDM subjects when assessed at the protein level (1, 3, 8, 9).

In this study, we developed and applied a new peptide-based insulin receptor radioimmunoassay (RIA) that is able to precisely quantitate total content of the two receptor protein isoforms and their relative distribution in samples of human tissues.

MATERIAL AND METHODS

Two peptides were synthesized as previously described (10). One peptide (Pep-12) corresponds to residues encoded by exon 11, and the other peptide (Pep-13) corresponding to residues 702-719 (numbered according to Ullrich et al.) (11) is derived from a C-terminal sequence of the α-subunit which is common to both HIR-A and HIR-B form. Polyclonal antibodies (PA-12 and PA-13) were raised in rabbits as previously described (10). Peptides were iodinated using the IODOGEN method, and monoiodinated peptides were purified by reverse-phase HPLC.The peptides were also used as standard in the RIA. NIH3T3 fibroblasts transfected with the HIR-B form were kindly provided by Dr. J. Whittaker (Stony Brook, NY, USA). NIH3T3 fibroblasts transfected with the HIR-A isoform were prepared as previously described (8). Human placentae were obtained from normal subjects after full term vaginal deliveries. Tissue samples of liver were obtained from nondiabetic subjects undergoing surgery for gallstone disease. Samples of subcutaneous adipose tissue were obtained from 6 nonobese controls, 6 obese nondiabetic, and 5 NIDDM patients during elective abdominal surgery. Consent was obtained from all subjects after the nature of the procedure was explained. Extracts from tissues were prepared by solubilization in 50 mM Hepes buffer, pH 7.6, containing 150 mM NaCl, 1% Triton X-100, 1 mg/ml bacitracin, 2 mM PMSF, 1000 units/ml aprotinin for 60 min at 4°C. Insoluble material was removed by centrifugation at 100.000 *g* for 60 min at 4°C. Placenta membranes or confluent NIH3T3 fibroblasts transfected the HIR-B form were solubilized and insulin receptors were purified to homogeneity by using sequential monoclonal antibody-agarose and wheat germ agglutinin-agarose affinity chromatography. Receptor number was determined by Scatchard analysis of insulin binding.

Multiple dilutions of sample, highly purified insulin receptors or unlabeled peptides (Pep-12 or Pep-13) were incubated in assay buffer containing 50 mM Hepes, 150 mM NaCl, 0.1% Triton X-100, 1 mM PMSF, 0.1% BSA, pH 7.6, for 16 h at 4°C with either PA-12 or PA-13. ^{125}I-Pep-12 or ^{125}I-Pep-13 at tracer concentration were added, and samples were incubated for an additional 24 h at 4°C. Goat anti-rabbit immunoglobulins were then added. After 16 h at 4°C, mixtures were centrifuged at 3000 *g* for 30 min at 4°C, pellets were washed once with assay buffer and bound radioactivity was counted.

RESULTS AND DISCUSSION

The binding of labeled peptides to the corresponding antibodies was completely inhibited at 10^{-10} mole/0.3 ml. For both peptides, a detectable inhibition of binding was seen at 10^{-14} mole/0.3 ml, whereas half-maximal displacement was observed at 2 x 10^{-13} mole/0.3 ml. The displacement curve produced by highly purified receptors from placenta which is known to contain both the HIR-A and the HIR-B form was parallel to the standard curve produced by Pep-13. Similarly, highly purified receptors from NIH3T3 fibroblasts expressing the HIR-B form produced competition curve that was parallel to the standard curve produced by Pep-12. A good correlation was observed between the moles of purified receptor calculated by Scatchard analysis of insulin binding and the molar equivalents to Pep-12 or Pep-13 measured in the RIA, thus indicating that insulin receptor and peptide ligand are seen as equimolar in the RIA. The specificity of both Pep-12- and Pep-13-based RIA was investigated by using NIH3T3 cells transfected with either the HIR-A or the HIR-B isoform. Cell lysates from either source competed with ^{125}I-Pep-13 for the corresponding antiserum, and competition-inhibition curves were parallel to the peptide standard. In contrast, only cellular extract from NIH3T3 transfectants expressing the HIR-B isoform was able to compete with ^{125}I-Pep-12 for the corresponding antiserum and its competition-inhibition curve was parallel to the peptide standard.

We measured both the absolute content and the relative abundance of the two isoforms in various human tissues. Displacement curves produced by multiple dilutions of tissue extracts were parallel to standard curves produced by both Pep-12 and Pep-13. Total HIR and HIR-B isoform amounts in tissue extracts expressed as pmole receptor/ 1 mg protein are shown in Table 1. The relative abundance of the two isoforms was expressed as the percentage of the HIR-B form content measured by Pep-12-based RIA vs total receptor content measured by Pep-13-based RIA.

Table 1. *Total content and relative abundance of the two isoforms in human tissues*

Tissue	Total HIR pmole/mg protein	HIR-B pmole/mg protein	HIR-B/Total HIR (%)
Placenta	3.9±1	2.0±0.6	51
Liver	3.5±1.2	3.1±1.2	88
Muscle	2.2±0.5	1.1±0.4	50
Fat	2.7±0.9	1.4±0.5	52

We employed RIA to quantitate the relative abundance of the two isoforms in samples of adipose tissue from nonobese controls, obese nondiabetic, and NIDDM subjects. The mean percentage of the HIR-B isoform content vs. total receptor content was significantly higher in adipose tissue from 6 obese nondiabetic (74±10%, p<0.01) and 5 NIDDM subjects (69±11%, p<0.03) than in 6 nonobese normal subjects (51±7%).

In conclusion, this study demonstrates the feasibility of using the present dual peptide-based radioimmunoassay to precisely quantitate the two insulin receptor isoforms in human tissues and its applicability to study changes of the relative abundance of the two receptor species in different metabolic states.

REFERENCES

1. Benecke H., Flier J.S. and Moller D.E. (1992): J. Clin. Invest. 89: 2066-2070.
2. Ebina Y., Ellis L., Jarnagin K., Edery M., Graf L., Clauser E., Ou J.H., Masiarz F., Kan Y.W., Goldfine I.D., Roth R.A and Rutter W.J. (1985): Cell 40: 747-758.
3. Kellerer M., Sesti G., Seffer E., Obermaier-Kusser B., Pongratz D.E., Mosthaf L. and Haring H.U. (1993): Diabetologia 36: 628-632.
4. McClain D.A. (1991): Mol. Endocrinol. 5: 734-739.
5. Mosthaf L., Grako D., Dull T.J., Coussens L., Ullrich A. and McClain D.A. (1990): EMBO J. 9: 2409-2413.
6. Mosthaf L., Vogt B., Haring H.U. and Ullrich A. (1991): Proc. Natl. Acad. Sci. USA 88: 4728-4730.
7. Mosthaf L., Eriksson J., Haring H.U., Groop L., Widen E. and Ullrich A. (1993): Proc. Natl. Acad. Sci. USA 90: 2633-2635.
8. Sesti G., Marini M.A., Tullio A.N., Montemurro A., Borboni P., Fusco A., Accili D. and Lauro R. (1991): Biochem. Biophys. Res. Comm. 181: 1419-1424.
9. Sesti G., Marini M.A., Montemurro A., Condorelli L., Borboni P., Haring H.U., Ullrich A., Goldfine I.D., De Pirro R. and Lauro R. (1992): Diabetes 41: 6-11.
10. Sesti G., Tullio A.N., Marini M.A., Manera E., Borboni P., Accili D., Longhi R., Fusco A., Lauro R. and Montemurro A. Mol. Cell Endocrinol. (in press).
11. Ullrich A., Bell J.R., Chen E.Y., Herrera R., Petruzzelli L.M., Dull T.J., Gray A., Coussens L., Liao Y.C., Tsubokawa M., Moson A., Seeburg P.H., Grunfeld C., Rosen O.M. and Ramachandran J. (1985): Nature (Lond.) 313: 756-761.

Frontiers in Endocrinology
Volume 9 - 1994

Phosphorylation and Signalling of the Insulin Receptor are controlled by a Basic Aminoacid Motif

C. Miele, P. Formisano, M. Pianese, M. Caruso, G. Bifulco, F. Tripodi, G. De Novellis, A. Oliva, F. Oriente, G. Palumbo and F. Beguinot

CNR Center of Experimental Endocrinology and Oncology; Department of Cellular and Molecular Biology and Pathology, University of Naples Medical School, Via Pansini 5, 80131 Naples, Italy

INTRODUCTION

The naturally occurring Arg_{1152}-Gln mutation alters a basic amino acid motif (RK motif) immediately next to the key tyrosine phosphorylation sites of the insulin receptor (IR) and constitutively activates its kinase and metabolic signalling (3, 4, 8). These functional alterations may be directly produced through mutation-induced structural receptor changes, may depend on abnormal interaction of the mutant receptor with receptor-regulatory proteins such as serine/threonine kinases, or depend on both factors.

RESULTS AND DISCUSSION

The possibility that the abnormal signalling properties of the mutant receptor (IR_{1152}) may depend on mutation-caused altered interactions with intracellular proteins was first investigated. Since substrate phosphorylation by most serine/threonine kinases require 1-3 basic aminoacid residues near the phosphoacceptor group (6), we hypothesized that the Arg_{1152}-Gln substitution impaired insulin receptor interaction with protein kinase A and C (PKA and PKC) (*in vitro* and *in vivo* receptor phosphorylation by these kinases has already been reported to turn the insulin receptor kinase off (2, 5, 9)).

To address this issue, NIH-3T3 cells overexpressing wild type and mutant insulin receptors were metabolically labelled with ^{32}P-orthophosphate and incubated with either tetradecanoylphorbol-13 acetate (TPA) or 8-bromo-cyclicAMP (8-Br-cAMP) (these agents activate PKC and PKA in cells). Receptor phosphorylation was then quantified upon immunoprecipitation and polyacrylamide gel electrophoresis (PAGE).

As shown in Figure 1, both PKC and PKA increased phosphorylation of the wild-type receptors by ≥ 2-fold. In contrast, almost no effect was observed with the mutated receptors. Treatment of the gel with 2N NaOH for 40 min at 50 C determined almost complete disappearance of radioactivity bound to the wild-type receptors (not shown in the figure), indicating ^{32}P association with serine/threonine rather than tyrosine residues in the receptor. Consistent with these findings, purified preparations of both PKC and PKA phosphorylated *in vitro* the wild-type but not the mutant insulin receptor. The addition of a synthetic peptide of the insulin receptor including 8 and 7 residues up- and downstream the intact RK motif, inhibited *in vitro* phosphorylation of the wild-type receptor by both PKC and PKA. Thus, the Arg-Gln substitution impaired insulin receptor interaction and subsequent phosphorylation by both PKC and PKA.

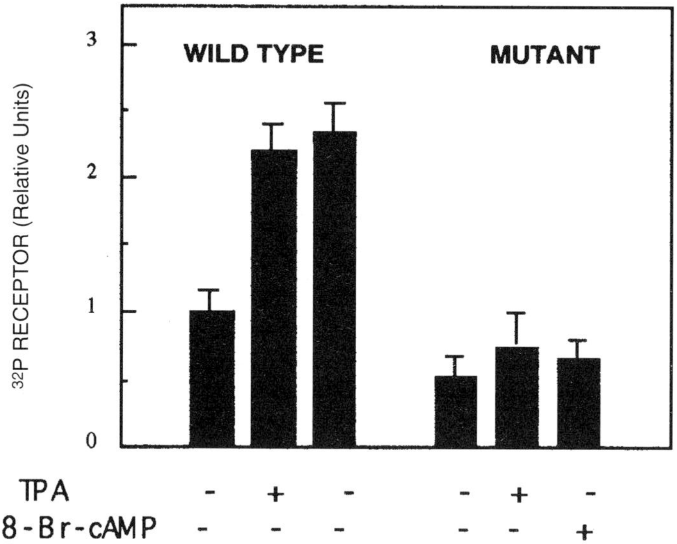

FIG.1. Phosphorylation of wild type and Arg_{1152}-Gln I_R by PKA and PKC in intact cells. Confluent NIH-3T3 cells overexpressing either the wild-type or the mutant insulin receptor were equilibrium labelled with ^{32}P-orthophosphate and then further treated with 0.2 mM TPA or 10 mM 8-Br-cAMP for 30 min. Cells were solubilized, insulin receptors were precipitated with receptor antibodies and analyzed by PAGE and autoradiography. Receptor phosphorylation was quantified by densitometry. Error bars represent S.D. of the means from at least three separate experiments.

Next, we have analyzed the structure of a 90 amino acid peptide of the insulin receptor including 50 and 40 residues up- and downstream the RK motif, respectively. The algorithms of Chou and Fasman and Kyte and Doolittle (1, 7) were used for secondary structure prediction of the peptide. By these methods, the region surrounding position 1152 in the receptor, i.e., the mutated region, exhibited a high probability of α-helix arrangement. Structural analysis by computer protein modelling of this sequence stretch revealed a possible further stabilization due to a strong electrostatic interaction between the positively charged Arg_{1152} and the negatively charged Asp_{1147} (the interaction is possible, however, even in the case of a less probable β-strand arrangement of the region including the mutation site).

This stabilization is absent in the mutant since the Arg_{1152} has been substituted by glutamine (Fig. 2.). Indeed, glutamine is a neutral amino acid with a large uncharged side chain. Due to possible unfavorable steric interactions with Asp_{1147}, glutamine may consequently act as a local structure destabilizer. Thus, the Arg_{1152}-Gln substitution has the potential to alter insulin receptor structure in a region which is relevant for controlling receptor interaction with PKC and A.

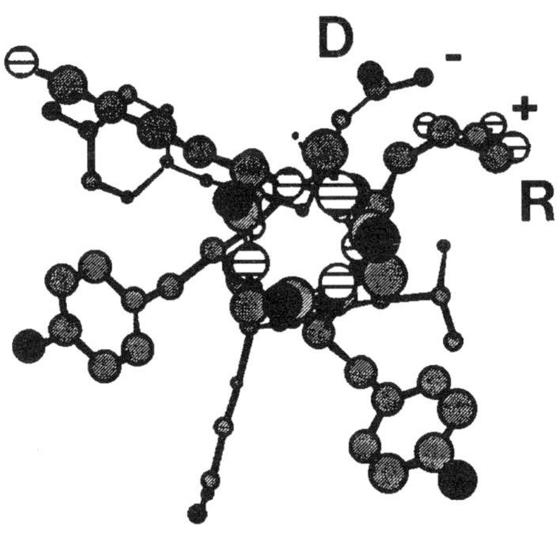

FIG. 2. a-helix arrangement of the sequence ...YETDYYRKGG... (end view). This helix is further stabilized by electrostatic interaction between the positively charged guanidinium group of arginine (R) and the negatively charged carboxylate group of Asp (D). Such stabilizing effect is absent in the mutated sequence.

We conclude that the Arg_{1152} residue in the RK motif is relevant in constraining insulin receptor kinase and metabolic signalling. At least in part, this regulatory role is exerted by allowing proper receptor interaction with protein kinase A and C. This, in turn, may result from the Arg_{1152} stabilizing effect on receptor secondary structure.

ACKNOWLEDGEMENTS

C. Miele - Recipient of a fellowship from the Associazione Italiana per la Ricerca sul Cancro.

REFERENCES

1. Argos P., Haney M. and Garavito R.M. (1978): FEBS Lett. 93: 19-28.
2. Bollag G.E., Roth R., Beaudion J., Mohely-Rosen D. and Koshland D.E. (1986): Proc. Natl. Acad. Sci. USA 83: 5822-5824.
3. Cocozza S., Porcellini A., Riccardi G., Monticelli A., Condorelli G.L., Ferrara A.M., Pianese L., Miele C., Capaldo B., Beguinot F. and Varrone S. (1991): Diabetes 41: 521-526.
4. Fomisano P., Sohn K.-J., Miele C., DiFinizio B., Petruzziello A., Riccardi G., Beguinot L. and Beguinot F. (1993): J. Biol. Chem. 268: 5241-5248.
5. Karasik A., Rotenberg P.L., Yamada K., White M.F. and Kahn C.R. (1990): J. Biol. Chem. 265: 10226-10231.
6. Kennelly P.J. and Krebs E.G. (1991): J. Biol. Chem. 266: 15555-15558.
7. Kyte J. and Doolittle R.F. (1982): J. Mol. Biol. 157: 105-113.
8. Petruzziello A., Formisano P., Miele C., Di Finizio B., Riccardi G., Ferrara A.M., Beguinot L. and Beguinot F. (1993): J. Clin. Endocrinol. Metab. 77: 409-412.
9. Stadtmauer L. and Rosen O. (1986): J. Biol. Chem. 261: 3402-3407.

Frontiers in Endocrinology
Volume 9 - 1994

Insulin-like Growth Factor-I (IGF-I) Action and Signal Transduction Pathways in Skeletal Muscle Cells

F. Giorgino* and R.J. Smith

Research Division, Joslin Diabetes Center, and Department of Medicine, Brigham and Women's Hospital, Harvard Medical School, Boston, Massachusetts 02215, USA

INTRODUCTION

Insulin-like growth factor (IGF)-I is a potent stimulator of cell growth and differentiation in several cell types (10). In human fibroblasts, glucocorticoids have been shown to enhance IGF-I stimulation of cell growth, without affecting the basal rates of cell proliferation (6, 7). The mechanism by which glucocorticoids enhance the action of IGF-I has not been clarified.

IGF-I actions are mediated by specific cell-surface receptors consisting of two α- and two β-subunits (20). IGF-I binding to the receptor results in activation of the receptor tyrosine kinase, and subsequent phosphorylation of both the receptor and intracellular substrate proteins (4, 12). Two distinct proteins have recently been characterized as direct substrates of the IGF-I receptor kinase, i.e., the insulin receptor substrate-1 (IRS-1) (19, 15), and the Shc proteins, which include three widely expressed SH2 domain-containing species of 46, 52, and 66 kD (16, 17). Tyrosine phosphorylation of IRS-1 results in the specific association of this protein with the SH2 domains of the 85 kD subunit of the phosphatidylinositol (PI) 3-kinase, leading to activation of the enzyme and production of 3'-phosphorylated products (1, 15, 19). It has been suggested that both the IRS-1/PI 3-kinase and the Shc pathways may mediate mitogenic responses to insulin and IGF-I (16, 21).

The objectives of this study were: to investigate the effects of the glucocorticoid dexamethasone on mitogenic responses to IGF-I and

*Present Address: Istituto di Clinica Medica, Endocrinologia e Malattie Metaboliche, University of Bari Medical School, 70124 Bari, Italy

determine in cultured muscle cell; the mechanism of the glucocorticoid-induced augmentation of IGF-I action. For this purpose, we used L6 rat skeletal muscle cells because these cells express a relatively high number of IGF-I receptors (2) and are markedly responsive to the growth-stimulating effects of IGF-I (2, 8, 9).

MATERIAL AND METHODS

L6 rat skeletal muscle cells were grown in MEM supplemented with 10% donor calf bovine serum (DCBS). When the cells were about 60% confluent, the medium was replaced with serum-free MEM containing 0.5% BSA, and cells were incubated in the presence or absence of 1 μM dexamethasone for 72 h. All experiments were carried out with undifferentiated myoblasts. IGF-I-stimulated DNA synthesis was measured by determining the rates of [^{3}H] thymidine incorporation into DNA, as previously described (2).

To study IGF-I signaling, quiescent cells were stimulated with 100 nM IGF-I for 10 min, and lysed in Tris buffer containing 1% Nonidet P-40, and various protease and phosphatase inhibitors. The cell lysate was then adjusted to a protein concentration of 2 mg/ml and used for immunoprecipitation. To determine tyrosine phosphorylation of the IGF-I receptors, IRS-1, and Shc, cell lysates were immunoprecipitated with antibodies specific to these proteins. The resulting immunoprecipitates were resolved by reducing SDS-PAGE, blotted with phosphotyrosine antibodies and ^{125}I-protein A, and subjected to autoradiography (11). Autoradiographic images were quantified by optical densitometry and data expressed using arbitrary units after normalizing to control values within each gel. PI 3-kinase activity was determined in IRS-1 immunoprecipitates by using an *in vitro* assay with ^{32}P-ATP and PI (19). All data are presented as mean±SE. Statistical analyses were performed by paired Student t test.

RESULTS AND DISCUSSION

Dexamethasone effects on cell proliferation Table 1 shows the effects of IGF-I on DNA synthesis in undifferentiated L6 skeletal muscle cells, as determined by measuring the rates of [^{3}H] thymidine incorporation into DNA. In control cells, IGF-I induced a small but significant dose-dependent increase in DNA synthesis. In contrast, in cells treated with 1 μM dexamethasone for 72 h, IGF-I stimulation of DNA synthesis was markedly enhanced (by approx. 4-fold). Dexamethasone did not affect basal rates of DNA synthesis. Dexamethasone treatment also increased IGF-I stimulation of L6 cell proliferation (data not shown).

Table 1. *^{3}[H] Thymidine incorporation into DNA (% of control basal)*

	Control	Dexamethasone
Basal	100	102±3
IGF-I	150±14*	280±15*#
LongR^{3}IGF-I	147±15*	285±10*#

Mean±SE. *p<0.05 vs Basal; #p<0.05 vs Control.

In addition, dexamethasone markedly augmented the stimulation of DNA synthesis by longR^{3}IGF-I, an IGF-I analog that has a very low affinity for IGF binding proteins (5), indicating that the increase in IGF-I responsiveness induced by dexamethasone cannot be explained by changes in the levels of IGF binding proteins.

Dexamethasone effects on tyrosine phosphorylation and content of IGF-I receptors and IRS-1 To investigate the influence of dexamethasone on tyrosine phosphorylation of IGF-I receptors and IRS-1, L6 cells were stimulated with a maximally active dose of IGF-I (100 nM) for 10 min, and the levels of tyrosine phosphorylation of IGF-I receptors and IRS-1 were determined as described in the Methods. Table 2 shows the quantitation of multiple experiments. The total amount of IGF-I-stimulated IGF-I receptor tyrosine phosphorylation was increased modestly but significantly in dexamethasone-treated cells. Dexamethasone also increased IGF-I receptor content in L6 cells by approx. 60%. On the other hand, the total amount of IRS-1 tyrosine phosphorylation was decreased by approx. 30% in dexamethasone-treated cells compared with control cells. Incubation of L6 cells with dexamethasone also resulted in a marked decrease in IRS-1 protein content (40% of control). Thus, the effects of dexamethasone on IRS-1 expression and tyrosine phosphorylation differed from the effects on expression and phosphorylation of IGF-I receptors.

Table 2. *Tyrosine phosphorylation and content of IGF-I receptors and IRS-1*

	Control	Dexamethasone
Tyrosine phosphorylation		
IGF-I Receptors	100	140±9*
IRS-1	100	75±4*
Protein content		
IGF-I Receptors	100	175±8*
IRS-1	100	41±3*

Data are expressed as % of Control. *p<0.05 vs Control.

Dexamethasone effects on IRS-1-associated PI 3-kinase activity IGF-I stimulation of intact cells results in the activation of PI 3-kinase (15). In L6 cells, a low level of PI 3-kinase activity was present in anti-IRS-1 immunoprecipitates in the basal state. After IGF-I stimulation, there was a rapid and marked 42-fold increase in the amount of PI 3-kinase activity associated with IRS-1 (Table 3). In cells treated with 1 μM dexamethasone for 72 h, there was no difference in the basal level of PI 3-kinase activity. However, IGF-1 stimulated IRS-1-associated PI 3-kinase activity by only 23-fold, so that the levels of IGF-I-stimulated PI 3-kinase activity associated with IRS-1 were reduced by 45% in cells treated with dexamethasone compared with control.

Table 3. *IRS-1-associated PI 3-kinase activity (% of basal)*

	Control	Dexamethasone
Basal	100	106±9
IGF-I	4250±630*	2310±340*#

Mean±SE. *p<0.05 vs Basal; #p<0.05 vs Control.

These results correlate with the decrease in tyrosine phosphorylation and expression of the IRS-1 protein and suggest that the IRS-1/PI 3-kinase signaling pathway is not involved in the mechanism of augmentation of IGF-I action by dexamethasone. In a recent study, Waters et al. found that inhibition of IRS-1 expression in CHO cells by an antisense IRS-1 RNA results in 40% decrease in insulin-stimulated IRS-1 tyrosine phosphorylation, coordinate decrease in IRS-1-associated PI 3-kinase activity, and marked inhibition of insulin-stimulated DNA synthesis and transcriptional activation of the c-Fos promoter (21). Although IRS-1 may play an essential role in the control of insulin and/or IGF-I-stimulated cell proliferation in certain cell types and conditions, this mechanism does not appear to be as important in L6 cells.

Dexamethasone effects on Shc tyrosine phosphorylation To investigate an alternative intracellular pathway distinct from IRS-1 and of potential relevance for the glucocorticoid response, we investigated tyrosine phosphorylation of the Shc proteins in response to IGF-I. The Shc proteins in the total lysate from L6 cells were immunoprecipitated with polyclonal Shc antibodies, and the levels of Shc tyrosine phosphorylation was determined by immunoblotting with phosphotyrosine antibodies. Stimulation of L6 cells with 100 nM IGF-I induced tyrosine phosphorylation of three proteins of 46, 52, and 66 kD, respectively, identified as the Shc proteins $p46^{shc}$, $p52^{shc}$, and $p66^{shc}$ (data not shown). The levels of Shc tyrosine phosphorylation following stimulation with IGF-I peaked after 5 min and then slowly returned to basal after 60 min. When cells were treated with dexamethasone for 72 h, the level of IGF-I-stimulated tyrosine phosphorylation of all three Shc proteins was approx. 2-fold higher than in control cells (data not shown). In addition, Shc tyrosine phosphorylation persisted at these high levels for as long as 180 min following stimulation with IGF-I. These results indicate that the increase in IGF-I-stimulated mitogenesis induced by dexamethasone is associated with higher and more sustained levels of Shc tyrosine phosphorylation.

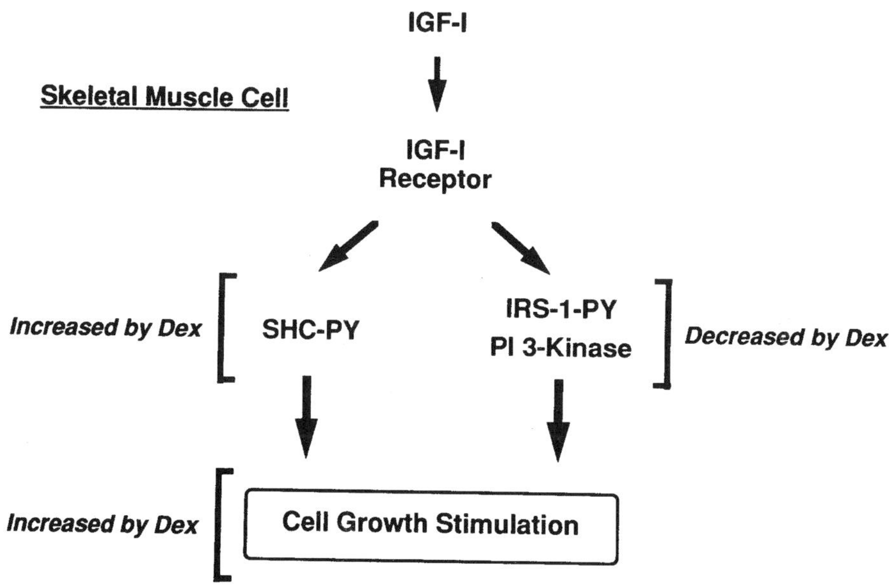

FIG. 1. Dexamethasone regulation of IGF-I action and signaling pathways in skeletal muscle cells.

The increased activity of the Shc signaling pathway in dexamethasone-treated cells is particularly important considering the mitogenic and/or transforming capabilities of these proteins. Indeed, overexpression of Shc in

NIH 3T3 mouse fibroblasts induces malignant transformation (16), and "constitutive" tyrosine phosphorylation of the Shc proteins is found in cells transformed by the oncogenic tyrosine kinases v-src, v-fps, and erbB-2 (14, 18). The increase in the maximal amount of Shc tyrosine phosphorylation and the prolongation of Shc phosphorylation after IGF-I stimulation observed in dexamethasone-treated cells suggest that the Shc signaling pathway could potentially explain the augmentation of IGF-I action by dexamethasone.

In conclusion, dexamethasone differentially regulates two distinct pathways involved in intracellular IGF-I signaling, i.e., the IRS-1/PI 3-kinase pathway and the Shc pathway. IRS-1 tyrosine phosphorylation and activation of PI 3-kinase are decreased whereas tyrosine phosphorylation of Shc is increased by dexamethasone. Since the increase in tyrosine phosphorylation of the Shc proteins correlates with the augmentation of IGF-I-stimulated mitogenesis in L6 cells, the results of this study suggest that augmentation of IGF-I-mediated mitogenesis by dexamethasone may occur via increased activity of the Shc signaling pathway (Fig. 1).

ACKNOWLEDGEMENTS

This work was supported in part by grants from the Juvenile Diabetes Foundation, and the National Institute of Health (Grant DK43038, Trauma Center Grant GM36428, and DERC Grant DK36836). F. Giorgino was supported by postdoctoral fellowships from the Juvenile Diabetes Foundation International and the Mary K. Iacocca Foundation. The Author sacknowledge Velta Ramolins and Karen Pickardt for their excellent technical support.

REFERENCES

1. Backer J.M., Myers Jr. M.G., Shoelson S.E. and Chin D.J. et al. (1992): EMBO J. 11: 3469-79.
2. Beguinot F., Kahn C.R., Moses A.C. and Smith R. J. (1985): J. Biol. Chem. 260: 15892-98.
3. Beguinot F., Kahn C.R., Moses A.C. and Smith R.J. (1986): Endocrinology 118: 446-55.
4. Beguinot F., Kahn C.R., Moses A.C., White M.F. and Smith R.J. (1989): Endocrinology 125: 1599-1605.
5. Clemmons D.R., Cascieri M.A., Camacho-Hubner C., McCusker R.H. and Bayne M.L. (1990): J. Biol. Chem. 265: 12210-16.
6. Conover C.A., Dollar L.A., Hintz R.L. and Rosenfeld R.G., (1983): J. Cell Physiol. 116: 191-197.
7. Conover C.A., Rosenfeld R.G. and Hintz R.L. (1989): In Vitro Cell Dev. Biol. 25: 521-27.
8. Ewton D.Z., Falen S.L. and Florini J.R. (1987): Endocrinology 120: 115-24.
9. Florini J.R., (1987): Muscle Nerve 7: 577-98.
10. Froesch E.R., Schmid C., Schwander J. and Zapf J. (1985): Annu. Rev. Physiol. 47: 443-67.
11. Giorgino F., Almahfouz A., Goodyear L.J. and Smith R.J. (1993): J. Clin. Invest. 91: 2020-30.
12. Jacobs S., Kull Jr., F.C., Earp H.S., Svoboda M.E., Van Wyk J.J. and Cuatrecasas P. (1983): J. Biol. Chem. 258: 9581-84.
13. Jin P., Sejersen T. and Ringertz N. R. (1991): J. Biol. Chem. 266: 1245-49.

14. McGlade J., Cheng A., Pelicci G., Pelicci P.G. and Pawson T. (1992): Proc. Natl. Acad. Sci. USA 89: 8869-73.
15. Myers Jr., M.G., Sun X.-J., Cheatham B. and Jachna B. et al. (1993): Endocrinology 132: 1421-30.
16. Pelicci G., Lanfrancone L., Grignani F. and McGlade J. et al.(1992): Cell 70: 93-104.
17. Pronk G.J., McGlade J., Pelicci G., Pawson T. and Bos J.L. (1993): J. Biol. Chem. 268: 5748-53.
18. Segatto O., Pelicci G., Giuli S. and Digiesi G. et al. (1993): Oncogene 8: 2105-12.
19. Sun X.-J., Rothenberg P., Kahn C.R. and Backer J.M. et al. (1991): Nature 352: 73-77.
20. Ullrich A., Gray A., Tam A.W. and Yang-Feng T. et al. (1986): EMBO J. 5: 2503-12.
21. Waters S.B., Yamaguchi K. and Pessin J.E. (1993): J. Biol. Chem. 268: 22231-34.

Frontiers in Endocrinology
Volume 9 - 1994

Functional Importance of Insulin-like Growth Factor I Receptor COOH-Terminal Region Tyrosine Phosphorylation Sites

G. Condorelli, C.G. Tocchetti, F. Andreozzi, A. Caiola, E. Crescenzi, F. Beguinot and [1]R.J. Smith

Department of Cellular and Molecular Biology and Pathology. CNR Center of Experimental Endocrinology and Oncology. Federico II University of Naples Medical School, via Pansini, 5, 80131 Naples, Italy;
[1]Joslin Diabetes Center, Harvard Medical School, Boston, 20115 MA, USA

INTRODUCTION

Insulin and IGF I receptors (I_R and IGF I_R) share close similarities in structure and function (7). Both receptors have a tyrosine kinase activity located in the receptor ß-subunit that is activated upon hormone binding to the α-subunit. This tyrosine kinase activity is believed to be important for insulin and IGF I signaling (1). Insulin and IGF I both stimulate the phosphorylation of the cellular substrate, insulin-receptor substrate-1 (IRS-1) (2, 6). Once phosphorylated, IRS-1 associates with other intracellular signaling molecules and thus activates post-receptor pathways (8). Although insulin and IGF I promote a similar hormone action, insulin is believed to preferentially transmit metabolic signals, while IGF I transmits mostly mitogenic effects. The role of the receptors in establishing functional specificity of the hormones is not yet known. The C-terminal domains of the IGF I_R and I_R differ in primary structure (only 43% identity) suggesting that this region could have a role in determining hormone specificity. The biological functions of the C-terminal domain of the I_R has been extensively investigated while less is known about the homologous region of the IGF I_R. Mutagenesis studies have shown that substitution of C-terminal phosphorylation sites in the I_R (Y1316 and Y1322) with phenylalanine increases mitogenic activity without affecting autophosphorylation, kinase activity or endocytosis (5). Homologous sites in the IGF I_R are occupied by phenylalanine (F1310) and tyrosine (Y1316) (Fig.1).

IR	W.T.	1316 1322 Y...........Y
IR	Y2	1316 1322 F...........F

IGFI R	W.T.	1310 1316 F...........Y
IGFI R	Y1310	1310 1316 Y...........Y
IGFI R	F1316	1310 1316 F...........F

FIG. 1. Insulin and IGF I receptor COOH-terminal phosphorylation sites in WT and mutant receptors.

RESULTS AND CONCLUSIONS

We generated two human IGF I_R mutants by site-directed mutagenesis. In the first, phenylalanine 1310 was substituted with tyrosine (IGF I_R Y1310); in the second mutant, tyrosine 1316 was replaced with phenylalanine (IGF I_R F1316) (Fig.1). Mutant and wild type (IGF I_R WT) cDNAs were transfected into CHO cells, and multiple clones expressing 0.5-0.8 x 10^6 receptors/cell were selected. The receptors exhibited similar IGF I binding affinity (Kd= 2x 10^{-9} M). In intact cells, IGF I stimulated receptor phosphorylation and IRS-1 phosphorylation was significantly reduced in IGF I_R F1316 compared to IGF I_R WT (54 ± 6% and 67 ± 11%, respectively) (Fig. 2 A, B). In IGF I_R Y1310, IGF I-stimulated receptor phosphorylation was increased 2-fold when compared to IGF I_R WT, and IRS-1 phosphorylation was unchanged (Fig. 2 A, B). Thus, mutagenesis of IGF I_R C-terminal phosphorylation sites alters autophosphorylation and kinase activity. To further investigate biological differences of the C-terminal mutants, we analyzed IGF I_R internalization. Cells were incubated for 0-10 min with ^{125}I-IGF I at 37°C, rapidly cooled to 4°C, and washed in neutral (pH 7.5) or acidic (pH 2.75) PBS to determine total cell associated or internalized radioactivity, respectively. The IGF I_R internalization rate in the two mutants was markedly reduced compared to the IGF I_R WT (k_e= 0.075 in IGF I_R WT,

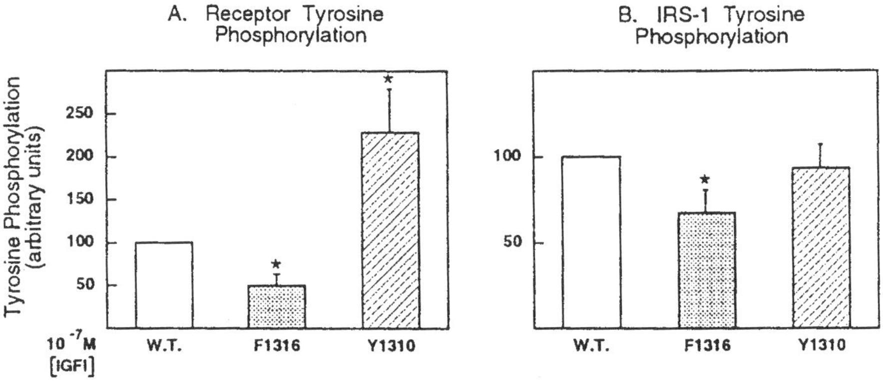

FIG. 2. IGF I stimulation of tyrosine phosphorylation in intact transfected CHO cells. Autoradiographs derived from immunoblots with anti-phosphotyrosine antibody and ^{125}I-protein. A were analyzed by densitometry. Data represent mean ± SE from multiple experiments normalized to percent of the mean value in WT transfected cells stimulated with 10^{-7} M IGFI.

0.033 in IGF I_R F1316, and 0.036 in IGF I_R Y1310) (Fig. 3). Thus, in constrast to the I_R, the C-terminal region of IGF I_R contains information regulating receptor internalization. Both C-terminal modified IGF I receptors have a decreased internalization rate, although different

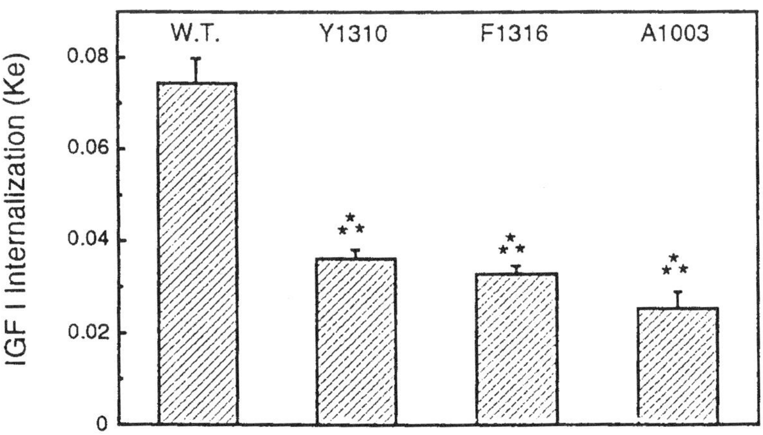

FIG. 3. ^{125}I-IGF I internalization in CHO cells. Cells were incubated for 0-10 min at 37° C with ^{125}I-IGF I. Internalized radioactivity was determined by washing at pH 2.75 and total cell associated radioactivity by washing at pH 7.5. Data represent the mean±SE of multiple experiments conducted on different clones for each receptor type.

changes in kinase activity. We conclude that autophosphorylation is not the only determinant of receptor endocytosis. Cytoplasmic terminal domains of other receptors are believed to contain crucial residues for efficient receptor endocytosis (3) and may represent recognition signals for components of the endocytotic compartment such as adaptins (4). We suggest that, differences in IGF I_R Y1310, F1316 and WT endocytosis could be explained by their different interactions with components of the endocytotic compartment.

REFERENCES

1. Kato H., Faria T.N., Stannard B., Roberts C.T. and LeRoith D. (1993): J. Biol.Chem. 268: 2655-2661.
2. Myers M.G., Sun X.J., Cheatham B., Jachina B.R., Glasheen E., Backer J.M. and White M.F. (1993): Endocrinology 132: 1421-1430.
3. Pearce B.M.F. and Robinson M.S. (1990): Annu. Rev. Cell Biol. 6: 151-71.
4. Sorkin A. and Carpenter G. (1993): Science 261: 612-15.
5. Sun X.J., Rotemberg P., Kahn C.R., Baker J.M., Araki E., Wilden P.A., Cahill D.A., Goldstein B.J. and White M.F. (1991): Nature 352: 73-77
6. Takata Y.,Webster N.J.G. and Olefsky J.M. (1991): J. Biol. Chem. 266: 9135-9139.
7. Ullrich A., Gray A., Tam A.W., Yang-Feng T., Tsubokawa M., Collins C., Henzel W., Le Bon T., Kathuria S., Chen E., Jacobs S., Francke U., Ramachandran J. and Fujita-Yamaguchi Y. (1986): EMBO J. 5: 2503-2512
8. White M.F. and Kahn R.C. (1994): J. Biol. Chem. 269: 1-4

Frontiers in Endocrinology
Volume 9 - 1994

Glucose Sensing and Islet Architecture in Isolated Porcine Pancreatic Islets

A.M. Rabuazzo, F. Purrello, A.M. Davalli[1], M. Buscema, C. Socci[1], M. Anello, F. Bertuzzi[1], G. Pozza[1] and R. Vigneri

Institute of Internal Medicine, Metabolism and Endocrinology, University of Catania Medical School, Piazza S. Maria di Gesù, 95123 Catania;
[1]San Raffaele Institute, Milan, Italy

INTRODUCTION

Porcine islets have been proposed as a future donor source for human transplantation, mainly because structure and biological activity of porcine insulin is similar to human insulin. However, their secretory function *in vitro* in response to glucose has been reported as low or absent (3, 1) if compared to rat or mouse islets. The reason(s) for their hampered response to glucose are unknown.

In the present study, therefore, we investigated, in isolated porcine pancreatic islets, the possible mechanisms responsible for impaired insulin release.

MATERIAL AND METHODS

Pig islet isolation and culture Islets were isolated from female pigs weighing 250-300 Kg. After purification, an average of 3380 ± 679 islets per gram of pancreas was obtained.

Metabolic studies In isolated porcine pancreatic islets we studied: a) glucose transport (measured by 3-O-[$^{+3}$H]-methylglucose uptake), b) glucose phosphorylation (determined by fluorimetric method) and c) glucose utilization (measured by formation of ^3H_2O from (5-^{3}H)-glucose) (5).

Morphologic studies The ultrastructure of B cells was evaluated by electron microscopy in sections of islet material fixed with 1% osmium tetroxide and embedded in epoxy resin. Immuno-histochemistry for insulin, glucagon, pancreatic-polypeptide and somatostatin were performed in a portion of pig pancreas or in the sample of the islet preparations fixed in Bouin's solution.

RESULTS

METABOLIC STUDIES

a) glucose transport Glucose transport in porcine pancreatic cells increased with increasing glucose concentrations up to 20 mmol/l. In agreement with previous studies in rat pancreatic islets (2, 5), the kinetic characteristics of glucose uptake in porcine pancreatic cells, calculated according to the Eadie-Hofstee plot, indicated the presence of two kinetically distinct components. The low affinity component had an apparent Michaelis constant (K_m) of 11.8±1.9 mmol/l and a Vmax (maximal capacity) of 0.48±0.08 nmol/μg DNA/15 sec. (n=5) (Table 1); the high affinity component had an apparent K_m of 1.2±0.6 mmol/l and a Vmax of 15-20 % of the total capacity.

b) glucose phosphorylation Glucose-6-P formation was used to calculate porcine islet hexokinase and glucokinase activity Vmax and Km according to the Eadie-Hofstee plot (Table 1).

Table 1. *Comparison of glucose transport, phosphorylation and utilization between rat and pig pancreatic islets*

	Transport		Phosphorylation		Utilization	
	Km	Vmax	Km	Vmax	Km	Vmax
	mM	nM/μg DNA/15"	mM	nM/μg DNA/h	mM	nM/μg DNA/h
Pig islets	11.8	0.48	8.3	8.0	7.7	6.9
Rat islets	16.6	0.32	9.7	8.7	8.9	7.6

c) glucose utilization In porcine islets cultured at glucose 5.5 mmol/l, glucose utilization increased from 1.79±0.34 nmol/μg DNA/2h at glucose 5 mmol/l to 5.97±0.16 and 6.19±0.29 at glucose 20 and 30 mmol/l, respectively (Fig. 1), with a calculated Vmax of 6.9±0.33 and a Km of 7.7±1.4 mmol/l (m±SE, n=5).

Values of glucose transport, phosphorylation and utilization in porcine islets were then compared to values obtained in previous experiments in rat islets (5) using the same procedures (Table 1). No significant difference was present except in the glucose transport K_m ($p<0.05$).

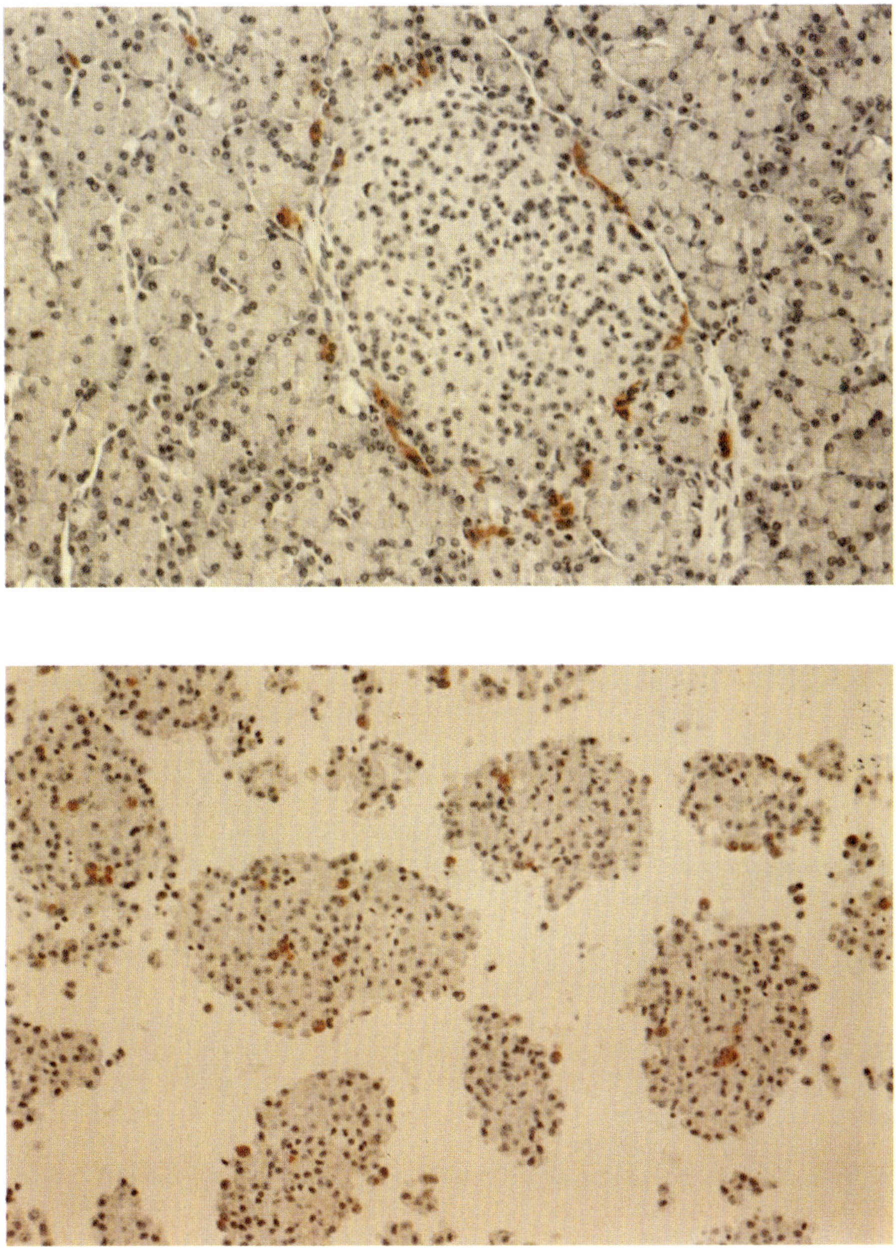

FIG. 1. Immuno-histochemical studies: In situ (upper panel) and freshly isolated (lower panel) porcine islets immunostained to show glucagon producing A-cells. Most porcine islets show usual mantle-core arrangement of peripheral A-cells and central B-cells, but some show a more complex arrangement with glucagon-positive cells more centrally located. At the end of isolation, most peripherally located A-cells were lost in porcine islets.

STRUCTURAL STUDIES

Cultured (48 h) porcine pancreatic islets were small and irregular aggregates of cells, mostly Beta cells. Beta-cells were large (up to 14 μm in diameter) and characterized by a voluminous nucleus, irregular in profile, with dispersed chromatin and a large nucleolus. The cytoplasm contained an abundant rough endoplasmic reticulum (RER), arranged in parallel or curvilinear cisternae, and one or more hypertrophic Golgi complexes with a tubulo-vesicular shape. Many mitochondria, small aggregates of glycogen and several lipid vacuoles and lisosomal structures were present in some Beta cells. In the Golgi area, small round clear vesicles were observed, sometimes with a thick membrane and combined with round secretory granules, 150-300 nm in diameter, with a round and regular inner core of variable electrondensity (pro-insulin granules). Some mature insulin granules with the typical lucent halo and crystalline core were present next to the cytoplasmic membrane.

Immuno-histochemistry Sections of pig native pancreas stained with a rabbit anti-glucagon polyclonal antibody are shown in Figure 1 (upper panel). Figure 1 also shows pig islets at the end of the isolation procedure (lower panel). Note that pig islets have lost most of the Alpha cells located peripherally but not the few Alpha cells located at the centre of the islet.

DISCUSSION

We have investigated certain functional and structural characteristics of isolated porcine islets that may be responsible for the hampered response to glucose *in vitro*. Among these:

1. the function of the first steps of glucose signalling and metabolism in Beta cells;
2. the ultrastructural characteristics of Beta cells;
3. the islet architecture.

Our data indicate that no alteration of either glucose transport, phosphorylation or utilization was present in isolated porcine islets. All these functions appeared both qualitatively and quantitatively similar to those observed in rat islets. Since values for glucose phosphorylation and utilization in porcine islets are comparable to those found in rat islets, it seems unlikely that the *in vitro* hampered response to glucose of porcine islets is due to differences in the glucose sensing mechanism of Beta cells, both due to species characteristics and to functional damage during the isolation procedure.

The electron microscopy observation shows that porcine pancreatic Beta cells in culture have a well preserved ultrastructure with intact plasma membrane and intracellular organelles. Therefore, as for glucose transport and metabolism, the cell ultrastructural characteristics could not account for the poor functional response of porcine islets to glucose.

At immunocytochemistry, glucagon producing Alpha cells appeared mainly located at the islet periphery when islets were studied in porcine pancreas sections, even if sparse Alpha cells may also be observed at the core of the islet. After the isolation procedure, however, most Alpha cells at the islet periphery had disappeared, and only the few Alpha cells observed at the islet core were present. These data raise the possibility that the loss of most glucagon-producing cells may also contribute to the hampered *in vitro* insulin secretory response to glucose of isolated porcine islets. Endogenously released glucagon is believed to be responsible for maintaining Beta cell cyclic AMP levels sufficiently high to allow glucose to exert its insulin-releasing action in isolated islets (4). Isolated Beta cells, in fact, have a blunted capacity to secrete insulin in response to glucose and this secretory defect can be reversed by either recombining Alpha and Beta cells, or adding exogenous db-cyclic AMP (4).

In conclusion, the present study demonstrates that isolated porcine islets have a normal glucose sensing mechanism and a normal insulin storage and secretory machine. The only abnormality that we have found associated with the poor glucose-induced insulin release is the damaged islet architecture, including the loss of peripherally-located Alpha cells.

REFERENCES

1. Crowther N.J., Gotfredsen C.F., Moody A.J. and Green I.C. (1990): J. Endocr. 126: 43-49.
2. Johnson J.H., Newgard C.B., Milburn J.L., Lodish H.F. and Thorens B. (1990): J. Biol. Chem. 265: 6548-51.
3. Marchetti P., Zappella A., Giannarelli R., Masiello P., Masoni A., Casanovi E., Gattai V., Pozzolini L., Marchetti A. and Navalesi R. (1988): Transplantation Proc. 20: 707-708.
4. Pipeleers D.G., Schuit F.C., In't Veld P.A., Maes E., Hooghe-Peters E.L., Van de Winkel M. and Gepts W. (1985): Endocrinology 117: 824-833.
5. Purrello F., Buscema M., Rabuazzo A.M., Caltabiano V., Forte F., Vinci C., Vetri M. and Vigner R. (1993): Diabetes 42: 199-205.

Frontiers in Endocrinology
Volume 9 - 1994

Novel Method for the Determination of Hepatic Glycogenolysis and Gluconeogenesis *in vivo* in Rats: Preliminary Results in Hypoglycemia

A. Buongiorno, L. Morviducci[1], D. Zorretta, F. Leonetti[1]
G. Tamburrano[1] and A. Giaccari

Division of Immunometrics, Clinical Biochemistry Department, Istituto Superiore di Sanità, Viale Regina Elena 299, 00161 Rome; [1]Endocrinology, II Institute of Clinical Medicine, University of Rome La Sapienza, Viale del Policlinico 155, 00161 Rome, Italy

INTRODUCTION

A rapid and efficient isocratic high-performance liquid chromatographic method for studying the metabolism of phosphoenolpyruvate and uridinediphosphate-glucose has been developed. For each compound this method can measure tissue concentrations in the range 0.1-1000 nmol/g of tissue and determine specific radioactivity. All measurements can be performed in 200 mg of tissue. The recoveries of uridinediphosphate (UDP) [6-^{3}H]-glucose and phosphoenol[1-^{14}C]-pyruvate (PEP) from liver tissue homogenates were 97% and 99%, respectively. Following intra-arterial infusion of [3-^{3}H]-glucose and [U-^{14}C]-lactate in conscious rat, the concentration and specific radioactivity of phosphoenolpyruvate and UDP-glucose were determined in rat liver.

Briefly, the first is performed on a solid-phase, strong anion-exchange cartridge, with the use of phosphate buffers of increasing molarity. This first purification allows us to partially separate the two compounds of interest from all non polar and most of the polar intracellular substrates with optimal recoveries. The second step is a reversed phase, ion pairing HPLC isocratic method, on a C18 column.

In order to provide evidence for the identity and purity of the chromatographic peaks, specific precolumn enzymatic conversions of UDPglucose and PEP were carried out. When these samples were injected into the HPLC system, no interfering peaks were eluted within the retention volumes of both PEP and UDP-glucose. The method was applied to experimentation in small animals using radiolabeled precursors, in order to quantitate *in vivo* the glycogenic and gluconeogenic fluxes.

It is now well established that in the presence of euglycemia (such as during a euglycemic hyperinsulinemic clamp), insulin completely suppresses hepatic glucose production, and this effect is mainly determined through a reduction in liver glycogenolysis (1, 6, 7). However, when blood glucose is clamped at a lower concentration, hypoglycemia markedly stimulates hepatic glucose production, mainly through a large increase, at least in the early phase, in liver glycogenolysis (1, 2, 5). Insulin-induced hypoglycemia, therefore, is a combination of either stimulus or suppression on hepatic glycogenolysis, in which insulin and glucose plasma concentrations play a major role.

It is the aim of the present study to evaluate the effect of insulin concentration per se on hepatic glycogenolysis and gluconeogenesis under identical conditions of hypoglycemia.

MATERIAL AND METHODS

For this purpose, we studied three groups of male Sprague Dawley rats during a hypoglycemic clamp with:

1) phloridzin, which is an inhibitor of glucose reabsorption (8) at kidney tubular level (at a dose of 3.0 mg/kg·min).

2) low insulin dose (4.0 mU/kg·min), with a plasma insulin concentration of about 100 μU/ml.

3) high insulin dose (20 mU/kg·min), with a plasma insulin concentration of about 500 μU/ml.

In order to completely suppress glucagon response to hypoglycemia, octreotide was infused at a rate of 100 ng/kg·min. Plasma glucose concentration was maintained constant at 60 mg/dl with a variable 10% glucose infusion. [3-^{3}H]-glucose infusion was given as a bolus of 30 μCi followed by a constant infusion of 1 μCi/min throughout the study, while [U-^{14}C]-lactate was given as a bolus of 0.5 μCi followed by a constant infusion of 0.1 μCi/min during the last 8 minutes of the study. At the end of each study, all rats were anesthetized and liver tissue samples quickly freeze-clamped in liquid nitrogen and subsequently processed with an HPLC method (3) for the determination of ^{14}C-^{3}H-UDPG specific activities and ^{14}C-PEP specific activity. Gluconeogenesis was estimated from the specific activities of ^{14}C-labelled UDPglucose and PEP and ^{3}H-labeled plasma glucose and liver UDPglucose following the infusion of

[U-^{14}C]-lactate and [3-^{3}H]-glucose. UDPG specific activities (both ^{14}C and ^{3}H) may be assumed as representing glucose-6-phosphate specific activities and, consequently, composed in percent by glucose recycling with plasma (^{3}H-UDPG s.a. / ^{3}H-glucose s.a. ratio) from gluconeogenesis (^{14}C-UDPG s.a. / 2 x ^{14}C-PEP s.a.) and from glycogenolysis (% of non labeled UDPG). Since [3-^{3}H]-glucose recycling is not measured in the calculation of hepatic glucose production, but may be measured as % of glucose-6-phosphate specific activity, total glucose output may also be estimated.

Therefore, gluconeogenesis may be calculated according to the following formula (4):

$$\text{Gluconeogenesis} = \frac{\text{HGP x } {}^{14}\text{C-UDPG s.a. x } {}^{3}\text{H-glucose s.a.}}{2 \text{ x } {}^{14}\text{C-PEP s.a. x } ({}^{3}\text{H-glucose s.a. - } {}^{3}\text{H-UDPG s.a.})}$$

RESULTS AND DISCUSSION

The calculated hepatic glucose production in the phloridzin, infused rats (group 1) and in the low insulin rats (group 2) were both about 10.5 mg/kg·min. On the contrary, hepatic glucose production was significantly reduced in the rats infused with 20 mU/kg·min of insulin (group 3). Although overall hepatic glucose production was similar in groups 1 and 2, a significant stimulation of the relative contribution of gluconeogenesis was present, and it further increased with the high dose of insulin (group 3). Therefore, even if the low dose of insulin (group 1 vs group 2) had no effect on overall hepatic glucose production, a suppressive effect was present on glycogenolysis. This result is evident also when considering the data as actual fluxes. It is clearly evident that the infusion of a low dose of insulin determined an increase in the gluconeogenic flux, while the infusion of the high dose of insulin suppressed gluconeogenesis again.

To summarize the data, it may be observed that the infusion of the low dose of insulin (4.0 mU/kg·min, with a plasma insulin concentration of about 100 μU/ml) did not affect overall hepatic glucose production. However, a relative decrease in liver glycogenolysis was observed. On the contrary, the infusion of the high dose of insulin (20 mU/kg·min, with a plasma insulin concentration of about 500 μU/ml), finally reduced overall hepatic glucose production, and this result is determined by a decrease in both gluconeogenesis and glycogenolysis.

In conclusion, it may be suggested that, in the presence of identical conditions of hypoglycemia, insulin concentration is a potent determinant of the relative contribution of gluconeogenesis and glycogenolysis to overall hepatic glucose production.

REFERENCES

1. Amiel S.A., Tamborlane W.V., Saccà L. and Sherwin R.S. (1988): Diabetes/Metabol. Rev. 4: 71-89.
2. Frizzel T.R., Campbell P.J. and Cherrington A.D. (1988): Diabetes/Metabol. Rev. 4: 51-70.
3. Giaccari A. and Rossetti L. (1989): J. Chromat. 497: 69-78.
4. Giaccari A. and Rossetti L. (1992): J. Clin. Invest. 89: 36-45.
5. Hansen I., Firth R., Haymond M., Cryer P. and Rizza R. (1986): Diabetes, 35: 186-191.
6. Rizza R.A., Mandarino L.J. and Gerich J.E. (1981): Am. J. Physiol. 240: E630-639.
7. Rossetti L. and Giaccari A. (1990 a): J. Clin. Invest. 85: 1785-1792.
8. Rossetti L., Giaccari A. and DeFronzo R.A. (1990 b): Diabetes Care 13: 610-630.

Frontiers in Endocrinology
Volume 9 - 1994

Development of Obesity and Insulin Resistance Syndrome by icv Neuropeptide Y (NPY) Administration to Normal Rats

R.Vettor[1], N. Zarjevski, I. Cusin, F. Rohner-Jeanrenaud and B. Jeanrenaud

Laboratoires de Recherches Métaboliques, Faculty and Department of Medicine, University of Geneva, 64 Avenue de la Roseraie,1211 Geneva 4, Switzerland;
[1]Institute of Semeiotica Medica, Patologia Medica III, University of Padua, Via Ospedale 105, 35128 Padua, Italy

INTRODUCTION

Obesity is a pathological condition characterized by an imbalance between caloric intake and energy expenditure. Hyperinsulinaemia and insulin resistance are also major features of this syndrome. The initial cause in the series of events leading to obesity are yet to be determined. Studies in genetically or ventromedial hypothalamus lesioned obese rats showed decreased sympathetic activity leading to decreased energy expenditure (4) and an increased parasympathetic tone responsible for hyperinsulinaemia (6). These observations suggest that the early event producing changes in ß-cell secretion, decreased energy expenditure and obesity could be present in the central nervous system. The discovery of Neuropeptide Y (NPY) and its peripheral hormonal as well as metabolic effects when administered icv further support this hypothesis. This 36 amino acid neuropeptide has been found in the central nervous system (3). Intracerebroventricularly administered NPY stimulates food intake, reduces energy expenditure (2), produces hyperinsulinaemia, and increases lipogenetic activity (8). Moreover hypothalamic NPY mRNA and protein levels were both increasing during the dynamic phase of these syndromes (1).

The aim of our work was to verify whether NPY could play a role in the development and maintenance of obesity syndrome. Therefore we administered NPY icv to normal rats and subsequently the treatment was stopped and the hormonal-metabolic changes were determined.

MATERIAL AND METHODS

Lean female rats of the Zucker (FA/?) strain were used throughout the study. Body weight, food intake, basal plasma insulin, glucose, triglycerides and FFA were then measured daily. Guiding cannulas were placed in anesthetized rats into the right lateral cerebral ventricle. After one week recovery cannulas were connected to osmotic minipumps. The animals were infused icv with 10 μg/day of NPY for 7 days. Three groups of rats were used: administered with icv NPY or its vehicle for 7 days and rats after 7 days cessation of NPY administration. All animals were submitted to euglycaemic-hyperinsulinaemic clamps. Primed-continuous infusion of U-^{14}C D-glucose (10 μCi/hour), was initiated to establish a steady state of glucose turnover. Hepatic glucose production (HGP) and rate of total glucose utilization (Rd) in basal conditions and at the end of clamp were then calculated (7). The glucose utilization index of inguinal white adipose tissue (WAT) as well as that of muscle (red and white gastrocnemius-rGAST and wGAST), was measured in the same group of animals, during the euglycaemic hyperinsulinaemic clamps associated with the 2-deoxy-D-[1^{3}H]-glucose technique. After iv injection of 2-deoxy-D-[1^{3}H]-glucose (30 μCi) at the end of clamp, the content in 2-deoxy-D-[1^{3}H]-glucose-6-phosphate was determined in white adipose tissue and muscle to measure the glucose utilization index. Protein concentration and DNA content in the membrane preparation was measured in sampled tissues. RNA was extracted electrophoresed, blotted and then hybridized to cRNA probe specific for GLUT 4. Western blots were also performed in order to measure the relative abundance of GLUT 4 protein using the polyclonal antibody against GLUT 4 R820.

Values are expressed as mean ± SEM. Statistical analysis was performed by ANOVA.

RESULTS

icv NPY administration to normal rats resulted in a sustained increase in food intake relative to controls (7th day, 55 ± 5 vs 18 ± 0.4g ; $p < 0.0001$). Indeed, within one day of NPY withdrawal, food intake returned to control values. Increased food intake resulted in a progressive increase in body weight in the icv NPY-treated group relative to controls. After stopping of central NPY administration, body weight progressively returned to normal control values. Significant increases in basal plasma insulin (1.7 ± 0.1 vs 7.9 ±

1.3 ng/ml; p< 0.001) and triglyceride levels (86 ± 11 vs 137 ± 12 mg/dl; p<0.001) were found in icv NPY-treated rats compared to controls. The increased plasma insulin and triglyceride levels of the icv NPY-administered animals returned to normal values seven days after stopping of icv NPY administration. In the euglycemic hyperinsulinemic clamp studies all groups were compared at similar steady-state levels of glycaemia and insulinaemia. Insulin inhibited HGP in all groups. At the end of the clamp Rd was, however, significantly decreased in the group of rats that was administered with icv NPY for seven days compared to respective controls (22 ± 1 vs 19 ± 1 $mg.\cdot Kg^{-1}.min^{-1}$; p<0.05). The decrease in Rd returned to normal values after stopping of NPY administration. The insulin-stimulated *in vivo* glucose uptake as measured by the labelled 2-deoxy-D-glucose technique by adipose tissue is shown by Table 1. Adipose tissue from 7 day icv NPY-treated rats

Table 1. *Glucose utilization index (ng/mg x min)*

	WAT	RGAST	WGAST
Control	3.1±0.4	40.5±3.3	16.4±2.6
NPY	21.0±1.8 **	12.2±1.7**	5.2±0.8**
Cessation	3.3±0.3	39.5±2	16.0±1.6

** p<0.01 vs control.

was much more insulin responsive than that of controls. This was accompanied by an analogous change in the GLUT 4 mRNA levels and total amount of the insulin responsive glucose transporter (GLUT 4) protein (data not shown). The return to control values of both *in vivo* adipose tissue glucose uptake and adipose tissue GLUT 4 protein levels seven days after stopping NPY administration was observed.The insulin-induced glucose utilization index observed in the muscles obtained from icv NPY-treated rats was significantly decreased in respect to muscle obtained from vehicle-infused rats (Table 1). However, it was normalized seven days after withdrawal of NPY administration. The changes observed in muscles from icv NPY-treated rats were not accompanied by any alteration in the level of GLUT 4 mRNA and GLUT 4 protein (data not shown).

CONCLUSIONS

The present study shows that icv NPY administration to normal rats produced many of the hormonal and metabolic changes observed during the dynamic phase of hypothalamic or genetic obesity (5). These changes were hyperphagia, increased body weight gain, hyperinsulinaemia, increased white adipose tissue metabolic activity as well as increased levels of GLUT 4 protein. At the same time the presence of an insulin resistant state at the level of the muscle tissue appeared. The icv NPY-induced effects are in agreement with other results obtained by lesioning the ventromedial hypothalamic area (5). During euglycaemic-hyperinsulinaemic clamps, a significant decrease in glucose utilization at maximal insulin levels supported the conclusion of a NPY-induced decreased insulin responsiveness. The HGP remained normally insulin responsive as often is the case in the dynamic phase of hypothalamic or genetic obesity (5). These data might be better interpreted when the *in vivo* 2-3H deoxy-glucose uptake by individual tissues is measured. Glucose uptake was more insulin responsive in white adipose tissue, but was insulin resistant in muscle of the NPY-treated animals compared to controls. The decreased rate of Rd in icv NPY-treated rats thus have been due to the decreased insulin responsiveness in muscles. The mechanisms underlying the divergent effects of insulin on adipose tissue and muscles were only partly understood. In adipose tissue, it was related to an increase in the amount of GLUT 4 protein as well as GLUT 4 expression while GLUT 4 protein was unchanged in muscles. This suggests that the overall expression of GLUT 4 was not implicated in muscular insulin resistance. The present study shows also the full reversibility of all changes induced by NPY administration after stopping icv peptide infusion. The increased insulin sensitivity of adipose tissue, the resistance to insulin action in muscles and hyperinsulinaemia returned to normal values 7 days after stopping icv NPY administration. As genetically obese rats are characterized by early increases in their hypothalamic NPY protein and mRNA levels (1) the present data together suggest that hypothalamic NPY may be one of the neuropeptide candidates responsible for the development or maintenance of obesity syndrome.

REFERENCES

1. Bchini-Hooft van Huijsduijnen O., Rohner-Jeanrenaud F. and Jeanrenaud B. (1993): Neuroendocrinol. 5: 381-386.
2. Billington C.J., Briggs J.E., Grace M. and Levine A.S. (1991): Am. J. Physiol. 260: R321-327.
3. Gray T.S. and Morley J.E. (1986): Life Sci. 38: 389-401.
4. Jeanrenaud B.,Halimi S. and van de Werve G. (1985): Diab. Metabol. Rev. 1: 261-291.
5. Penicaud L., Rohner-Jeanrenaud F. and Jeanrenaud B. (1986): Am. J. Physiol. 250: E662-E668.
6. Rohner-Jeanrenaud F. and Jeanrenaud B. (1985): Endocrinology 116: 830-834.
7. Terretaz J. and Jeanrenaud B. (1983): Endocrinology 112: 1346-1351.
8. Zarjevsky N., Cusin I., Vettor R., Rohner-Jeanrenaud F. and Jeanrenaud B. (1993): Endocrinology 133: 1753-1758.

Frontiers in Endocrinology
Volume 9 - 1994

Metabolic Effects of Metformin

A. Tiengo, S. Del Prato and P. Tessari

Cattedra di Malattie del Metabolismo, University of Padova,
Via Giustiniani, 2, 35128 Padova, Italy

Metformin represents one of the very few drugs available in clinical practice for the treatment of "insulin resistance syndrome", characterized by central obesity, non-insulin-dependent diabetes, hypertriglyceridemia and hypertension.

The fact that the antihyperglycemic effect of metformin occurs in the absence of a stimulation insulin concentration allows us to consider this drug among the insulin-sensitizer substances. However, metformin may also act on lipid metabolism by reducing hyperglyceridemia and, in some cases, it may diminish hypertension in obese diabetic patients. By means of these different positive effects metformin could be considered a useful therapeutic approach in the plurimetabolic syndrome.

GLUCOSE METABOLISM

The antihyperglycemic effect of metformin cannot be attributed to increased insulin concentrations. Insulin concentrations in the basal state and after an oral glucose challenge, as well as during day profiles, are unchanged or only slightly reduced during metformin therapy in obese and nonobese non-insulin-dependent diabetes mellitus (NIDDM) patients (5, 16).

Metformin may reduce hyperglycemia in NIDDM through three putative mechanisms: suppression of the excessive rate of hepatic glucose production in NIDDM, stimulation of glucose utilization and glycolysis, and reduced intestinal glucose absorption. However, this last mechanism has not been confirmed in NIDDM even if Bailey (1) demonstrated in animals that metformin slows the rate of intestinal glucose absorption and increases intestinal glucose utilisation.

In vitro studies demonstrated that metformin increases hepatic insulin sensitivity, suppresses gluconeogenesis and stimulates insulin-mediated glucose transport in insulin sensitive (1) and in insulin-insensitive tissues (19).

In the clinical condition of hyperglycemia of non-insulin-dependent diabetic patients the acute administration of metformin induces a significant decrease of hepatic glucose production (-30%), a slight decrease of glucose oxidation without modifying either glucose uptake or non oxidative glucose metabolism (17).

However, after chronic treatment, metformin was able to decrease basal hepatic glucose output (16), probably by increasing the sensitivity of the liver to the antigluconeogenic action of insulin. Therapeutic concentrations of metformin act synergistically with insulin to reduce gluconeogenesis in isolated rat hepatocytes (25). According to De Fronzo (9) the major effect of metformin on the liver seems to be an inhibition of glycogenolysis since gluconeogenesis was unchanged; neither lactate turnover nor the amount of glucose derived from lactate were altered. Moreover, metformin improves insulin metabolism in the liver without significant modification of regional blood flow through a direct effect on insulin post-receptor events in the liver (23).

However, the main cause of decreased basal glycemia during metformin therapy seems to be due to an increase in glucose utilization. Improved glucose tolerance without increased insulin suggests that metformin enhances insulin-mediated glucose disposal (2). Clamp studies carried out in NIDDM patients and reported by Bailey (1) generally confirmed this hypothesis and showed that metformin increases glucose disposal at submaximal and maximal insulin concentrations.

In particular, our results indicate that 4 weeks of metformin treatment improves peripheral removal of glucose in type II diabetes, mainly improving insulin action at a postreceptor step since a significant increase of maximal glucose disposal rate was observed without any change in insulin binding in circulating cells (16). Recently we confirmed (22) that metformin induces an improvement in glucose metabolism both in the basal and in the insulin-stimulated state. The improvement in glucose disposal, observed in NIDDM patients submitted to metformin treatment, is entirely due to an increase of non-oxidative glucose metabolism without a significant modification of glucose oxidation.

According to Perriello et al. (17) the improvement of insulin-mediated glucose utilization, observed after chronic metformin treatment, may be due to a better glycemic control and to the removal of glucotoxicity rather than to a specific effect of the drug. Consistent with our results are not only previous reports that metformin increases insulin-mediated glucose disposal in NIDDM (18, 3, 4, 26), but also the findings obtained in diabetic rats (13). In these animals the drug was able to normalize insulin-mediated glucose disposal and muscle glycogen synthesis. Non-oxidative glucose metabolism is mainly represented by glycogen synthesis. Therefore, also in humans, the main post-receptor event of insulin action stimulated by metformin treatment seems to be the glycogenic pathway.

LIPID METABOLISM

Metformin decreases plasma FFA both acutely (17) and during chronic treatment both in obese and non obese diabetic patients (22).

Lipid oxidation was decreased after acute administration of metformin at baseline and at the low-dose insulin step of an hyperinsulinemic glucose clamp (17). Plasma FFA turnover rate and FFA oxidation were also lower after chronic metformin treatment (22). In our experiments euglycemic hyperinsulinemia was followed, on the other hand, by a reduction in plasma FFA concentration turnover rate that remained the same before and after metformin therapy.

The fact that the reduction in FFA and total lipid oxidation was present only in the basal state and not in the insulin-stimulated condition could be explained by the different concentrations of plasma insulin. In the post-absorptive condition, basal insulin still allows a significant flow of FFA from lipolysis, therefore metformin can exhibit its inhibition on FFA oxidation. In the presence of hyperinsulinemia, the rate of lipolysis is almost completely suppressed. Therefore, the inhibitory effect of metformin on FFA oxidation would be expected to be minimized.

Table 1. *Metabolic effects of metformin*

Suppression of hepatic glucose production
– ↓ gluconeogenesis
– ↓ glucogenolysis
Stimulation of peripheral glucose uptake
– ↑ non oxidative glucose metabolism
Reduction of FFA and lipid oxidation
Reduction of plasma VLDL-triglyceride
No interference on amino acid and protein metabolism

The suppression of lipid oxidation after metformin could be due, only in part, to decreased availability of plasma FFA and it was largely the consequence of a direct suppression of oxidation of the intracellular FFA pool (17, 27).

According to Perriello et al. (17) the decrease in plasma FFA after metformin could be attributed to increased FFA reesterification rather than suppressed lipolysis. In fact, at least *in vitro* metformin does not possess an antilipolytic effect (7).

Metformin may also decrease plasma triglyceride, VLDL-triglyceride, cholesterol and VLDL-cholesterol (26). Many years ago and more recently we ourselves confirmed these data (22) in diabetic and non diabetic patients.

The reduction of triglycerides is more consistent in hypertriglyceridemia patients with up to 50%. This is largely due to a decrease in VLDL-triglyceride and studies in metformin-treated fructose-fed rats have shown a decreased rate of VLDL production (28). Moreover, it has been shown that postprandial concentrations of TG-rich lipoproteins of intestinal origin were dramatically lower after metformin treatment (21). A hypocholesterolemic effect of metformin is less important and frequent and, where observed, it has been attributed to a decrease in LDL-cholesterol or VLDL cholesterol (26). A small increase in HDL has been observed in non diabetic subjects and in NIDDM patients treated with metformin, although no effect has been noted in other clinical and animal studies.

PROTEIN METABOLISM

Among the metabolic effects of biguanides, a possible interference on amino acid and protein metabolism could be proposed. Although amino acid turnover has been found to be normal in type 2 diabetes (4), both under fasting and fed conditions, metformin could theoretically worsen body protein kinetics in diabetes affecting some oxidative or non oxidative steps of amino acid metabolism. On the other hand, biguanides inhibit intestinal amino acid transport (6).

Groop et al. (12) observed a decreased lean body mass after 3 months of metformin treatment suggesting a decrease in body protein content. *In vivo* an increase of only alanine concentration in type II diabetic patients has been reported following metformin treatment (14). However, in an acute study, metformin administration did not affect either protein oxidation or total energy expenditure (17).

In particular, these authors showed that protein oxidation, estimated by total urinary nitrogen excretion, was not affected by metformin.

In a very recent study, our group (24) has demonstrated that metformin treatment for four weeks did not affect fasting or postprandial protein turnover in mild NIDDM subjects. In fact, as compared to the pretreatment period, metformin administration did not change total phenylalanine rate of appearance, dietary and endogenous phenylalanine rate of appearance, dietary phenylalanine oxidation and splanchnic uptake, after a mixed meal. Therefore, endogenous breakdown was not affected.

CONCLUSIONS

Our results, as well as data in the literature show that chronic metformin treatment induces an improvement in glucose metabolism both in the basal and insulin-stimulated state. In basal conditions, but not during euglycemic hyperinsulinemia, this improvement is associated with a reduction in FFA oxidation and an increase in the oxidative metabolism of glucose. During the insulin-stimulated condition, the increase in non-oxidative glucose metabolism is the main cause of the improvement in glucose disposal.

On the other hand, it seems that the primary antihyperglycemic effect of metformin in NIDDM, after acute treatment, is represented by the suppression of hepatic glucose production in the absence of an increase in peripheral or portal plasma insulin concentration. The suppression of FFA oxidation and FFA plasma concentration induced by metformin seems to be the principal mechanism of metformin enhancement of hepatic and whole body glucose metabolism.

With respect to this concept, more and more data have been gathered to indicate that the alteration of the oxidative and non oxidative glucose metabolism in NIDDM, at least in part, may be attributed to a concomitant increase in FFA oxidation which, through Randle's cycle, would reduce glucose oxidation and disposal (20, 8).

On the other hand, in NIDDM the excessive rate of hepatic glucose production in the postabsorptive state is attributed primarily to increased gluconeogenesis that, in turn, is enhanced by FFA and intrahepatic lipid oxidation (10). A positive correlation between the rate of hepatic glucose production and of lipid oxidation has been demonstrated by Perriello et al. (17) in NIDDM patients after placebo or metformin administration, before and during the low-dose insulin of the hyperinsulinemic-isoglycemic clamp.

The suppression of lipid oxidation, induced by metformin, and the decreased availability of the substrate plasma FFA seems to be a crucial mechanism, which improves glucose disposal and reduces hepatic glucose production in NIDDM patients.

It is very comforting and reassuring that prolonged metformin administration does not interfere with protein and amino acid metabolism (24).

The positive effect of metformin on the lipoprotein profile, by reducing VLDL and LDL triglycerides, and the recent observations of its favorable action on PAI-1 activity and on arterial blood pressure (15, 11) indicate that metformin not only improves glycemic control and lowers insulin resistance but also corrects other risk factors for cardiovascular disease. Thus, metformin could be considered positive in the treatment of plurimetabolic syndrome.

REFERENCES

1. Bailey C. (1992): Diab. Care 15, 755-772.
2. Bailey C.J. (1988): Diab. Med. 5, 315-320.
3. Benzi L., Trischitta V., Ciccarone A., Cecchetti P., Brunetti A., Squatrito S., Marchetti P., Vigneri R. and Navalesi R.(1990): Diabetes 39, 844-849.
4. Biolo G., Tessari P., Inchiostro S., Bruttomesso D., Sabadini L., Fongher C., Panebianco G., Frattoni M.G. and Tiengo A. (1992): Am. J. Physiol. 263: E877-E883.
5. Campbell I.W., Duncan C.D., Patton N.W., Bradhead T., Tucker G.T. and Woods H.F. (1987): Diab. Med. 4, 337-41.
6. Caspary W. and Creutzfeld W. (1973): Diabetologia 9, 6-12.
7. Cigolini M., Bosello O., Zancanaro C., Orlandi P., Fezzi O. and Smith U. (1984): Diab. Metab. 10, 311-315.
8. De Fronzo R.A. (1988): Diabetes 37, 667-687.
9. De Fronzo R. Mechanism of metformin action: clinical studies in NIDDM. In: NIDDM: Prevention and Treatment. Heidelberg, September 25-26, 1994.
10. Fanelli C., Calderone S., Epifano L., De Vincenzo A., Modarelli F., Pampanelli S., Perriello G., De Feo P., Brunetti P., Gerich J.E. and Bolli G.B. (1993): J. Clin. Invest. 92, 1617-1622.
11. Giugliano D., Acampora R., De Rose N., Buonicanti R., Di Mario G., Martella R. and D'Onofrio F. (1993): Diab. Care 16, 1387-90.
12. Groop L., Widen E. and Fransilla-Kallunki A. (1989): Diabetologia 32, 599-605.
13. Jackson R.A., Hawa M.I., Jaspen J.B., Sim B.M., Di Silvio L., Flatherbe D. and Kurtz A.B. (1987): Diabetes 36, 632-640.
14. Marchetti P., Masiello P. and Benzi L. (1989): Drugs Exp. Clin. Res. 15, 565-570.
15. Nagi D.K. and Yudkin T. (1993): Diab. Care 16, 621-629.
16. Nosadini R., Avogaro A., Trevisan R., Valerio A., Tessari P., Duner E., Tiengo A., Velussi M., Del Prato S., De Kreutzenberg S., Muggeo M. and Crepaldi G. (1987): Diab. Care 10, 62-67.
17. Perriello G., Misericordia P., Volpi E., Santucci A., Santucci C., Ferrannini E., Ventura M.R., Santeusanio F., Brunetti P. and Bolli G. (1994): Diabetes 43, 920-928.
18. Prager R. and Schernthaner G. (1983): Diabetes 32, 1083-1086.
19. Purrello F., Gullo D., Brunetti A., Buscema M., Halia S., Goldfine I.D. and Vigneri R. (1987): Metabolism 36, 774-776.
20. Randle P.J., Garland P.B., Hales C.N. and Newshalme E.A. (1963): Lancet I, 785-89.
21. Reaven G. Clinical utility of metformin in different types of non-insulin-dependent diabetes mellitus. In: NIDDM: Prevention and treatment. Heidelberg, September 25-26, 1994.
22. Riccio A., Del Prato S., Vigili de Kreutzenberg S. and Tiengo A. (1991): Diab. Metab. 17, 180-184.
23. Signore A. and Pozzilli P. Metformin: modification of hepatic insulin metabolism and regional blood flow. In: NIDDM: Prevention and treatment. Heidelberg, September 25-26, 1994.
24. Tessari P., Biolo G., Bruttomesso D., Inchiostro S., Panebianco G., Vedovato M., Fongher C. and Tiengo A. (1994): J. Clin. Endocrinol. Metab.
25. Wollen N. and Bailey C.J. (1988): Biochem. Pharmacol. 37, 4353-58.
26. Wu M.S., Johnston P., Shen W.H.H., Hollenbeck C.B., Jeng C.Y., Goldfine I.D., Che Y.D. and Reaven G.M. (1990): Diab. Care 13, 1-8.
27. Yki-Jarvinen H.Z., Perhakainen I., Saloranta C., Groop L. and Taskinen M.R. (1991): Am. J. Physiol. 260, E680-689.
28. Zavaroni I., Dall'Aglio E., Bruschi F., Alpi C., Coscelli C. and Butturini U. (1984): Horm. Metab. Res. 16, 85-87.

ADRENALS

p. 397 - 414

Frontiers in Endocrinology
Volume 9 - 1994

Angiotensin II Receptors in Cortical and Medullary Adrenal Tumors

G. Opocher, S. Rocco, M. Cimolato, B. Vianello and [1]F. Mantero

Institute of Semeiotica Medica, University of Padua, via Ospedale 105, 35128 Padova;
[1]Endocrinology Clinic, University of Ancona, Ospedale di Torrette, 60100 Ancona, Italy

INTRODUCTION

Type 1 angiotensin II (AII) receptor (AT1) transduces most, if not all, the known actions of AII including the steroidogenic and trophic action on the adrenal gland as well as the vascular smooth muscle cells (VSMC) constriction (6). This receptor, which has been cloned also in humans, belongs to the seven transmembrane domains receptor family and is transduced by G proteins that inhibit cAMP and stimulates phospholipases.

Type 2 AII receptor (AT2) has been cloned in rat (3, 4) and is similar to AT1 although with different intracellular and extracellular tails. The only signal transduction so far described for rat AT2 is the inhibition of phosphotyrosine phosphatase. A strong element in favour of an important role in the control of the growth is the high density of AT2 during foetal development (2), nonetheless its exact biological role remains unclear. Evidence suggests that AII is not only a steroidogenic and vasoactive peptide but also a mitogenic agent (7) and despite the lack of definite knowledge on the action transduced by AT2 receptor, a link between AII receptors and tumors of target tissues, particularly adrenal gland, cannot be excluded.

AII receptors have been located not only in the zona glomerulosa but also in the zona fasciculata (5) and in the adrenal medulla (1); only in the latter is there a prevalence of AT2 receptors. In contrast to the zona glomerulosa, the effect of AII receptors in the zona fasciculata and in the medulla is yet to be clarified.

MATERIAL AND METHODS

To address the question whether in different adrenal tumors, density, affinity and subtype of AII receptors are comparable to non tumorous adrenal cortex, we have studied AII receptors in cell membranes obtained from 8 aldosterone producing adenomas (APA), 4 Cushing's adrenal adenomas (Cush), 6 adrenal pheochromocytomas (Pheo) and 9 normal adrenal cortex (zona glomerulosa plus zona fasciculata).

Methods Tissue was homogenized by Polytron, stirred on ice for 20 min, filtered through a nylon gauze and centrifuged at 100 g for 10 min. The supernatant was centrifuged for 30 min at 30.000 g. The pellet was resuspended and homogenized with a glass/teflon homogenizer. Binding capacity of adrenal cellular membranes (100-150 µg protein) was assayed by incubation with 0.15 nM ^{125}I-Angiotensin II (native hormone) (Amersham, UK) and increasing doses of cold AII (10^{-8}-10^{-10} M). Non-specific binding was determined in the presence of 1 µM cold AII. Subtype characterisation was performed using Dup 753 and CGP 42112 (10^{-6}-10^{-8} M) as selective AT1 and AT2 antagonists, respectively. After incubation (45 min at 22°), bound radioactivity was separated by centrifugation and counted.

Data were computed using the Ligand software.

RESULTS AND DISCUSSION

The results (Table 1) indicate that the mean receptor density and affinity of AII receptors are not significantly different in APA and in normal adrenal cortex although in selected APAs AII receptor number was 5-10 fold higher than in normals. In patients with aldosteronoma a resistance to AII is frequently seen *in vivo* and partially also *in vitro*: our results are consistent with the hypothesis of a defect of the signal transduction machinery rather than to receptor structural changes. The high variability of receptor density in APA does not exclude a direct link with the tumor growth although the ratio AT1/AT2 is fairly normal and, in many cases, receptor density and affinity were comparable to the normals.

Table 1. *Receptor density, affinity and subtype of angiotensin II receptors in adrenal tumors*

		Density (fmol/mg)	K_D (nM)	Subtype (%) AT1	(%) AT2
APA	n. 8	178.5±88.4	0.9±0.1	73.0±5.9	27.0±5.9
Cush	n. 4	20.1±5.2*	0.7±0.1	62.8±22.1	37.2±22.1
Pheo	n. 4**	5.0±1.8*	1.0±0.3	94.2±7.2	5.8±7.2
Normal	n. 9	54.6±9.3	0.6±0.08	79.0±8.2	21.2±8.2

* $p < 0.05$ vs normal. **Undetectable in two additional cases.

The finding of a measurable receptor density of AII receptors although below the normal in Cush, is consistent with the presence of a discrete number of AII receptors in zona fasciculata (5). Most interestingly, in two patients, the AT2 was the prevalent subtype: this observation is new and can be relevant in the understanding of a role of AII in the control of cell growth in these particular tumors.

In pheochromocytomas, AII receptor density is very low (undetectable in 2 cases) and affinity lower than normal adrenal cortex: this confims, in a relatively large number of cases, previous studies (1). In spite of the lack of an appropriate internal control, as would be normal adrenal medulla, this finding is important since autoradiographic studies showed a high density of AT2 receptors in normal medulla and AT2 have been cloned even from rat pheochromocytoma cells: thus, for, as yet, unknown reasons AII receptors disappear in human pheochromocytoma.

In conclusion, the study of AII receptor binding in adrenal tumors provides useful information, although further investigations on the expression and functional characterization of AII receptors are required to better clarify its possible role in adrenal tumorigenesis.

REFERENCES

1. Gonzales-Garcia C. and Keiser H.R., (1990): J. Hypertens. 8: 433-441.
2. Grady E.F., Sechi L.A., Griffin C.A., Schambelan M. and Kalinyak J.E. (1991): J. Clin. Invest. 88: 921-933.
3. Kambayashi Y., Bardhan S., Takahashi K., Tsuzuki S., Inui H., Hamakubo T. and Inagami T. (1993): J. Biol. Chem. 25: 24543-24546.
4. Mukoyama M., Nakajima M., Horiuchi M., Sasamura H., Pratt R.E. and Dzau V.J. (1993): J. Biol. Chem. 25: 24539-24542.
5. Naville D., Lebrethon M.C., Kermabon A.Y., Rouer E., Benarous R. and Saez J.M. (1993): FEBS 321: 184-188.
6. Peach M.J. and Dostal D.E. (1990): J. Cardiovasc. Pharmacol. 16 (suppl 4): S25-S30.
7. Schelling P., Fischer H. and Ganten D. (1991): J. Hypertens. 9: 3-15.

Frontiers in Endocrinology
Volume 9 - 1994

Abnormality of Aldosterone and Cortisol Late Pathways in Glucocorticoid-Remediable Aldosteronism

F. Fallo, M. Pistorello, U. Kuhnle[1] and N. Sonino

Division of Endocrinology, University of Padova,
Via Ospedale 105, 35128 Padova, Italy;
[1]Universitätskinderklinik, D-8000 München 2, Germany

INTRODUCTION

Glucocorticoid-remediable aldosteronism (GRA) is an ACTH-dependent autosomal dominant form of mineralocorticoid hypertension in which the excessive aldosterone (ALDO) production and clinical syndrome are corrected by the administration of glucocorticoids (1). The genetic abnormality has recently been described (4), the mutation resulting from fusion of the genes encoding steroid 11β-hydroxylase and ALDO synthase. In the adrenal zona fasciculata, this may lead to ectopic expression under ACTH control of ALDO synthase activity, which normally catalizes in the zona glomerulosa both corticosterone (B) and 18-OHB methyl oxidations. A specific biochemical abnormality of this disease is, in fact, the overproduction of cortisol (F) C-18 oxidation metabolites (8). Scattered data are available on precursor steroids of ALDO and F in this disease.

We studied 3 patients with GRA assessing mineralocorticoid and glucocorticoid pathways both in baseline conditions and after ACTH stimulation.

MATERIAL AND METHODS

Three siblings (patient 1, female aged 19 years, and patients 2 and 3, males aged 23 and 35 years, respectively) in a family with 9 siblings were shown to have GRA. Family pedigree and a detailed biochemical and hormonal assessment of all family members has been previously published (2). The chimaeric bands analyzed by Southern blot in leukocyte DNA indicating the genetic abnormality in patients 1 and 2 have been reported (5); in patient 3 this genetic study was not performed. All 3 patients were hypertensive and hypokalemic at the time of the study. As previously reported (8), they had very high urinary excretion of cortisol C-18 oxidation products 18-oxoF and 18-OHF, measured by gas chromatography/mass spectrometry.

Hormonal evaluation was conducted before glucocorticoid treatment. Plasma levels of progesterone (P), 11-deoxycorticosterone (DOC), B, ALDO, and of 17α-hydroxyprogesterone (17-OHP), 11-deoxycortisol (S), F, were measured at 0900 h in the supine position, before and 60 min after ACTH- (1-24) (Synacthen, Ciba, Switzerland) 250 μg as an iv bolus.

Twenty healthy subjects (10 males and 10 females, aged 17-44 years) were used as normal controls. All plasma steroids were measured by the method of Sippell et al. (7) using a mechanised Sephadex LH-20 multiple column chromatography and specific RIA.

For normal values see Table 1.

Table 1. *Plasma steroid levels in the 3 patients with GRA and in normal controls (n=20; mean values) before and after ACTH*

	P nmol/L	DOC nmol/L	B nmol/L	ALDO pmol/L	17-OHP nmol/L	S nmol/L	F nmol/L
Pat. 1							
Baseline	0.58	0.37	9.02	416.8	2.3	13.2	221.2
ACTH	2.49	4.55	87.1	1156	7.0	43.1	594.0
Pat. 2							
Baseline	0.66	0.46	8.82	341.2	3.7	14.1	181.8
ACTH	2.27	5.72	47.9	890.2	11.0	78.3	380.7
Pat. 3							
Baseline	0.28	0.37	4.46	205.4	2.6	14.5	178.8
ACTH	1.80	5.22	52.4	818.3	8.7	77.7	525.0
Normals							
Baseline	0.45	0.13	8.42	124.2	2.4	1.65	281.4
ACTH	1.51	1.54	97.4	196.8	6.4	6.7	642.8

RESULTS

Plasma steroid results are reported in Table 1. Baseline P, B, 17-OHP and F were normal in all 3 patients, and responded normally to ACTH standard stimulation test. Baseline and ACTH-stimulated DOC, ALDO and S were above normal. Both baseline B/DOC and F/S ratios, expressed on an equimolar basis, were abnormally low (24, 19, 12 vs a normal range of 46-78, and 17, 13, 12 vs a normal range of 158-210, respectively), and decreased further after ACTH-(1-24) (19, 8, 10 vs a normal range of 52-84, and 14, 5, 7 vs a normal range of 104-153, respectively).

DISCUSSION AND CONCLUSIONS

Recently, fusion genes generated by unequal crossover were identified as the underlying cause of GRA in 16 kindreds, including ours (5). The biochemical consequence of the genetic rearrangement in GRA is the formation of ALDO under ACTH drive by the zona fasciculata, together with 18-OHF and 18-oxoF formation from the methyl oxidation of F. Interestingly, both baseline and ACTH-stimulated DOC and S were above normal in our cases, suggesting a hyperresponsivity of the zona fasciculata to ACTH involving multiple steroidogenic steps. Overproduction of sodium-retaining steroids other than ALDO has been advocated to explain the dramatic effect in increasing blood pressure in these patients after prolonged ACTH administration (6). However, due to abnormal adrenal zonation, it is not possible to separate mineralocorticoid and glucocorticoid pathways in the absence of glucocorticoid treatment. Ratios of plasma concentrations of B to DOC and F to S are considered an indirect assessment of 11β-hydroxylase activity (3). Both these ratios were below normal in our patients, in whom an accelerated metabolism of B and F, due to abnormal sensitivity of 11β-hydroxylase/ALDO synthase to endogenous ACTH, seems to occur. Moreover, exogenous ACTH administration further lowered both B/DOC and F/S ratios, confirming the marked ACTH dependence of F metabolites and ALDO as a typical feature of GRA. In conclusion, our data are in agreement with a hyperfunction of the 11β-hydroxylase/ALDO synthase complex in the adrenal zona fasciculata, induced by the new chimaeric gene, in this disorder.

REFERENCES

1. Fallo F. and Mantero F. (1990) In: Endocrine Hypertension, edited by E.G. Biglieri and J.C. Melby, pp. 87-98. Raven Press. New York.
2. Fallo F., Sonino N., Armanini D., Luzzi T., Pedini F., Pasini C. and Mantero F. (1985): Clin. Endocrinol. 22: 777-785.
3. Gangul A., Meikle A.W., Tyler F.H. and West C.D. (1977): J. Clin. Endocrinol. Metab. 44: 560-568.
4. Lifton R.B., Dluhy R.G., Powers M., Rich G.M., Cook S., Ulick S. and Lalouel J.M. (1992): Nature 35: 262-265.
5. Lifton R.P., Dluhy R.G., Powers M., Rich G.M., Gutkin M., Fallo F., Gill J.R. Jr., Feld L., Ganguly A., Laidlaw J.C., Murnaghan D.J., Kaufman C., Stockigt J.R., Ulick S. and Lalouel J.M. (1992): Nature Genetics 2: 66-74.

6. New M.I., Peterson R.E., Saenger P. and Levine L.S. (1976): J. Clin. Endocrinol. Metab. 43: 1283-1293.
7. Sippell W.G., Bidlingmaier F., Becker H., Brunig T., Dorr H., Hahn H., Golder W., Hollmann G. and Knorr D. (1978): J. Steroid Biochem. 9: 63-78.
8. Ulick S., Chan C.K., Gill J.R., Jr, Gutkin M., Letcher L., Mantero F. and New M.I. (1990): J. Clin. Endocrinol. Metab. 71: 1151-1157.

Frontiers in Endocrinology
Volume 9 - 1994

Clinical Reliability and Minimal Invasiveness of Laparoscopic Adrenalectomy: first 16 Cases

G. Guazzoni, F. Montorsi, A. Centemero, P. Rigatti, R. Lanzi[1] and A.E. Pontiroli[1]

Departments of Urology and [1]Internal Medicine, Istituto Scientifico San Raffaele, Via Olgettina 60, 20132 Milan, Italy

INTRODUCTION

Surgical laparoscopy is becoming an increasingly common procedure in the treatment of abdominal diseases, in the light of its therapeutic efficacy associated with minimal invasiveness (2, 7). In particular, as far as concerns retroperitoneal ablative surgery, favourable results have been reported for laparoscopic nephrectomies, performed both for benign and malignant kidney diseases (1, 2).

The present study aimed to assess both the feasibility and the efficacy of laparoscopic adrenalectomy for the treatment of monolateral hypersecreting benign adrenal tumors.

MATERIAL AND METHODS

Subjects The study protocol was approved by the local Ethics Committee. During the period September 1992 - December 1993, sixteen patients with a unilateral hypersecreting adrenal tumor were considered eligible for laparoscopic surgery. Clinical details of patients are shown in Table 1.

Informed consent was obtained from the patients regarding the laparoscopic technique and the possible need to convert this approach to open field surgery. Preoperative pharmacological management of the patients varied according to their clinical and hormonal picture.

Table1. *Clinical and pathological details of the patients*

Pat.	Sex	Age	Path.	Size mm	Side	Pat.	Sex	Age	Path.	Size mm	Side
1	F	41	Conn	15x20	Left	9	F	51	Pheo.	60x55	Left
2	F	38	Conn	20x15	Left	10	F	60	Conn	15x10	Left
3	M	28	Conn	15x20	Right	11	F	36	Cush.	35x35	Right
4	M	65	Conn	20x15	Left	12	F	36	Pheo.	40x40	Right
5	F	46	Pheo.	55x45	Left	13	F	36	Cush.	10x15	Left
6	F	41	Cush.	20x25	Right	14	F	47	Conn	30x20	Right
7	F	47	Conn	15x25	Left	15	M	51	Pheo.	25x35	Left
8	M	36	Conn	15x25	Left	16	F	34	Conn	25x20	Right

Pat.: patient number; Path.: pathology; Conn: Conn's disease; Pheo.: Pheochromocytoma; Cush.: Cushing's syndrome.

All patients underwent a mechanic and antibiotic bowel preparation, and, at induction of anesthesia, received a dose of a broad spectrum cephalosporin, which was continued until the first postoperative day. All patients pre-deposited two units of their blood at least 10 days before surgery, and were typed and cross matched for 3 further units of blood. Under general anesthesia, they were placed on a 45-degree flank position with the bed tilted 30 degrees to increase the surgical field between the ribs and the iliac crest. A 10-degree reverse-Trendelemburg position was used to mobilize the intestines away from the surgical area. A Vereness needle was inserted through a small incision of the umbilicus and CO_2 was insufflated to achieve a 13-15 mm Hg pneumoperitoneum. The trocars were positioned according to a modification of the scheme described by Clayman et al. (1) for laparoscopic nephrectomy. The first 10 mm trocar was inserted through the umbilical incision and was used for the laparoscope. The second 10 mm trocar was inserted on the mamillary line, 1 to 3 cm above the transverse umbilical line, and the third just lateral to the midline, 2 to 4 cm over the transverse umbilical line. A 5 mm trocar was placed in the anterior axillary line between the tip of the 12th rib and the iliac crest. The location and size of the fifth trocar differed according to the side of the adrenal mass. For right sided lesions, a 10 mm trocar was positioned just lateral to the midline, and 1 cm below the costal margin, while, on the left side, a 5 mm trocar was positioned on the mamillary line, just below the costal margin. Different techniques were followed to reach and to remove the affected adrenal gland, according to its right or left location, as previously reported (4). At the end of the excision, the gland was entrapped in a specifically designed sac, which was removed from the abdomen through the umbilical incision, slightly enlarged in cases of the larger masses. All trocars were removed under direct vision, and the anterior fascia of the larger trocar sites were closed with a no. 1 absorbable suture; finally, all carbon dioxide was removed from the peritoneal cavity. Tape strips were used to close the skin incisions. The sequential stockings were left in place until the patient was ambulatory, i.e. usually on the first postoperative day. Clear liquids were given on the day after surgery, and an oral antibiotic preparation was continued for 7 days after completion of the intravenous course.

Abdominal ultrasonography was performed before discharge from hospital, to detect fluid or blood collections.

RESULTS

The affected adrenal gland was succesfully removed in all cases.The operative time varied from 130 to 370 minutes (185 ± 52 min, mean ± SEM). Intraoperative surgical and anesthesiological complications were never encountered, and blood transfusions were never required.

All patients were able to walk on the morning of the first postoperative day; during the first 2-3 postoperative days, they complained of diffuse abdominal pain, that was easily controlled with small doses of analgesic drugs. Mean postoperative time of hospitalization after surgery was 3.5 ± 0.9 days (range 2 to 5 days). Working activity was started by all patients within the first 15 postoperative days.

Pathological analysis of the specimens removed confirmed the clinical diagnosis of adrenal adenoma (12 cases) and pheochromocytoma (4 cases). In the 3 patients with Cushing's syndrome, glucocorticoid replacement therapy was started on the day of surgery, and maintained as indicated. Two months after surgery, none of the patients showed clinical, biochemical or hormonal evidence of recurrence or persistence of the disease. At that time, only patient n. 4 (Conn's disease) required low dose anti-hypertensive therapy, while the 2 patients with Cushing's syndrome were still under glucocorticoid replacement therapy. In patients undergoing left laparoscopic adrenalectomy, pancreatic function was not affected postoperatively, as revealed by the normal values of plasma pancreatic enzymes.

DISCUSSION

Traditional approaches to adrenal surgery, including the anterior transabdominal, the posterior flank and the thoracoabdominal procedures, are burdened by the need to make large incisions (especially in relation to the small size of the adrenal gland), long postoperative hospitalization, and long recovery times (5).

The results of the present study, together with those of previous reports

(3, 6, 8), indicate that laparoscopic surgery is a feasible, effective and safe alternative for the treatment of monolateral hypersecreting benign adrenal tumors. In fact, in all 16 cases here reported, the adrenal gland was successfully removed, with no intraoperative surgical or anesthesiological complications, and with no need for blood transfusions. Neither the size nor the side, left or right of the affected gland, were limiting factors for the laparoscopic technique. In terms of morbidity, mean operative time, postsurgical recovery, hospitalization, convalescence and return to working activity, these were markedly reduced as compared to those observed in our latest 16 open adrenalectomies. The efficacy of the laparoscopic approach was confirmed in all patients by the clinical, hormonal and metabolic picture observed two months after surgery, showing no persistence or recurrence of the disease.

This experience demonstrates that laparoscopic adrenalectomy is a safe, effective and minimally invasive procedure for the treatment of hyperfunctioning adrenal tumors.

REFERENCES

1. Clayman R., Kavoussi L.R., McDougall E.M., Soper N.J., Figenshau R.S., Chandhoke P.S. and Albala D.M. (1992): Surg. Laparosc. Endosc. 2: 29-34.
2. Coptoat M.J. (1992): Br. J. Urol. 69: 561-567.
3. Gagner M., Lacroix A. and Bolté E. (1992): N. Engl. J. Med. 327: 1033.
4. Guazzoni G., Montorsi F., Bergamaschi F., Rigatti P., Cornaggia G., Lanzi R. and Pontiroli A.E. (1994): J. Urol. (in press).
5. Guz B.V., Straffon R.A. and Novik A.C. (1989): Urol. Clin. North Am. 16: 527-534.
6. Higashihara E., Tanaka Y., Horie S., Aruga S., Nutahara K., Minowada S. and Aso Y. (1993): J. Urol. 149: 973-976.
7. Manyak M.J. (1992): Semin. Urol. 10: 205-212.
8. Sardi A. and McKinnon W. (1993): JAMA 269: 989-990.

Frontiers in Endocrinology
Volume 9 - 1994

Glucocorticoids Inhibit Gonadotropin-Releasing Hormone Secretion from Explanted Male Rat Hypothalamus

N. Burrello, F. Bonaffini, R.F.A. Weber[1] and A.E. Calogero

First Department of Internal Medicine, Chair of Andrology, University of Catania, 95123 Catania, Italy; [1]Department of Internal Medicine III, Erasmus University, Rotterdam, The Netherlands

INTRODUCTION

Women with psychogenic cause of amenorrhea (14), including anorexia nervosa (4), also have chronically elevated serum cortisol levels. Long distance runners commonly have elevated serum cortisol levels and alteration of the hypothalamic-pituitary-gonadal (HPG) axis (16). In different experimental models, each of the various hormonal components of the HPA axis has been suggested as the factor responsible for causing the hypogonadal state (11). Since adrenalectomy has been shown to abolish hypothalamic-pituitary-adrenal (HPA) axis-induced suppression of gonadotropin secretion (8), glucocorticoid (GLC) excess per se may be the common denominator of the hypogonadism which occurs during the hyperactivation of the HPA axis. However, the mechanism(s) and sites whereby GLC act to induce hypogonadism remain controversial. In the rat, it has been shown that GLCs suppress basal and gonadotropin-releasing hormone (GnRH)-stimulated pituitary gonadotropin release (6, 10, 12). However, it has also been postulated that GLCs inhibit hypothalamic GnRH release (9, 12).

The purpose of this study was to evaluate the effects of GLCs on hypothalamic GnRH release. To accomplish this, we tested the effects of corticosterone (B) and dexamethasone (DEX) on basal and potassium chloride (KCl)-stimulated immunoreactive GnRH (iGnRH) release. Because of the reported relationship between gonadal steroids and GLCs (1,

13, 17), we evaluated whether testosterone (T) or dihydro-testosterone (DHT) could influence the effects of B on iGnRH release.

MATERIAL AND METHODS

Experiments were performed using intact male Sprague-Dawley rats weighing 200-225 g (Charles River, Calco, CO, Italy) as previously reported (3). iGnRH release was evaluated from singularly incubated hemi-hypothalami (1 hemi-hypothalamus/well/0.5 ml) according to the following protocols:

Protocol 1 was designed to evaluate the effects of GLCs on basal iGnRH release. To this end, each hemi-hypothalamus was incubated in medium without test substance in the first two wells and exposed to vehicle or graded concentrations of B or DEX in the third well.

Protocol 2 was designed to evaluate the effects of GLCs on KCl-stimulated iGnRH release. To this aim, the hemi-hypothalami were incubated in plain medium in the first well and in placebo, 100 nM B or 10 nM DEX in the second and third well. KCl at the concentration of 30 mM was added in the third well.

Protocol 3 was designed to evaluate whether T or DHT modulate the inhibitory effect of B on iGnRH release. To this end, the tissues were incubated in plain medium in the first well and in vehicle, 0.1 nM T or 0.01 nM DHT in the second and third well. B at the concentration of 100 nM was added in the third well.

The concentration of iGnRH in the incubation medium was measured by RIA as previously reported (3). The sensitivity (ED_{90}) of the assay was 2.66±0.2 pg/ml (1.33±0.1 pg/well). The intraassay and interassay coefficients of variation were 2.84±0.36% and 15.76%, respectively.

Results (mean±SEM), shown as percentage of basal iGnRH release, were analyzed using the ANOVA followed by the Duncan multiple range test.

RESULTS AND DISCUSSION

Basal iGnRH release was 9.27±0.8 pg/hemi-hypothalamus/0.5 ml and the exposure to 60 mM KCl increased its release by about 3-fold. Both B and DEX inhibited basal GnRH release in a concentration-dependent fashion (Table 1).

B was effective at concentrations that can be regarded as physiological in the rat (2). According to its greater GLC activity, DEX was more potent than B in suppressing iGnRH release, but lost its effect at the concentration of 100 nM. B and DEX had no effect on the release of GnRH stimulated by 30 mM KCl.

Table 1. *Effects of B and DEX on basal hypothalamic iGnRH release*

	0	1	10	100	1000
B (nM)	120±6.7 n = 11	102±11 n = 6	102±8.2 n = 8	83.5±9.5* n = 10	79±9.6* n = 7
DEX (nM)	120±6.7 n = 11	101±7.4 n = 9	64±8.7* n = 9	89.7±9.1 n = 9	NT

n = number of tissues tested; NT not tested; *p<0.05 vs Zero.

Previous studies have suggested that GLCs inhibit serum gonadotropin levels by acting at the hypothalamic level. In the male rat, DEX suppresses post-castration gonadotropin rise and the number of GnRH receptors at the pituitary level (12). Also in humans there is indirect evidence that GLCs act on the hypothalamus to inhibit gonadotropin release. Indeed, Melis et al. (9) showed that DEX, given at the dose of 2.25 mg/day for a week, reduced the postcastration rise in serum gonadotropin in women, whereas it does not have any effect on basal or GnRH-stimulated gonadotropin serum levels in normal cycling female (5, 7, 15).

A relationship between gonadal steroids and GLCs on gonadotropin secretion has been reported. For example, GLCs block estrogen-induced LH surges in female rats (1) and women (13) and enhance the inhibitory feedback of small doses of T on LH secretion in the male rat (17). To evaluate whether androgens may influence the effects of B on iGnRH release, we tested the effects of B (100 nM) in the presence of low concentrations of T (0.1 nM) or DHT (0.01 nM) (3). T alone did not have any statistically significant effect, whereas DHT suppressed slightly, but significantly, basal iGnRH release ($p<0.05$). These two androgens did not have any effect on B-suppressed iGnRH release, suggesting that androgens do not modulate the effects of B.

In conclusion, we found that GLCs inhibit hypothalamic GnRH release and that this effect is not modulated by androgens, at least under these experimental conditions. We suggest that the hypothalamus is another site for the complex interplay between GLCs and the HPG axis.

REFERENCES

1. Baldwin D.M. (1979): Endocrinology 105: 120-128.
2. Calogero A.E., Kamilaris T.C., Johnson E.O., Tartaglia M.E. and Chrousos G.P. (1990): Endocrinology 127: 1574-1579.
3. Calogero A.E., Weber R.F.A. and D'Agata R. (1993): Neuroendocrinology 57: 152-158.
4. Casper R.C., Chatterton R.T. Jr. and Davis J.M. (1979): J. Clin. Endocrinol. Metab. 49: 406-411.

5. Georgitis W.J., Treece G.L. and Hofeldt F.D. (1983): Clin. Endocrinol. (Oxf.) 19: 319-324.
6. Kamel F. and Kubajak C.L. (1987): Endocrinology 121: 561-568.
7. Lachelin G.C.L., Judd H.L., Swanson S.C., Hauck M.E., Parker D.C. and Yen S.S.C. (1982): J. Clin. Endocrinol. Metab. 55: 768-773.
8. Mann D.R., Evans D., Edoimioya F., Kamel F. and Butlerstein G.M. (1985): Neuroendocrinology 40: 297-302.
9. Melis G.B., Mais V., Gambacciani M., Paoletti A.M., Antinori D. and Fioretti P. (1987): J. Clin. Endocrinol. Metab. 65: 237-241.
10. Padmanabhan V., Keech C. and Convey E.M. (1983): Endocrinology 112: 1782-1787.
11. Rivier C. and Rivest S. (1991): Biol. Reprod. 45: 523-532.
12. Rosen H., Jameel M.L. and Barkan A.L. (1988): Endocrinology 122: 2873-2880.
13. Sowers J.R., Rice B.F. and Blanchard S. (1979): Horm. Metab. Res. 11: 478.
14. Suh B.Y., Liu J.H., Berga S.L., Laughlin G.A. and Yen S.S.C. (1988): J. Clin. Endocrinol. Metab. 66: 733-739.
15. Vierhapper H., Waldhausl W. and Nowotny P. (1981): J. Endocrinol. 91: 399-403.
16. Villanueva A.L., Schlosser C., Hopper B., Liu J.H., Hoffman D.I. and Rebar R.W. (1986): J. Clin. Endocrinol. Metab. 63: 133-136.
17. Vreeburg J.T.M., de Greef W.J., Ooms M.P., van Wouw P. and Weber R.F.A. (1984): Endocrinology 115: 977-983.

DIAGNOSTIC PROCEDURES

p. 415 - 436

Management of Out-Patients in the Endocrine Laboratory: Use of the Fully Automated Random Access Assay System (AxSYM) (Workshop)

p. 415 - 436

SOCIETA'
ITALIANA
DI ENDOCRINOLOGIA

Frontiers in Endocrinology
Volume 9 - 1994

INTRODUCTION

Automated Assays in Clinical Investigations

F. Trimarchi

Chair of Endocrinology, Policlinico Universitario,
Via Consolare Valeria, 98125 Messina, Italy

Hormone assays in human blood are no longer requested only by the specialist in Clinical Endocrinology, but have become almost a matter of routine in many fields of Clinical Medicine.

Of the various hormone measurements performed, thyroid function tests hold a very important place from a statistical point of view, inasmuch as evaluation of thyroid function accounts for some 25% of all routine endocrine laboratory investigations.

This means that, today, reliable and feasible methods are necessary to guarantee precise and rapid results and which also provide a more efficient cost/benefit ratio. As far as concerns this latter aspect, attention should be focused on obtaining reliable results in the shortest possible time, thus avoiding useless delay and, indeed, the frequent need to repeat the hormone assay.

Radioimmunoassay and immunoradiometric methods have led to remarkable progress in hormone measurement. However, in carrying out these hormone assays, a calibration curve was necessary for a single assay, and from the point of view of costs, it was necessary, in each run, to measure several samples. Furthermore, intra-assay controls had to be made on account of the far from negligible intra-assay variability.

Over the last few years, the various new technological approaches developed have been aimed at reducing to a minimum any interference on the precision of the assay by means of fully automated and an extremely stable calibration curve. The development of new technologies progressively substituted radio-active markers with chemiluminescent or fluorescent tracers, thus contributing also to a more prolonged stability and consequently the possiblity of longer storage of the reagents.

In this Workshop a novel fully automated analyzer (AxSYM, Abbott) is presented. This instrument, which makes use of two well-known techniques, namely Fluorescence Polarized Immuno-Assay (FPIA) and Microparticle Enzyme Immuno-Assay (MEIA), has been fully evaluated by two groups of investigators, led, respectively, by F. Minuto in Genova and G. Messeri in Florence.

The studies presented in this Workshop demonstrate that results obtained with this fully automated system are both reliable and reproducible, and comparable to those obtained with the conventional radioimmunometric methods, but with the added advantage offered by the possibility of random access and by the possibility of having results of a very large number of assays available within a very short time.

Moreover, imprecision investigations based on computing imprecision profiles and inter-assay and intra-assay imprecision confirmed the reliability of the system for clinical use with only the very slight limitation due to the discriminating ability for low thyrotropin values. The calibration curve also appeared to be stable for the period claimed by the manufacturer and the results obtained using a stored calibration curve were better than those obtained using a calibration curve for each run.

On the basis of the reports presented in this Workshop, and since the criteria currently used for evaluating an assay system to be used for clinical purposes are met, the AxSYM analyser may be defined as more than satisfactory.

Frontiers in Endocrinology
Volume 9 - 1994

Evaluation of a New Fully Automated Immunoassay System for Thyroid Function

L. Fazzuoli, M. Ballerini[1], P. Bellati[1] and F. Minuto

Department of Endocrinology and Metabolism, University of Genova,
Viale Benedetto XV 6, 16132 Genova;
[1]Abbott S.p.A., Divisione Diagnostici,
Via Mar della Cina 262, 00144 Rome, Italy

INTRODUCTION

In 1993 more than 10,000 patients were tested and about 64,000 assays were performed in our laboratory. The laboratory deals with hormonal assays (Fertility, Thyroid, Growth-hormone-IGF-I, Bone metabolism Adrenals). The patients tested are mostly from the Division of Endocrinology of the Department of Endocrinology and Metabolism (15.7% in-patients, 24.7% out-patients, 24.9% day hospital), 12.8% from the same hospital, 19.5% from other hospitals in our town and 2.6% from other hospitals in Italy.

These data show that our laboratory is dedicated to the work of the specialist in endocrinology and acts as a reference for other laboratories in the area.

To date the methodology used is almost exclusively based on RIA or IRMA. The thyroid panel covers about 24% of the routine work.

A fully automated random access assay system (AxSYM, Abbott) based on microparticle enzyme immunoassay (MEIA) or on fluorescence polarization immunoassay (FPIA) has recently become available for thyroid hormones.

The various aspects of the technique have been compared with those of the classic RIA systems used in our laboratory.

MATERIAL AND METHODS

The AxSYM system was tested in the period December 1993 - February 1994. Aims of the study were the definition of the characteristics of the assays in terms of practical features, such as technical difficulties, performances, time required for calibration and testing, etc. and in terms of quality control, such as within and inter assay CVs, sensitivity, comparison of the results with the methods currently used in our Laboratory and with the Abbott IMx system.

Tests were performed in three different periods. In the first period, familiarization with the instrument, TT3, TT4 and fT4 were tested for two weeks. In the second period, TSH was tested. In the third period, results of TSH and TT4 in about 100 additional serum samples were compared between AxSYM, IMx and the method in use (Fig. 1).

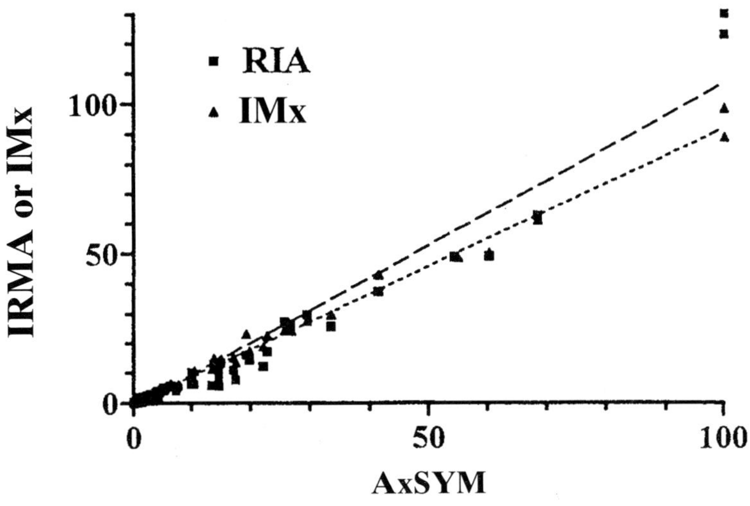

FIG. 1. Correlation of TSH values obtained in a series of 160 subjects by the AxSYM system and by IRMA or IMx (values are expressed as μIU/ml).

RESULTS AND DISCUSSION

TSH, Total T3 (TT3) and T4 (TT4) and free T4 (fT4) were assayed by this system in a zero concentration sample and, for each assay, in 5 samples at different concentrations ranging from low to high values with respect to the normal population. The RIA systems used for comparison were those in routine clinical use in our laboratory and particularly the coated-tube assays supplied by DPC (Los Angeles, CA, USA) for TSH, TT4 and TT3, and the two step coated tube assay provided by Incstar Corporation (Stillwater, MN, USA) for fT4. Sensitivity, intra and inter assays precision were evaluated on the basis of the results observed in 17 analytical sessions for a total of 1526 (1) tests (202 TSH, 447 TT4, 434 fT4, 443 TT3). Sensitivity was 0.013 μIU/ml for TSH, 0.54 μg/dl for TT4, 0.31 ng/dl for fT4 and 0.39 ng/ml for TT3 (0.25, 0.08 0.07, respectively, in the RIA assays tested). Percent inter and intra assay coefficients of variation at the different hormone concentrations are shown in Table. 1.

Table 1. *Percent inter and intra assay coefficients of variations at the different hormone concentrations*

	TSH			TT4			fT4			TT3	
μIU/ml	inter	intra	μg/dl	inter	intra	ng/dl	inter	intra	ng/ml	inter	intra
0.182	0.89	11.42	2.66	5.33	5.34	0.59	2.13	4.55	0.69	7.52	6.70
0.185	11.97	11.78	4.03	5.46	3.65	0.70	4.12	5.15	0.69	8.23	9.49
0.472	14.51	11.58	7.67	3.72	2.56	1.25	3.62	3.69	1.20	4.72	6.71
5.754	5.25	4.92	7.83	3.91	2.28	1.27	2.35	2.92	1.38	4.59	5.16
47.94	5.13	5.30	14.70	2.87	1.67	3.24	2.66	3.23	3.34	3.19	3.84

About 200 subjects presenting with different thyroid function and with other non thyroidal conditions were also analyzed and the results compared with the RIA (2).

Regression analysis revealed an r value of 0.982 for TSH, a slope of 0.88 and an intercept of –0.24 μIU/ml in a second series of 94 patients.

As far as concerns TT4 an r value of 0.88 was found, a slope of 0.96 and an intercept of 0.42 μg/dl in a first series of 102 samples. In a second series of 99 samples, r (0.96) was definitely higher compared with the first series of observations, while intercept and slope were nearly identical (1.60 and 0.93, respectively).

fT4 showed an r of 0.90, slope of 0.95 and intercept of 0.09 ng/dl.

TT3 showed an r of 0.80, slope of 0.74 intercept of 0.21 ng/ml.

Overall, a high reproducibility of the results is demonstrated for all three hormones tested, with values comparable as far as TSH, TT4 and fT4 are concerned, while TT3 showed a tendency of about 25% underestimation in the system tested with respect to RIA.

Other correlations are shown in Table 2 (double values represent two different series).

Table 2. *Thyroid tests: comparison between the different methods*

		RIA vs IMx	AxSYM vs RIA	AxSYM vs IMx
TSH (IRMA)	r	0.954, 0.985	0.956, 0.987	0.9819, 0.996
sensitivity 0.013 µIU/ml	slope	0.78, 1.03	1.05, 0.92	0.88, 0.97
	intercept	2.57, -0.01	-2.28, -0.16	0.02, -0.24
TT4	r	0.922, 0.889	0.876, 0.964	0.900, 0.941
sensitivity 0.54 µg/dl	slope	0.94, 0.89	0.80, 0.93	0.84, 0.92
	intercept	-0,24 -0.56	1.69, 1.60	0.49, 0.10
fT4	r	0.809	0.901	0.8721
sensitivity 0.31 ng/dl	slope	0.88	0.85	0.89
	intercept	0.09	0.26	0.12
TT3	r	0.624	0.799	0.649
sensitivity 0.39 ng/ml	slope	0.55	0.86	0.65
	intercept	0.86	0.37	0.81

CONCLUSIONS

In conclusion, this fully automated random access system is characterized not only by the possibility of carrying out a large number of assays per day with results available in less than an hour, but also by a precision unmatched by the classic RIA systems, with good reproducibility of the results.

The lower sensitivity does not seem to be of clinical importance since in TT4 and TT3 assays it is about one order of magnitude and in fT4, about three times lower than the low-normal ranges. Moreover, the high level of equivalence with RIA values, particularly for TT4 and fT4, makes these endocrine parameters comparable for nuclear medicine and clinical chemistry laboratories.

REFERENCES

1. Broughton P.M.G. and Bergonzi C. et al. (1987): Guidelines for the evaluation of diagnostic kits. Part. 2. General principles and oútlines procedures for the evaluation of kits for qualitative tests. ECCLS document.
2. Malvano R., Pilloton E. and Pizzocolo G. et al. (1991): Assessment of qualitative tests. Ann. Ist. Sup. Sanità 27: 437.

Frontiers in Endocrinology
Volume 9 - 1994

Evaluation of a Thyroid Test Panel on a Novel Immunoassay Analyser

S. Vannini, P. Tozzi, M. Ficarra and G. Messeri

Laboratory of Endocrinology, CTO, Careggi Hospital, Largo Palagi 1, 50139 Florence, Italy

INTRODUCTION

The present study was designed to evaluate the performance of the thyrotropin (TSH), thyroxine (tT4), triiodothyronine (tT3) and free thyroxine (fT4) immunoassay on the new AxSYM (Abbott) random access immunoassay analyser.

The T4 method is based on the Fluorescence Polarization Immuno-Assay technology, already used on the TDX (Abbott) batch analyser. All the other tests take advantage of the Microparticle Enzyme Immuno-Assay technology already used by the IMx (Abbott) batch analyser.

The calibration curve of all the tests can be stored and no additional calibrator is required in individual runs. The manufacturer claims that the calibration is stable for at least two weeks.

MATERIAL AND METHODS

Imprecision profiles were computed according to Sadler et al. (4) by replicating the measurement of six different serum pools or control samples over ten analytical series run on different days.

Intra-assay and intra-day imprecision were computed by measuring twenty replicates of three-level control samples in the course of the same run (intra-assay) or in the course of different runs carried out on the same day (intra-day).

Reliability of the calibration procedure was tested by processing a full set of calibrators during all the above-mentioned analytical runs. The values of serum pools were then computed by using both the stored and the "daily" calibration curve, and the results compared.

Comparison studies were performed by analysing about one hundred patient samples both by the AxSYM system and the previous Abbott batch analysers: TDX (tT4) and IMx (TSH, fT4, fT3).

The minimum detectable concentration (analytical) of TSH was measured by replicating the analysis of the zero calibrator and of three low content serum pools (0.2, 0.1 and 0.05 µIU/ml, respectively) on ten different runs over a fifteen-day interval. A TSH concentration as low as 0.05 µIU/ml could be significantly discriminated from the zero calibrator ($p<0.05$). The "functional sensitivity" (1) of TSH (concentration at interassay CV=20%) was derived from the interassay imprecision profile and found to be 0.15 µIU/ml.

Diagnostic accuracy (discrimination between normal and subnormal values) around a TSH cut-off of 0.3 µIU/ml was computed according to Pilo et al. (2).

RESULTS AND COMMENTS

The calibration curves are well positioned towards the reference interval of all the tests (Figs. 1-4).

The imprecision profiles (Figs. 5-8) approach the analytical goals proposed for the thyroid hormones (3).

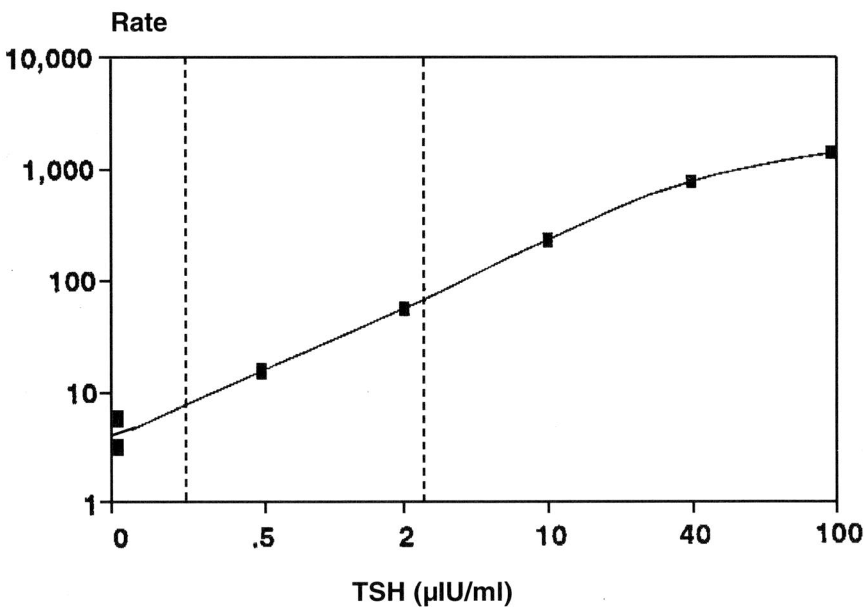

FIG. 1. TSH. AxSYM calibration curves. The line depicts the average values from ten different runs and the squares the mean ± SD. The dotted lines refer to the reference interval.

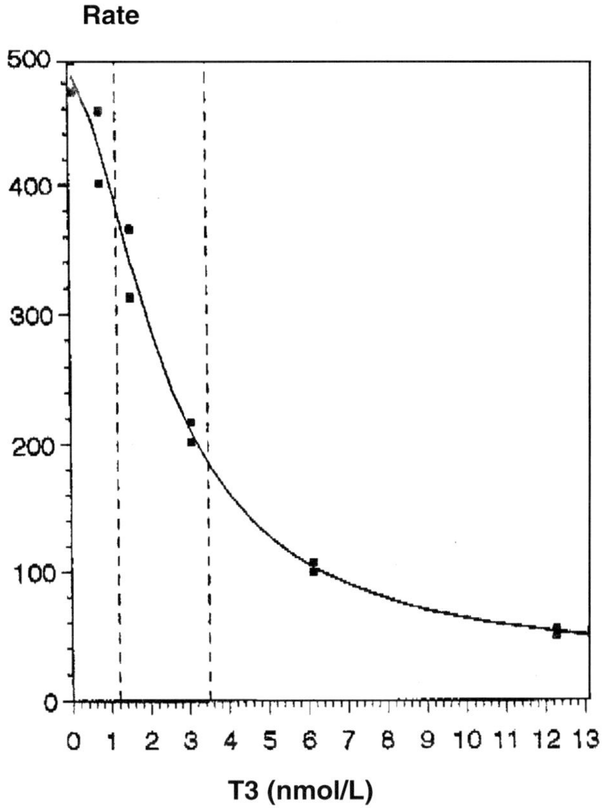

FIG. 2. T3. AxSYM calibration curves. The line depicts the average values from ten different runs and the squares the mean ± SD. The dotted lines refer to the reference interval.

Table 1. *Interassay imprecision computed from values obtained by the calibration procedure recommended by the manufacturer and by a full daily calibration*

	Stored mean	CV%	Daily mean	CV%
Total T4[1]				
Low	55.3	5.1	52.8	4.1
Medium	103.4	4.6	100.0	5.0
High	162.3	4.0	157.8	5.0
Free T4[2]				
Low	8.8	5.9	8.8	3.4
Medium	15.9	4.1	16.0	3.1
High	24.8	3.1	24.3	3.5

[1]nmol/L [2]pmol/L.

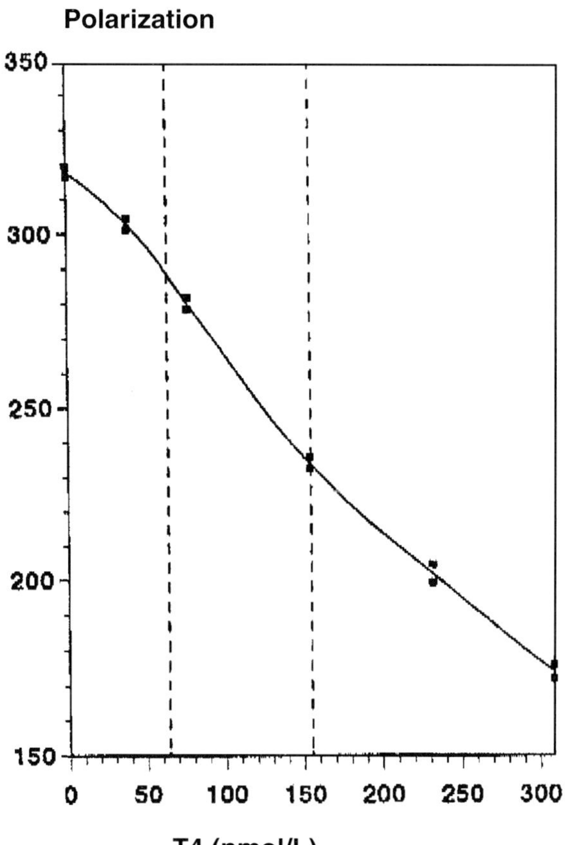

FIG. 3. T4. AxSYM calibration curves. The line depicts the average values from ten different runs and the squares the mean ± SD. The dotted lines refer to the reference interval.

Table 2. *Interassay imprecision computed from values obtained by the calibration procedure recommended by the manufacturer and by a full daily calibration*

	Stored mean	CV%	Daily mean	CV%
TSH[1]				
Low	0.10	23.1	0.11	31.4
Medium	1.16	6.4	1.03	8.2
High	2.43	6.0	2.36	5.6
Total T3[2]				
Low	1.22	4.1	1.45	4.7
Medium	1.63	5.8	1.88	5.6
High	2.61	5.4	2.79	3.9

[1]µIU/ml [2]nmol/L.

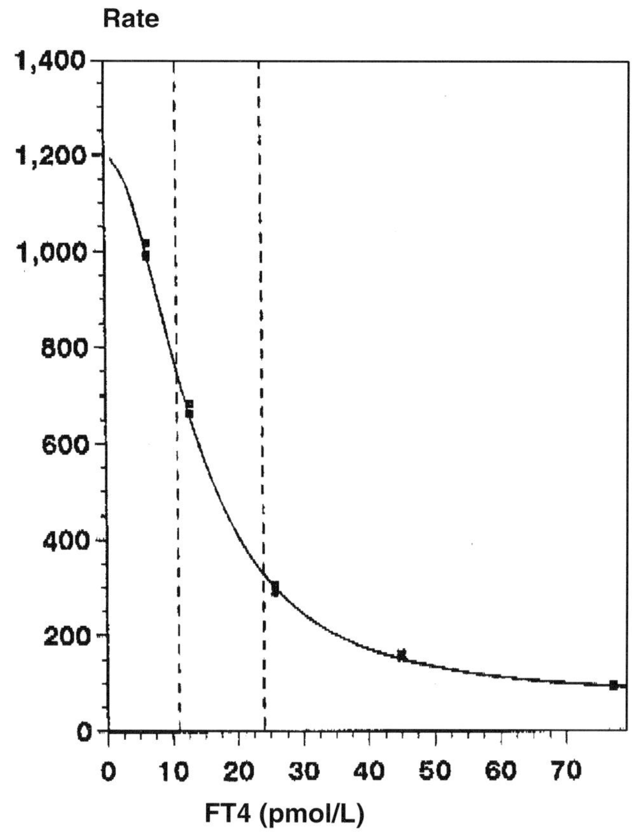

FIG. 4. FT4. AxSYM calibration curves. The line depicts the average values from ten different runs and the squares the mean ± SD. The dotted lines refer to the reference interval.

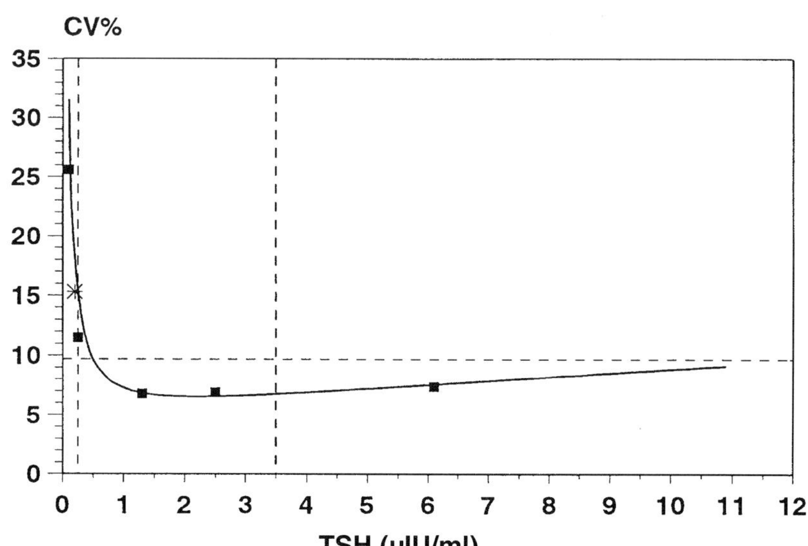

FIG. 5. TSH. Imprecision profiles computed according to Sadler from five serum pools replicated on ten runs performed on ten different days over a fifteen-day interval. The instrument was never recalibrated during the study interval. The horizontal dotted line represents the proposed «analytical goals» (3). The vertical dotted lines refer to the reference interval.

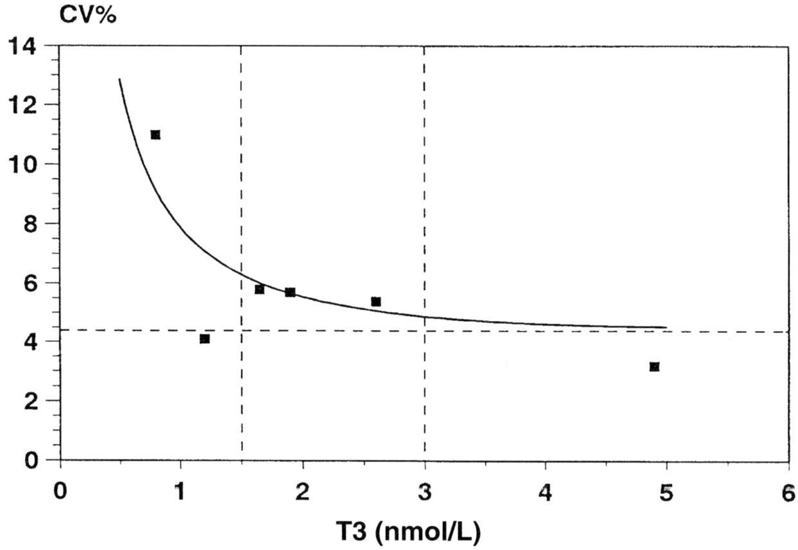

FIG. 6. T3. Imprecision profiles computed according to Sadler from five serum pools replicated on ten runs performed on ten different days over a fifteen-day interval. The instrument was never recalibrated during the study interval. The horizontal dotted line represents the proposed «analytical goals» (3). The vertical dotted lines refer to the reference interval.

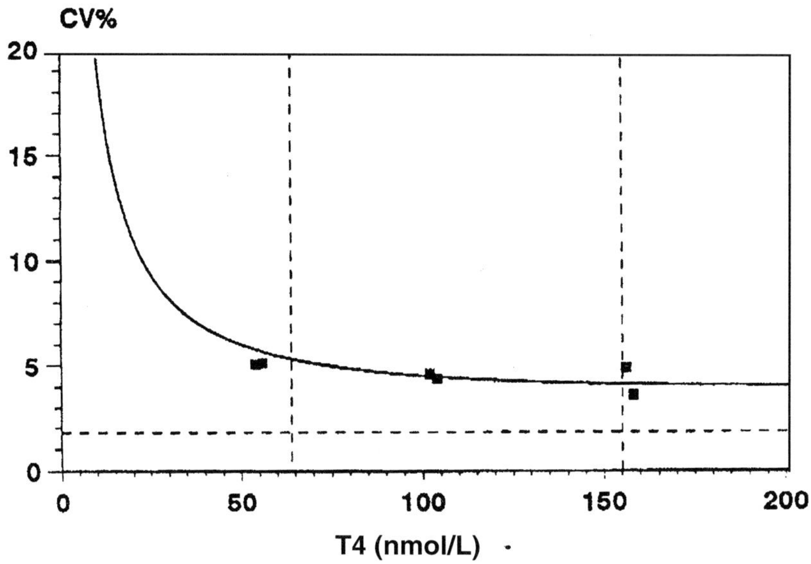

FIG. 7. T4. Imprecision profiles computed according to Sadler from five serum pools replicated on ten runs performed on ten different days over a fifteen-day interval. The instrument was never recalibrated during the study interval. The horizontal dotted line represents the proposed «analytical goals» (3). The vertical dotted lines refer to the reference interval.

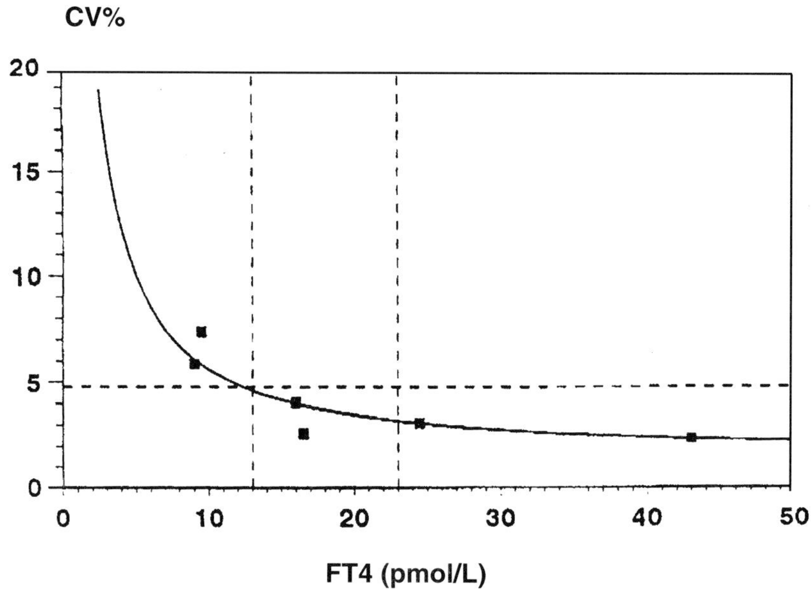

FIG. 8. FT4. Imprecision profiles computed according to Sadler from five serum pools replicated on ten runs performed on ten different days over a fifteen-day interval. The instrument was never recalibrated during the study interval. The horizontal dotted line represents the proposed «analytical goals» (3). The vertical dotted lines refer to the reference interval.

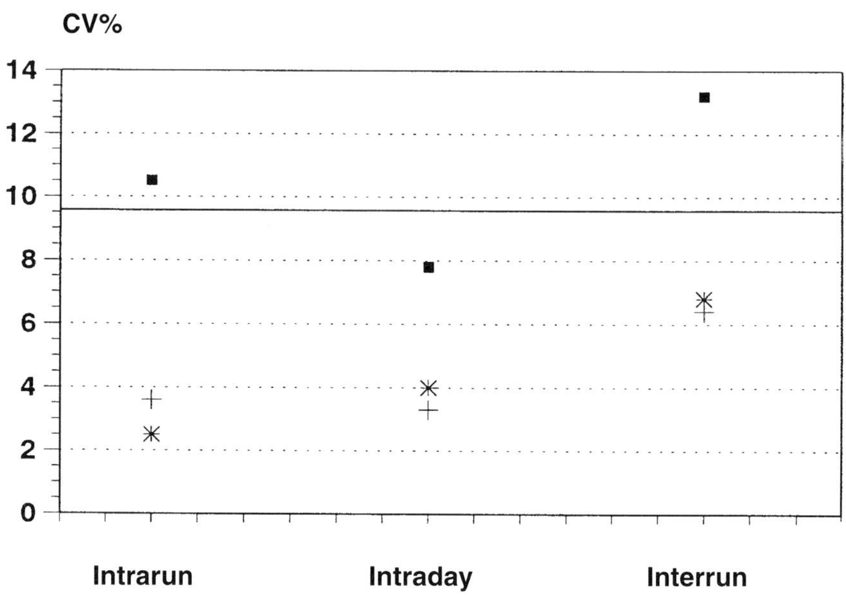

FIG. 9. TSH. ■ 0.25 μIU/ml + 6.0 μIU/ml ★ 50 μIU/ml.
Overall summary of imprecision studies.

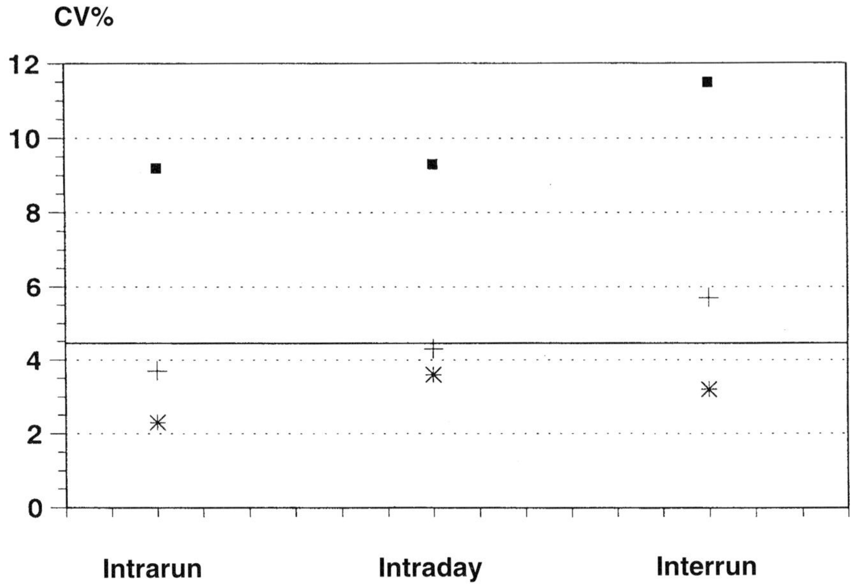

FIG. 10. T3. ■ 1.1 nmol/L + 2.3 nmol/L ★ 5.7 nmol/L.
Overall summary of imprecision studies.

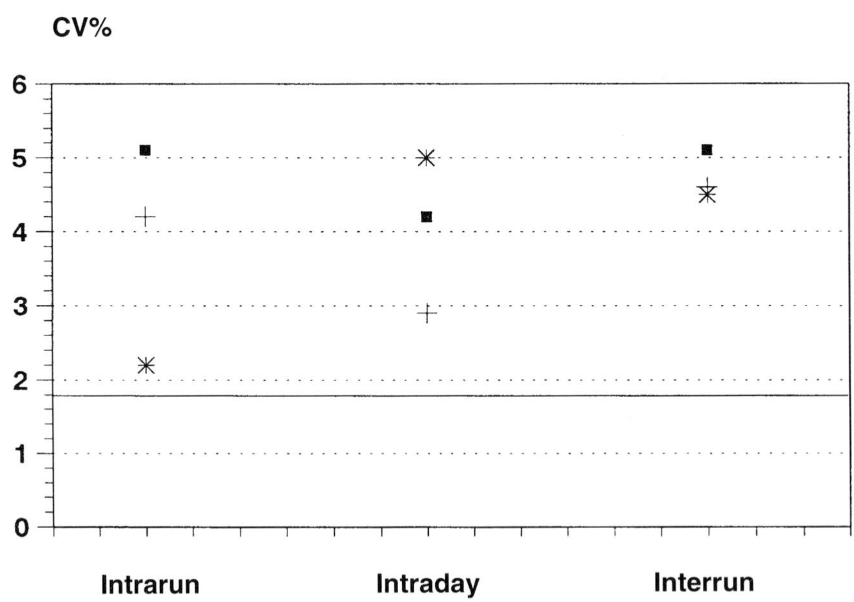

FIG. 11. T4. ■ 58 nmol/L + 103 nmol/L ★ 193 nmol/L.
Overall summary of imprecision studies.

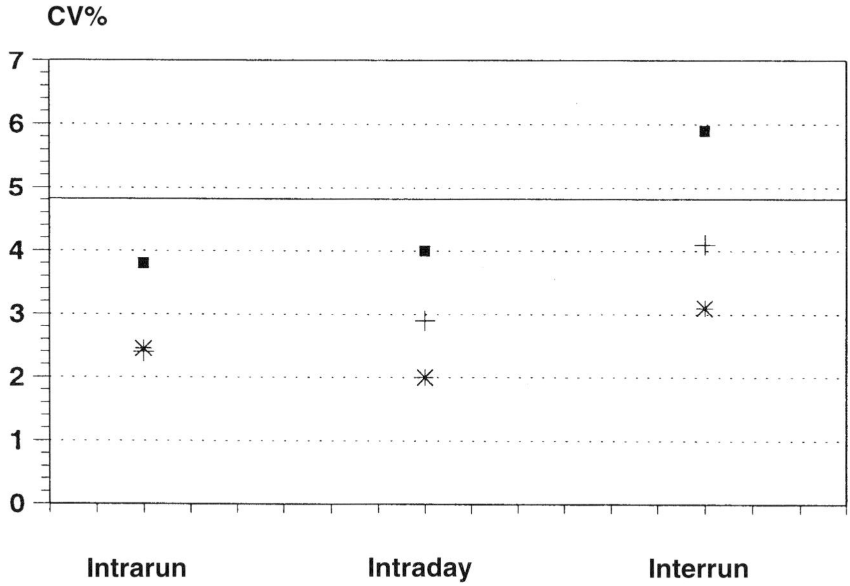

FIG. 12. FT4. ■ 9 pmol/L + 15 pmol/L ★ 39 pmol/L.
Overall summary of imprecision studies.

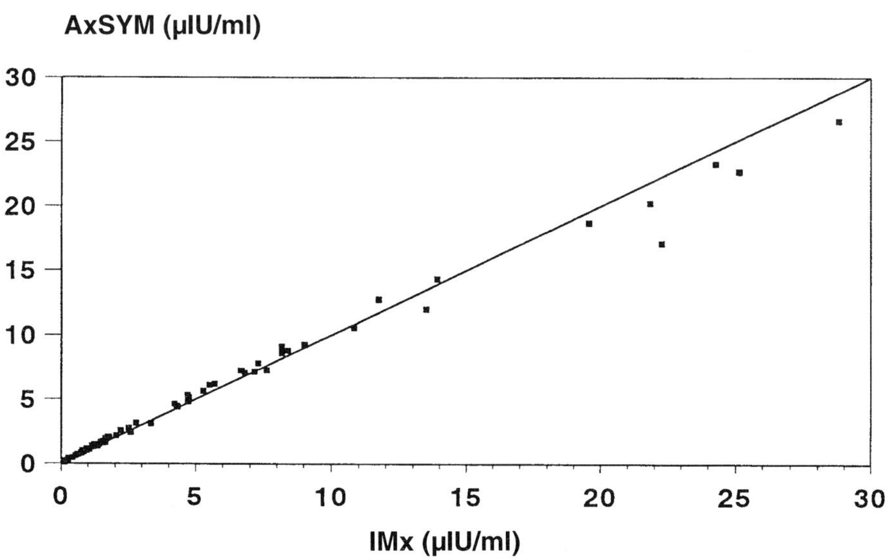

FIG. 13. TSH. y = 0.89x + 0.48, r=0.990.
Overall summary of imprecision studies.

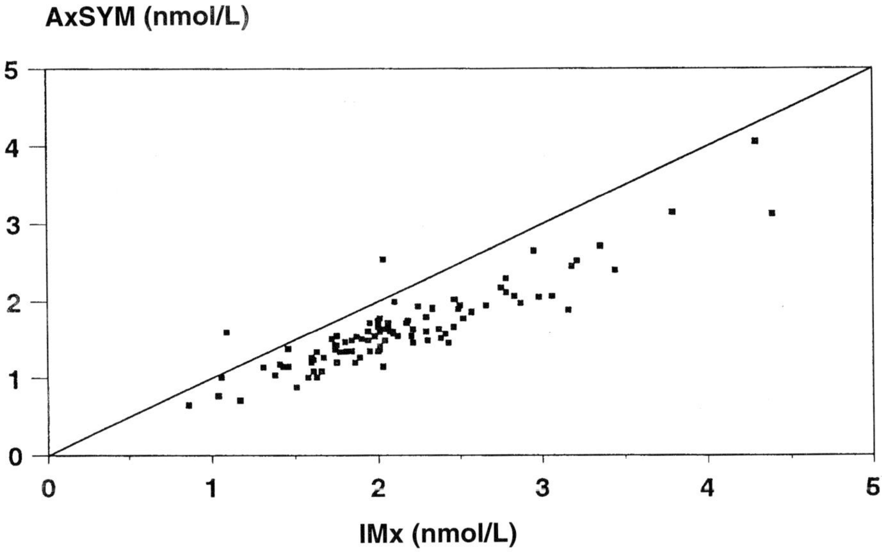

FIG. 14. T3. y = 0.75x + 0.04, r=0.90.
Comparison studies performed on 100 patient samples.

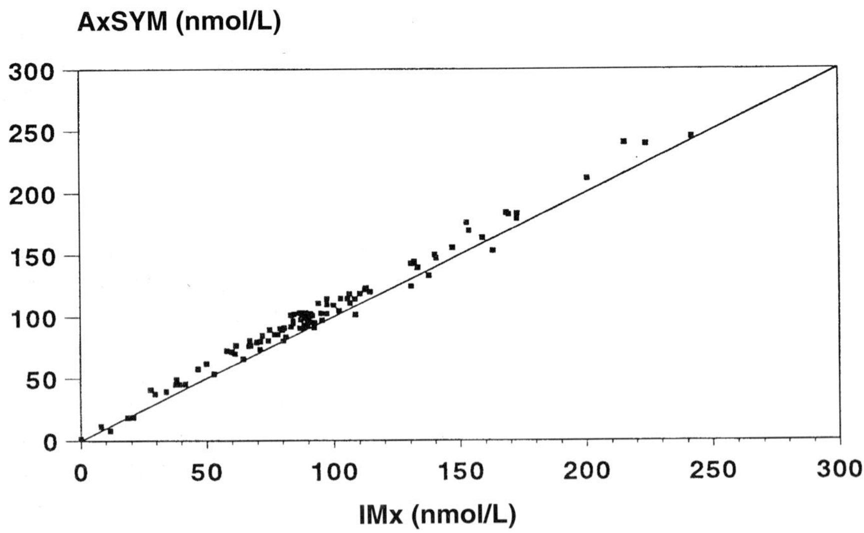

FIG. 15. Total T4. y = 1.01 + 2.3, r=0.989.
Comparison studies performed on 100 patient samples.

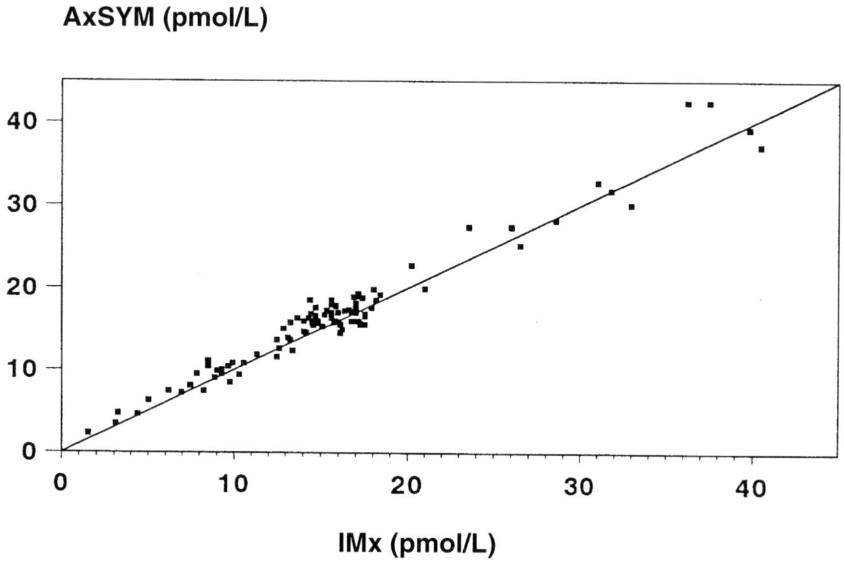

FIG. 16. Free T4. y = 0.94 + 1.63, r=0.976.
Comparison studies performed on 100 patient samples.

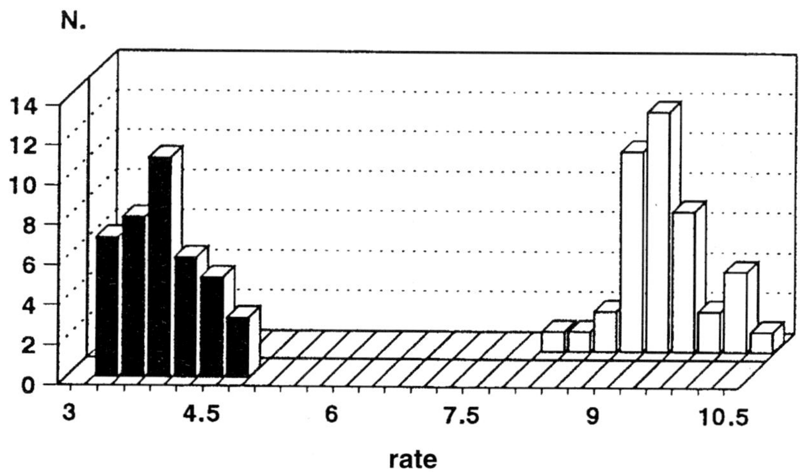

FIG. 17a. TSH (μIU/ml). ■ Cal. 0 □ Pool 0.20.
Distribution of the rates of the zero calibrator and of low content pools, analysed as five replicates over ten different runs.

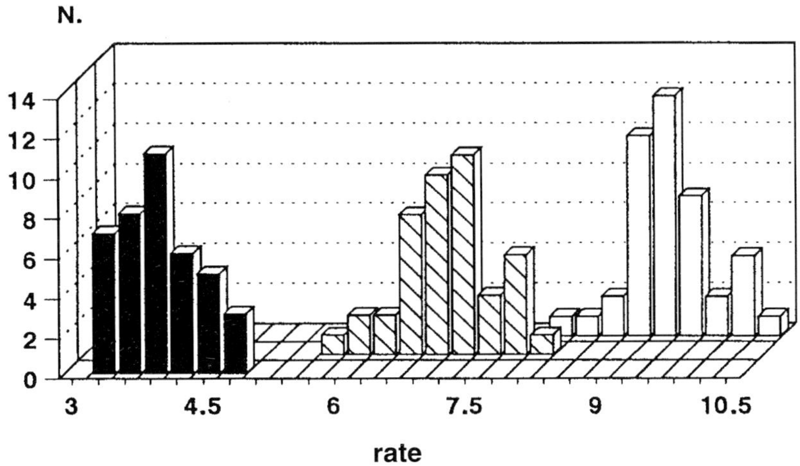

FIG. 17b. TSH (µIU/ml). ■ Cal. 0 ▧ Pool 0.10 □ Pool 0.20.
Distribution of the rates of the zero calibrator and of low content pools, analysed as five replicates over ten different runs.

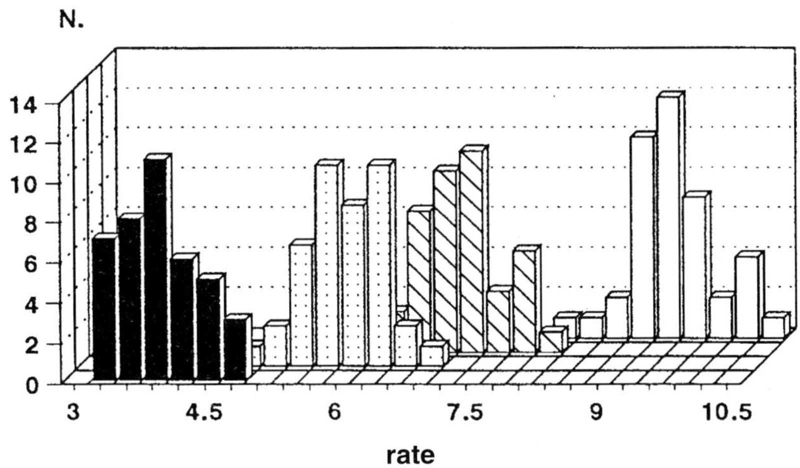

FIG. 17c. TSH (µIU/ml). ■ Cal. 0 ⬚ Pool 0.05 ▧ Pool 0.10 □ Pool 0.20.
Distribution of the rates of the zero calibrator and of low content pools, analysed as five replicates over ten different runs.

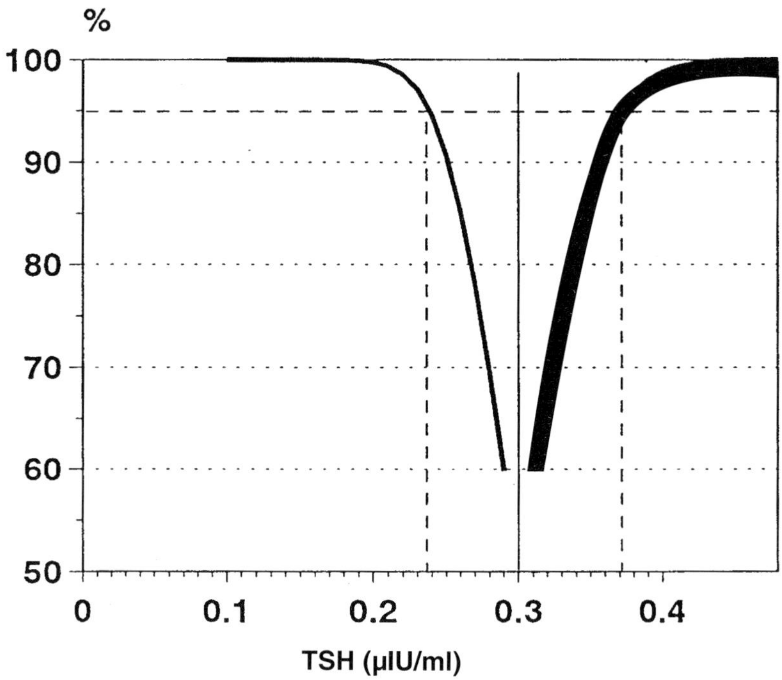

FIG. 18. Clinical accuracy. Cut-off 0.3 μIU/ml. — True Low % ■ True Normal %
TSH discrimination power around the cut-off 0.3 μIU/ml. At 95% accuracy, the undetermined interval around 0.3 was 0.23-0.37 μIU/ml.

Intra-assay, intra-day and inter-assay imprecision (Figs. 9-12) are very similar, as expected from an automatic machine.

The reduced intra-assay imprecision makes duplicating analysis of the samples unnecessary.

The calibration procedure seems to provide results which are even better than those obtained by calibrating on each run (Tables 1, 2).

The results are in a good agreement with those from the previous Abbott methods with the only exception of T3, which appeared to be markedly underestimated when measured by the AxSYM system (Figs. 13-16).

TSH minimum detectable concentration, derived from the replication of low content pools over ten different days (Fig. 17), was <0.05 μIU/ml. This is consistent with the claim of the "second generation method" (interassay CV at 0.25 μIU/ml <20%).

Following imprecision data derived from the interassay imprecision profile, the diagnostic accuracy (discrimination between normal and subnormal values) was computed in the low TSH range (Fig. 18). The reduced undetermined interval around the 0.3 μIU/ml confirms that the new test is adequate for clinical use.

REFERENCES

1. Chubb S.A.P., Davis J.A. and Wood A.T. (1987): Clin. Chem. 36: 1855.
2. Pilo A., Zucchelli G.C. and Malvano R. et al. (1992): Clin. Chem. 38(7): 1345-1349.
3. Ricos C. and Arobs M.A. (1990): Ann. Clin. Biochem. 27: 353-358.
4. Sadler W.A., Smith M.H. and Legge H.M. (1988): Clin. Chem. 6: 1058-1064.

AUTHOR INDEX - GLOSSARY

SUBJECT INDEX

Author Index

Glossary of Abbreviations

ACTH-OMA	adrenocorticotrophic adenoma
ADH	antidiuretic hormone
AITD	autoimmune thyroid disease
c-AMP	cyclic AMP
Anti-TPO	antiperoxidase autoantibodies
APS	autoimmune polyendocrine syndrome
AVP	arginin-vasopressin
ARE	androgen response element
AxSYM	automated random access assay system
CG	chorionic gonadotropin
CGβ	chorionic gonadotropin β subunit
CH	congenital hypothyroidism
CHO	Chinese hamster ovary cells
CT	computed tomography
DA	dopamine agonists
DES	diethylstilbestrol
DGGE	denaturing gradient gel electrophoresis
EGF	epidermal growth factor
ER	estrogen receptor
ERE	estrogen response element
ERT	estrogen replacement therapy
ET	endothelin
F IX	factor IX
F XII	factor XII
FNA	fine needle aspiration
FPIA	fluorescence polarized immunoassay
FSH	follicular stimulating hormone
GH	growth hormone
rGH	recombinant growth hormone
GHD	growth hormone deficiency
GHDA	growth hormone deficiency, adults
GH-OMA	somatotrophic adenoma
GHRH	growth hormone releasing hormone
GHRH-r	growth hormone releasing hormone receptor
GHRPs	growth hormone releasing peptides
GnRH	gonadotropin releasing hormone
GRA	glucocorticoid remediable aldosteronism
GRF	growth hormone releasing factors

HPA	hypothalamic pituitary adrenal axis
HPB	hypophysial portal blood
5 HT	serotonin
IGF	insulin-like growth factor
IPS	inferior petrosal sinuses
IQ	intelligence quotient
IR	insulin receptor
IRS	insulin receptor substrate
IVF	in vitro fertilization
Leu	leucine
LH	luteinizing hormone
LHRH	luteinizing hormone releasing hormone
MBP	myelin basic proteins
MEIA	microparticle enzyme immunoassay
MHC	major histocompatibility antigens
MRI	magnetic resonance imaging
MT	melatonin
NFPA	non functioning pituitary adenomas
NPY	neuropeptide Y
OCT	octreotide
PAF	platelet activating factor
PCO	polycystic ovary syndrome
PCR	polymerase chain reaction
PRL	prolactin
PTH	parathyroid hormone
PTHrP	parathyroid hormone related peptide
RTH	resistance to thyroid hormones
SIADH	syndrome of inappropriate secretion of antidiuretic hormone release
SS	somatostatin
SSA	somatostatin analogs
TCH	transient congenital hypothyroidism
TG Ab	thyroglobulin antibodies
TK	tyrosine kinase
TPO	thyroid peroxidase
TPO-Ab	antiperoxidase autoantibodies
TRAP	thyroid receptor auxiliary protein
TRE	thyroid response elements
TRH	thyrotropin releasing hormone
TSAb	thyroid stimulating antibodies
TSH	thyrotropin
TSH-B Ab	thyrotropin blocking antibodies
VIP	vasoactive intestinal peptide
VIP-R	vasoactive intestinal peptide receptor

Subject Index